EMERGENCY
MEDICINE
QUICK GLANCE

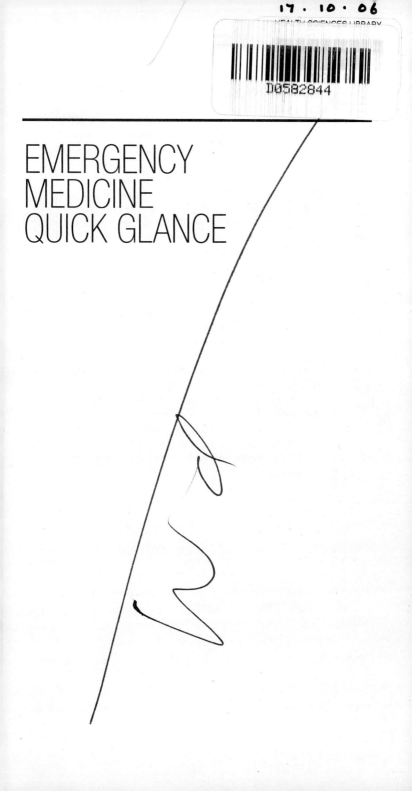

NOTICE

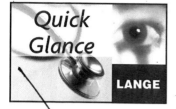

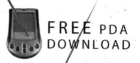

FREE PDA DOWNLOAD

EMERGENCY MEDICINE

Christopher R. H. Newton, MD • Rahul Khare, MD

FOLLOW THESE INSTRUCTIONS TO DOWNLOAD YOUR FREE PDA SOFTWARE

1) Use your Web browser to go to:
   http://books.mcgraw-hill.com/eb.php?i=0071448187

2) Register now

3) Fill in the required fields

4) Enter your unique registration code below

5) Download the free software and sync into your handheld device

Code Listed Here

e42898f8

Use this code to register and receive your free PDA software. See above for complete directions.

If you have any problems accessing your download, please visit: www.books.mcgraw-hill.com/techsupport

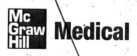

p/n 0-07-147700-4

www.mcgraw-hillmedical.com

EMERGENCY MEDICINE QUICK GLANCE

Edited by

Christopher R. H. Newton, MD

Assistant Medical Director
Department of Emergency Medicine
Saint Joseph Mercy Hospital
Adjunct Clinical Instructor
University of Michigan Medical Center
Ann Arbor, Michigan

Rahul K. Khare, MD

Assistant Professor
Department of Emergency Medicine
Feinberg School of Medicine
Northwestern University
Northwestern Memorial Hospital
Chicago, Illinois

McGraw-Hill
MEDICAL PUBLISHING DIVISION

New York / Chicago / San Francisco / Lisbon / London / Madrid / Mexico City
Milan / New Delhi / San Juan / Seoul / Singapore / Sydney / Toronto

Emergency Medicine Quick Glance

1 2 3 4 5 6 7 8 9 0 DOC/DOC 0 9 8 7 6

Set ISBN: 0-07-144818-7
Book ISBN: 0-07-147699-7
Card ISBN: 0-07-147700-4

The book was set in Palatino by Silverchair Science + Communications, Inc.
The editors were Martin J. Wonsiewicz, Karen Edmonson, and Penny Linskey.
The production supervisor was Catherine H. Saggese.
The book designer was Marsha Cohen.
The cover designer was Aimee Nordin.
The indexer was Rena Morse.
RR Donnelley was printer and binder.

This book is printed on acid-free paper.

Cataloging-in-Publication data for this title are on file with the Library of Congress.

INTERNATIONAL EDITION ISBN: 0-07-110077-6
Copyright © 2006, Exclusive rights by The McGraw-Hill Companies, Inc., for manufacture and export. This book cannot be re-exported from the country to which it is consigned by McGraw-Hill. The International Edition is not available in North America.

To my beautiful wife Mary, you provide me with love, happiness, and are my best friend. To my three energetic boys, Cameron, Jamie, and baby Newton, your enthusiasm gives me inspiration and makes every day something to look forward to.

To my family and friends in Scotland—I miss you all and look forward to my trips back home.

CRHN

To Amy, my supportive wife who has given me such inspiration and love. To Dylan, my beautiful son, who makes me smile and laugh every time I see him. To my loving parents, who continue to help guide me in my life. To all my mentors and my residents who continue to amaze me with their dedication and spirit.

RKK

CONTENTS

I: CARDIOVASCULAR EMERGENCIES

V: GENITOURINARY EMERGENCIES

VI: NEUROLOGIC EMERGENCIES
Edited by Robert Silbergleit, MD

IX: TRAUMATIC EMERGENCIES

X: TOXICOLOGIC EMERGENCIES
Edited by Brian D. McBeth, MD

XIII: ORTHOPEDIC EMERGENCIES

XVI: OTOLARYNGOLOGY EMERGENCIES

XVII: MISCELLANEOUS

CHIEF EDITOR

Christopher R. H. Newton, MD

Assistant Medical Director
Department of Emergency Medicine
Saint Joseph Mercy Hospital
Adjunct Clinical Instructor
University of Michigan Medical Center
Ann Arbor, Michigan

Chapter 5, Chapter 10, Chapter 11, Chapter 25, Chapter 41, Chapter 49, Chapter 117, Chapter 118, Chapter 130, Chapter 131, Chapter 154

ASSOCIATE EDITOR

Rahul K. Khare, MD

Assistant Professor
Department of Emergency Medicine
Feinberg School of Medicine
Northwestern University
Northwestern Memorial Hospital
Chicago, Illinois

Chapter 23, Chapter 35, Chapter 41, Chapter 80, Chapter 141, Chapter 169

ASSISTANT EDITORS

Andrew R. Barnosky, DO

Clinical Assistant Professor
Department of Emergency Medicine
University of Michigan Medical Center
Ann Arbor, Michigan

Chapter 36

Laura Roff Hopson, MD

Assistant Professor
Department of Emergency Medicine
University of Michigan Medical Center
Ann Arbor, Michigan

Chapter 15, Chapter 16, Chapter 32, Chapter 88

Terry Kowalenko, MD

Clinical Associate Professor
Emergency Medicine Residency Program Director
University of Michigan Medical Center/Saint Joseph Mercy Hospital
Ann Arbor, Michigan

Chapter 76

Brian D. McBeth, MD

Staff Physician
Regions Hospital
Assistant Professor
University of Minnesota
St. Paul, Minnesota

Section X (editor), Chapter 92, Chapter 94, Chapter 95, Chapter 99, Chapter 100, Chapter 101, Chapter 104, Chapter 109

Robert Silbergleit, MD

Assistant Professor
Department of Emergency Medicine
University of Michigan Medical Center
Ann Arbor, Michigan

Section VI (editor)

Rachel Stanley, MD

Clinical Assistant Professor
Department of Emergency Medicine/Pediatrics
University of Michigan Medical Center
Ann Arbor, Michigan

Section VIII (editor), Chapter 69

Brian Zink, MD

Associate Dean for Student Programs
University of Michigan Medical School
Associate Professor
Department of Emergency Medicine
University of Michigan Medical Center
Ann Arbor, Michigan

Nima Afshar, MD

Resident Physician
University of Michigan Medical
* Center/Saint Joseph Mercy*
* Hospital*
Ann Arbor, Michigan

Chapter 119

Amer Z. Aldeen, MD

Resident Physician
Feinberg School of Medicine
Northwestern University
Chicago, Illinois

Chapter 23, Chapter 103

Paige W. Archey, MD

Resident Physician
University of Michigan Medical
* Center/Saint Joseph Mercy*
* Hospital*
Ann Arbor, Michigan

Chapter 159, Chapter 160

Dan B. Avstreih, MD

Resident Physician
University of Michigan Medical
* Center/Saint Joseph Mercy*
* Hospital*
Ann Arbor, Michigan

Chapter 177, Chapter 178

Michael Baker, MD

Attending Physician
Saint Joseph Mercy Hospital
Ann Arbor, Michigan

Chapter 125

Andrew R. Barnosky, DO

Clinical Assistant Professor
Department of Emergency Medicine
University of Michigan Medical
* Center*
Ann Arbor, Michigan

Chapter 36

Dominic A. Borgialli, DO

Clinical Instructor
Hurley Medical Center
Flint, Michigan

Chapter 113

Nathaniel S. Bowler, MD

Resident Physician
University of Michigan Medical
* Center/Saint Joseph Mercy*
* Hospital*
Ann Arbor, Michigan

Chapter 33, Chapter 39, Chapter 58

Stuart A. Bradin, DO

Assistant Professor
Department of Emergency
* Medicine/Pediatrics*
University of Michigan Medical
* Center*
Ann Arbor, Michigan

Chapter 127

Jeffrey Callard, PA-C

Physician Assistant
Saint Joseph Mercy Hospital
Ann Arbor, Michigan

Chapter 21

Sara Chakel, MD

Resident Physician
University of Michigan Medical
* Center/Saint Joseph Mercy*
* Hospital*
Ann Arbor, Michigan

Chapter 48, Chapter 78, Chapter 146

Neal Chawla, MD

Resident Physician
University of Michigan Medical
* Center/Saint Joseph Mercy*
* Hospital*
Ann Arbor, Michigan

Chapter 44, Chapter 45

Jeremy L. Cooke, MD

Resident Physician
University of Michigan Medical
Center/Saint Joseph Mercy
Hospital
Ann Arbor, Michigan

Chapter 1, Chapter 6

Rebecca M. Cunningham, MD

Assistant Professor
University of Michigan Medical
Center
Ann Arbor, Michigan

Chapter 107

Thomas J. Deegan, MD

Assistant Professor
Department of Emergency
Medicine/Pediatrics
University of Michigan Medical
Center
Ann Arbor, Michigan

Chapter 65, Chapter 74

Robert M. Domeier, MD

Attending Physician
Saint Joseph Mercy Hospital
Ann Arbor, Michigan

Chapter 81

J. Jeff Downie, MBChB

Specialist Registrar
Department of Oral and
Maxillofacial Surgery
Southern General Hospital
Glasgow, Scotland

Chapter 79, Chapter 164

Constance J. Doyle, MD

Attending Physician
Saint Joseph Mercy Hospital
Ann Arbor, Michigan

Chapter 18, Chapter 114

George M. Elliott, MD

Resident Physician
University of Michigan Medical
Center/Saint Joseph Mercy
Hospital
Ann Arbor, Michigan

Chapter 118, Chapter 142,
Chapter 161

Kirsten G. Engel, MD

Clinical Lecturer
University of Michigan Medical
Center
Ann Arbor, Michigan

Chapter 18

John P. Erpelding, MD

Attending Physician
Saint Joseph Mercy Hospital
Ann Arbor, Michigan

Chapter 105, Chapter 112

Scott Ferguson, MD

Resident Physician
University of Michigan Medical
Center/Saint Joseph Mercy
Hospital
Ann Arbor, Michigan

Chapter 32, Chapter 117

James A. Freer, MD

Clinical Assistant Professor
University of Michigan Medical
Center
Ann Arbor, Michigan

Chapter 166

Nathan Goymerac, MD

Resident Physician
Feinberg School of Medicine
Northwestern University
Chicago, Illinois

Chapter 80, Chapter 83

Matthew J. Greenberg, MD

Resident Physician
University of Michigan Medical
  Center/Saint Joseph Mercy
  Hospital
Ann Arbor, Michigan

**Chapter 7, Chapter 17, Chapter 139,
Chapter 171**

Thomas G. Greidanus, MD

Attending Physician
Parkview Medical Center
Pueblo, Colorado

Chapter 10, Chapter 53

Colin F. Greineder, MD

Resident Physician
University of Michigan Medical
  Center/Saint Joseph Mercy
  Hospital
Ann Arbor, Michigan

**Chapter 43, Chapter 54, Chapter
137**

Geetika Gupta, MD

Attending Physician
Saint Joseph Mercy Hospital
Ann Arbor, Michigan

Chapter 59, Chapter 60

Joseph H. Hartmann, DO

Assistant Professor
University of Michigan Medical
  Center
Ann Arbor, Michigan

**Chapter 136, Chapter 172,
Chapter 173**

Ann Hess, MD

Attending Physician
Saint Joseph Mercy Hospital
Ann Arbor, Michigan

Chapter 24

Marquita N. Hicks, MD

Resident Physician
University of Michigan Medical
  Center/Saint Joseph Mercy
  Hospital
Ann Arbor, Michigan

Chapter 46, Chapter 47, Chapter 62

Victoria L. Hogan, MD

Resident Physician
University of Alabama
Birmingham, Alabama

Chapter 84

Stephanie Hollingsworth, MD

Resident Physician
University of Alabama
Birmingham, Alabama

Chapter 13

Jolie C. Holschen, MD

Clinical Assistant Professor
University of Michigan Medical
  Center
Ann Arbor, Michigan

Chapter 144

Laura Roff Hopson, MD

Assistant Professor
Department of Emergency Medicine
University of Michigan Medical
  Center
Ann Arbor, Michigan

**Chapter 15, Chapter 16,
Chapter 32, Chapter 88**

Matthew K. Hysell, MD

Resident Physician
University of Michigan Medical
  Center/Saint Joseph Mercy
  Hospital
Ann Arbor, Michigan

Chapter 28, Chapter 37, Chapter 138

John Kahler, MD

Clinical Instructor
University of Michigan Medical
  Center
Ann Arbor, Michigan

Chapter 27, Chapter 28

Scott A. Kelley, MD

Resident Physician
University of Michigan Medical
  Center/Saint Joseph Mercy
  Hospital
Ann Arbor, Michigan

Chapter 16

Eugene Kenny, MD

Resident Physician
Froedtert Hospital and Medical
  College of Wisconsin
Milwaukee, Wisconsin

Chapter 14

Rahul K. Khare, MD

Assistant Professor
Department of Emergency Medicine
Feinberg School of Medicine
Northwestern University
Northwestern Memorial Hospital
Chicago, Illinois

Chapter 23, Chapter 35, Chapter 41,
Chapter 80, Chapter 141, Chapter 169

Erich C. Kickland, MD

Resident Physician
University of Michigan Medical
  Center/Saint Joseph Mercy
  Hospital
Ann Arbor, Michigan

Chapter 20, Chapter 86, Chapter 87

Kerry L. Kikuchi, MD

Attending Physician
Greater Houston Emergency
  Physicians
Houston, Texas

Chapter 162, Chapter 163

Jacques W. Kobersy, MD

Resident Physician
University of Michigan Medical
  Center/Saint Joseph Mercy
  Hospital
Ann Arbor, Michigan

Chapter 91, Chapter 120,
Chapter 121, Chapter 122

Keith E. Kocher, MD

Resident Physician
University of Michigan Medical
  Center/Saint Joseph Mercy
  Hospital
Ann Arbor, Michigan

Chapter 19, Chapter 170

Gregory Kowalenko, MD

Clinical Instructor
University of Michigan Medical
  Center
Ann Arbor, Michigan

Chapter 76

Terry Kowalenko, MD

Clinical Associate Professor
Emergency Medicine Residency
  Program Director
University of Michigan Medical
  Center/Saint Joseph Mercy
  Hospital
Ann Arbor, Michigan

Chapter 76

Diann M. Krywko, MD

Clinical Assistant Professor
Hurley Medical Center
Flint, Michigan

Chapter 31

Ari Leib, MD

Resident Physician
Feinberg School of Medicine
Northwestern University
Chicago, Illinois

Chapter 175

William E Lew, MD

Attending Physician
Saint Joseph Mercy Hospital
Ann Arbor, Michigan

Chapter 132, Chapter 149

Michael Lutes, MD

Assistant Professor
Froedtert Hospital and Medical
*   College of Wisconsin*
Milwaukee, Wisconsin

Chapter 14, Chapter 175

Jacob MacKenzie, PA-C

Physician Assistant
Saint Joseph Mercy Hospital
Ann Arbor, Michigan

Chapter 134, Chapter 145

Stephen P. R. MacLeod, MBChB

Attending Physician
Department of Oral and
*   Maxillofacial Surgery*
Hennipin County Medical Center
Minneapolis, Minnesota

Chapter 79, Chapter 164

Michelle Macy, MD

Pediatric Emergency Medicine
*   Fellowship*
University of Michigan Medical
*   Center*
Ann Arbor, Michigan

Chapter 68

Sanjeev Malik, MD

Resident Physician
Feinberg School of Medicine
Northwestern University
Chicago, Illinois

Chapter 85, Chapter 140

Swagata Mandal, MD

Resident Physician
Feinberg School of Medicine
Northwestern University
Chicago, Illinois

Chapter 97, Chapter 167

Elke G. Marksteiner, MD

Resident Physician
University of Michigan Medical
*   Center/Saint Joseph Mercy*
*   Hospital*
Ann Arbor, Michigan

Chapter 22, Chapter 30, Chapter 98

James Mattimore, MD

Attending Physician
Saint Joseph Mercy Hospital
Ann Arbor, Michigan

Chapter 20, Chapter 86, Chapter 87

Brian D. McBeth, MD

Staff Physician
Regions Hospital
Assistant Professor
University of Minnesota
St. Paul, Minnesota

**Section X (editor), Chapter 92,
Chapter 94, Chapter 95, Chapter 99,
Chapter 100, Chapter 101, Chapter
104, Chapter 109**

Robert F. McCurdy, MD

Medical Director
Saint Joseph Mercy Hospital
Ann Arbor, Michigan

Chapter 55

Robert H. McCurren IV, MD

Chairman/Medical Director
Saint Joseph Mercy Hospital-
*   Livingston*
Howell, Michigan

Chapter 2

Heather S. McLean, MD

Attending Physician
Saint Joseph Mercy Hospital
Ann Arbor, Michigan

Chapter 75

Samuel A. McLean, MD

Lecturer
University of Michigan Medical
*   Center*
Ann Arbor, Michigan

Chapter 176

Michael Mikhail, MD

Chairman
Saint Joseph Mercy Hospital
Ann Arbor, Michigan

Chapter 40

James C. Mitchiner, MD

Attending Physician
Saint Joseph Mercy Hospital
Ann Arbor, Michigan

Chapter 93, Chapter 96

David Moyer-Diener, MD

Attending Physician
Valley Baptist Medical Center
Harlingen, Texas

Chapter 89, Chapter 90

David E. Newcomb, MD

Resident Physician
University of Michigan Medical
*   Center/Saint Joseph Mercy*
*   Hospital*
Ann Arbor, Michigan

Chapter 4, Chapter 12, Chapter 35

Christopher R. H. Newton, MD

Assistant Medical Director
Department of Emergency Medicine
Saint Joseph Mercy Hospital
Adjunct Clinical Instructor
University of Michigan Medical
*   Center*
Ann Arbor, Michigan

Chapter 5, Chapter 10, Chapter 11,
Chapter 25, Chapter 41, Chapter 49,
Chapter 117, Chapter 118, Chapter
130, Chapter 131, Chapter 154

Manya Faith Newton, MD

Resident Physician
University of Michigan Medical
*   Center/Saint Joseph Mercy*
*   Hospital*
Ann Arbor, Michigan

Chapter 50, Chapter 150

Trac Xuan Nghiem, MD

Attending Physician
Feinberg School of Medicine
Northwestern University
Chicago, Illinois

Chapter 158

Stacey K. Noel, MD

Resident Physician
University of Michigan Medical
*   Center/Saint Joseph Mercy*
*   Hospital*
Ann Arbor, Michigan

Chapter 8, Chapter 9

Lynn Nutting, BA, MPA

Billing/Coding Director Healthcare
University of Michigan Medical
*   Center*
Ann Arbor, Michigan

Chapter 180

Michele Nypaver, MD

Pediatric Emergency Medicine
Fellowship
University of Michigan Medical
Center
Ann Arbor, Michigan

Chapter 66

Marc Olson, MD

Attending Physician
Saint Joseph Mercy Hospital
Ann Arbor, Michigan

Chapter 146, Chapter 148,
Chapter 156

Elaine Pomeranz, MD

Clinical Assistant Professor
Department of Emergency
Medicine/Pediatrics
University of Michigan Medical
Center
Ann Arbor, Michigan

Chapter 70

James Pribble, MD

Lecturer
University of Michigan Medical
Center
Ann Arbor, Michigan

Chapter 110, Chapter 111,
Chapter 135

Rahul Rastogi, MD

Attending Physician
Saint Joseph Mercy Hospital
Ann Arbor, Michigan

Chapter 26, Chapter 165

David Renken, MD

Attending Physician
Saint Joseph Mercy Hospital
Ann Arbor, Michigan

Chapter 42, Chapter 157

Clifford W. Robins, MD

Resident Physician
University of Michigan Medical
Center/Saint Joseph Mercy
Hospital
Ann Arbor, Michigan

Chapter 133

Victor S. Roth, MD

Adjunct Clinical Assistant Professor
University of Michigan Medical
Center
Ann Arbor, Michigan

Chapter 106

Christopher R. Schmelzer, MD

Resident Physician
University of Michigan Medical
Center/Saint Joseph Mercy
Hospital
Ann Arbor, Michigan

Chapter 49, Chapter 130, Chapter 131

Steven Schmidt, MD

Resident Physician
University of Michigan Medical
Center/Saint Joseph Mercy
Hospital
Ann Arbor, Michigan

Chapter 29, Chapter 77, Chapter 123

Carol H. Schultz, MD

Clinical Assistant Professor
University of Michigan Medical
Center
Ann Arbor, Michigan

Chapter 34

Lisa M. Schweigler, MD

Resident Physician
University of Michigan Medical
Center/Saint Joseph Mercy
Hospital
Ann Arbor, Michigan

Chapter 56, Chapter 57

Phillip A. Scott, MD

Assistant Professor
University of Michigan Medical
* Center*
Ann Arbor, Michigan

Chapter 51, Chapter 52

Jonathan Shenk, MD

Resident Physician
University of Michigan Medical
* Center/Saint Joseph Mercy*
* Hospital*
Ann Arbor, Michigan

Chapter 102, Chapter 168

Amy Shirk, MD

Pediatric Emergency Medicine
* Fellowship*
University of Michigan Medical
* Center*
Ann Arbor, Michigan

Chapter 64

Athina Sikavitsas, DO

Clinical Assistant Professor
Department of Emergency
* Medicine/Pediatrics*
University of Michigan Medical
* Center*
Ann Arbor, Michigan

Chapter 71

Stefanie Simmons, MD

Resident Physician
University of Michigan Medical
* Center/Saint Joseph Mercy*
* Hospital*
Ann Arbor, Michigan

Chapter 176

Troy Christian Sims, DO

Resident Physician
University of Michigan Medical
* Center/Saint Joseph Mercy*
* Hospital*
Ann Arbor, Michigan

Chapter 115, Chapter 116,
Chapter 128, Chapter 129

Joshua A. Small, MD

Resident Physician
University of Michigan Medical
* Center/Saint Joseph Mercy*
* Hospital*
Ann Arbor, Michigan

Chapter 99, Chapter 109

Candice A. Sobanski, MD

Resident Physician
University of Michigan Medical
* Center/Saint Joseph Mercy*
* Hospital*
Ann Arbor, Michigan

Chapter 124, Chapter 143

Cemal B. Sozener, MD

Resident Physician
University of Michigan Medical
* Center/Saint Joseph Mercy*
* Hospital*
Ann Arbor, Michigan

Chapter 38

Nicole S. Sroufe, MD

Pediatric Emergency Medicine
* Fellowship*
University of Michigan Medical
* Center*
Ann Arbor, Michigan

Chapter 72, Chapter 73

Rachel Stanley, MD

Clinical Assistant Professor
Department of Emergency
  Medicine/Pediatrics
University of Michigan Medical
  Center
Ann Arbor, Michigan

Section VIII (editor), Chapter 69

Richard G. Taylor, MD

Resident Physician
University of Michigan Medical
  Center/Saint Joseph Mercy
  Hospital
Ann Arbor, Michigan

Chapter 151, Chapter 153,
Chapter 155

J. Jeremy Thomas, MD

Resident Physician
University of Alabama
Birmingham, Alabama

Chapter 82

Joanne Torres, MD

Resident Physician
University of Michigan Medical
  Center/Saint Joseph Mercy
  Hospital
Ann Arbor, Michigan

Chapter 152, Chapter 154

Amit R. Trivedi, MD

Resident Physician
University of Michigan Medical
  Center/Saint Joseph Mercy
  Hospital
Ann Arbor, Michigan

Chapter 108

Hadar Tucker, MD

Attending Physician
Saint Joseph Mercy Hospital
Ann Arbor, Michigan

Chapter 63, Chapter 67

Brad J. Uren, MD

Resident Physician
University of Michigan Medical
  Center/Saint Joseph Mercy
  Hospital
Ann Arbor, Michigan

Chapter 11, Chapter 174, Chapter 179

Thomas E. VanHecke, MD

Attending Physician
Department of Internal Medicine
William Beaumont Hospital
Royal Oak, Michigan

Chapter 3

Diamond Vrocher III, MD

Assistant Professor
University of Alabama
Birmingham, Alabama

Chapter 13, Chapter 82, Chapter 84

Daniel R. Wachter, MD

Resident Physician
University of Michigan Medical
  Center/Saint Joseph Mercy
  Hospital
Ann Arbor, Michigan

Chapter 88

Ellen C. Walkling, MD

Resident Physician
University of Michigan Medical
  Center/Saint Joseph Mercy
  Hospital
Ann Arbor, Michigan

Chapter 61, Chapter 147

Edward Walton, MD

Clinical Assistant Professor
Department of Emergency
  Medicine/Pediatrics
University of Michigan Medical
  Center
Ann Arbor, Michigan

Chapter 126

Jim Edward Weber, MD

*Assistant Professor/Research
    Director*
Hurley Medical Center
Flint, Michigan

Chapter 3

Holly Weymouth, MD

Resident Physician
*University of Michigan Medical
    Center/Saint Joseph Mercy
    Hospital*
Ann Arbor, Michigan

Chapter 15

Emergency Medicine Quick Glance is a handbook written almost entirely by the faculty and residents of the combined University of Michigan/Saint Joseph Mercy Hospital Emergency Medicine Residency Program. This includes many current and potential future leaders in emergency medicine.

It is a rapid practical review of the broad spectrum of diseases that we see in the emergency department, but also provides enough detail to prevent the reader from having to search other sources for additional information. It includes the core content of emergency medicine as well as cutting edge chapters, such as bioterrorism, conventional explosives, and an approach to chronic pain and addiction. Drug doses have been included when possible to assist in making *Emergency Medicine Quick Glance* a single reference.

This handbook is aimed at the senior emergency medicine resident level, but it will be useful for experienced physicians, mid-level providers, and students who rotate through the emergency department. Many physicians now rely on their PDAs for their schedules and references, so this is the first emergency medicine handbook offered in a combined paper and PDA version.

Christopher R. H. Newton, MD
Editor

We would like to thank Dr. Brian Zink for his mentorship, oversight, and help in getting the book started. We would also like to thank Annaliese Peffer, whose administrative assistance was invaluable to completing the book.

We would like to thank department chairs Drs. Barsan and Mikhail, who supported the book and encouraged faculty to participate.

Finally, we would like to thank all the residents and faculty of the combined University of Michigan/Saint Joseph Mercy Hospital Emergency Medicine Residency Program who took time from their busy schedules to author and edit the many chapters in our handbook.

Christopher R. H. Newton, MD
Rahul K. Khare, MD

CHAPTER 1

APPROACH TO CHEST PAIN

Jeremy L. Cooke

- ▶ 1 in 20 ED patients presents with chest pain.
- ▶ ED chest pain evaluations exceed an annual cost of $3 billion.
- ▶ ~50% of deaths in the U.S. are due to CAD.
- ▶ 1–4% of patients with an AMI are sent home from the ED.
- ▶ ~650,000 deaths per year are due to PE.
- ▶ The diagnosis of PE is missed more than 400,000 times per year in the U.S.
- ▶ Missed thoracic aorta dissection is associated with a 90% mortality rate.
- ▶ Multiple etiologies can present with similar clinical pictures.

DIFFERENTIAL DIAGNOSIS

- ▶ Immediate life threats:
  - ACS, acute PE, aortic dissection, tension PTX, esophageal rupture
- ▶ Emergent diagnoses:
  - Acute chest syndrome, cocaine-related chest pain, myocarditis, pericarditis, PTX, mediastinitis, esophageal tear, cholecystitis, pancreatitis
- ▶ Non-emergent diagnoses:
  - Cardiovascular: valvular heart disease, aortic stenosis, MVP, hypertrophic cardiomyopathy
  - Pulmonary: pneumonia, pleuritis, tumor, pneumomediastinum
  - Gastrointestinal: esophageal spasm, esophageal reflux, peptic ulcer, biliary colic
  - Musculoskeletal: muscle strain, rib fracture, arthritis, tumor, costochondritis, non-specific chest wall pain
  - Neurologic: spinal root compression, thoracic outlet, herpes zoster, post-herpetic neuralgia
  - Other: panic disorder, hyperventilation

DIAGNOSTIC APPROACH

▶ After ensuring patient stability, the diagnostic approach proceeds with consideration of age, sex, clinical presentation, and risk factors for specific conditions.

▶ Abnormal vital signs, diaphoresis, vomiting, pallor, altered mental status, air hunger, severe pain, and anxiety should raise suspicion for serious conditions.

▶ IV access, O_2 administration, cardiac monitoring with pulse oximetry, and an immediate 12-lead ECG to be seen by an attending physician within 10 minutes of patient's arrival should be routine.

▶ Physical exam with particular attention to the cardiovascular and pulmonary systems is essential in identifying emergent conditions.

▶ 12-lead ECG is a mainstay of diagnosis for cardiac ischemia/infarction but can also suggest pericarditis, effusion, digoxin toxicity, or electrolyte abnormalities.

▶ The diagnostic value of cardiac troponins has been well established for detecting myocardial injury, but if negative, cannot be used alone to rule out ACS or other life-threatening diagnoses.

▶ Urine drug screens, if appropriate, may detect cocaine- or amphetamine-related causes of chest pain.

▶ Even in patients with a normal pulmonary exam, a CXR may provide a diagnosis. It is essential in the detection of PTX, heart failure, and pneumonia and may suggest aortic dissection. Mediastinal or subcutaneous air can suggest mediastinitis or esophageal rupture.

▶ V/Q scanning is useful for diagnosing PE but has significant limitations and can be largely influenced by the clinician's pre-test suspicion.

▶ D dimer assay, if negative in a patient with low pre-test probability, is supportive of an alternative diagnosis to PE.

▶ More advanced imaging modalities such as CT scanning, MRI, angiography, or echocardiography may be needed for diagnosis of certain clinical entities.

▶ TEE is sensitive and specific but usually impractical for ED diagnosis of aortic dissection. CT scanning is usually the imaging modality of choice in the ED setting.

TREATMENT AND DISPOSITION

► The majority of patients presenting to the ED with chest pain of a pulmonary or cardiac etiology are admitted to the hospital. Most cardiac patients at higher risk for ischemia and/or arrhythmia may benefit from a telemetry bed. Patients who are potentially unstable require ICU admission.

► Many of the patients with life-threatening and emergent causes of chest pain initially appear stable. Aggressive and rapid mobilization of diagnostic testing and treatment saves lives.

► All patients with consideration of ischemic chest pain should be started on ASA unless absolutely contraindicated.

► Patients with suspected ACS and myocardial injury pattern seen on ECG should have cardiology consult, beta-blocker, and pain treated with opiates and/or NTG. The work-up and initial treatment should not delay the cardiology consult and definitive treatment with cardiac catheterization or thrombolytics.

► Serial cardiac markers, continuous 12-lead ECGs, and early provocative testing (cardiac stress testing) can be accomplished in ED observation centers and are appropriate for patients at lower risk for ACS.

► Patients at low risk for the emergent and life-threatening causes of chest pain may be discharged if an alternative diagnosis has been found and close follow-up with adequate discharge instructions are understood.

◐ **PEARLS**

• The focus of the ED physician in patients who present with chest pain is not necessarily to make a specific diagnosis but instead to rule out life-threatening diagnoses.

• Specific attention should be given directly to acute cardiac ischemia or infarction, aortic dissection, PE, and, to a lesser extent, esophageal rupture. Delays in diagnosis of these often occult conditions are not rare but are potentially fatal.

• Because clinical features alone can rarely predict which patients may be discharged without further testing, liberal use of diagnostic tests, including CXR, ECG, and cardiac markers, is necessary.

• Normal cardiac enzymes or markers do not rule out the possibility of life-threatening illness or even acute cardiac syndromes. They may help with placing the patient into an appropriate risk group and guide triage decisions.

- Many patients with panic disorder present with chest pain. Although a diagnosis of exclusion, the vast majority of these patients do not receive adequate recognition or treatment for their underlying disorder despite negative cardiac investigations.

CHAPTER 2

APPROACH TO SYNCOPE

Robert H. McCurren IV

▶ Sudden LOC and postural tone with spontaneous recovery.
▶ Lifetime risk is 1:4. Likelihood varies with age and comorbidities.
▶ 1–2% of all ED visits.
▶ Difficult diagnostic dilemma:
  • Large differential diagnosis (trivial to life-threatening etiology).
  • Evaluations may be time-consuming and costly.
  • Often, the cause cannot be determined (up to 50%).
▶ Near-syncope and syncope are generally evaluated in the same manner.

PATHOPHYSIOLOGY

▶ Sudden CNS dysfunction.
  • Usually from decrease of cerebral blood flow.
▶ 35% decrease in cerebral blood flow causes unconsciousness.

CLINICAL PRESENTATION

History

▶ Important historical features:
  • Rate of onset, position, time of LOC (> 5 minutes suggests seizure).
  • Activity at onset: exercise/exertion worrisome for outflow obstruction.
  • Vagal stimulation? Aura?
  • Post-syncope symptoms: Post-ictal? Tongue biting, incontinence.
  • Associated symptoms: chest pain, SOB, palpitations.

- Past medical history: CAD, CHF, and structural heart disease are the most important risks for dysrhythmia or cardiac cause!
- Medications: review in detail.
▶ Classic neurocardiogenic (vasovagal) symptoms:
  - Upright/standing position.
  - Weakness/lightheadedness.
  - Pale/diaphoretic.
  - Blurry vision, loss of visual function, gray, tunnel vision.
  - Loss of muscle tone.
  - Brief apnea, hypotension, and bradycardia are common.
  - Myoclonic jerking or twitching is common (not a seizure).
  - Resumption of consciousness in 15–20 seconds.
▶ Symptoms worrisome for life-threatening cause:
  - Abrupt LOC, no warning symptoms
  - Sitting or supine position
  - Aura (seizure)
  - Exercise-related syncope
  - Family history of sudden cardiac death

Physical Exam

▶ Cardiac and neurologic exam is most important.
▶ Focus on additional systems based on presentation and patient history.
▶ Rectal exam for evidence of GI bleeding.

Differential Diagnosis

▶ See Tables 2-1 and 2-2.

EMERGENCY DEPARTMENT MANAGEMENT

▶ Stabilization: ABCs, ACLS, and spine protection if indicated
▶ Vital signs (orthostatic), monitor, IV, O_2, ECG, blood sugar
▶ Carotid sinus massage: > 50 years old (no bruit or previous CNS ischemia)
▶ Tests/studies:
  - **ECG is most important!** Rhythm, intervals (QT, WPW), ischemia.
  - CXR (screen for cardiomegaly).
  - Labs: **Limited use!** CBC, electrolytes, cardiac markers, HCG, UA (should be ordered selectively).

TABLE 2-1.
SERIOUS OR POTENTIALLY LIFE-THREATENING CAUSES OF SYNCOPE

Cardiac dysrhythmias
    Fast HR
        VT/VF
        Torsades
        WPW syndrome
    Slow HR
        Sinus node disease (sick sinus syndrome)
        High-grade AV block
    Electrocardiographic abnormalities
        Long QT syndrome
        Pacemaker/AICD malfunction
Cardiac ischemia/CHF
    AMI
    Cardiomyopathy
Cardiac outflow obstruction
    Mitral/aortic/pulmonic stenosis
    Hypertrophic cardiomyopathy
    Atrial myxoma
    Pulmonary HTN
    Tamponade
    Congenital heart disease
Acute cardiovascular events
    PE
    Aortic dissection/aneurysm
        Blood loss
            Trauma
            GI bleed
            Gynecologic: ectopic pregnancy
Acute CNS problems
    SAH
    CNS ischemia (bilateral or brainstem)
    Hypoglycemia
    Seizure
    Hypoxemia
Toxic/metabolic
    CO
    Electrolyte imbalance
Medication related
    Antidysrhythmic (QT prolonging)
    Hypoglycemic medications

- CT/LP: Only if history suggests SAH, CNS ischemia, seizure.
▶ Additional inpatient/outpatient testing:
  - Holter or event monitor
  - Pacemaker/AICD interrogation
  - Tilt table

TABLE 2-2.
BENIGN OR NON–LIFE-THREATENING CAUSES OF SYNCOPE

Supraventricular cardiac dysrhythmias
    SVT
CNS dysfunction or hypoperfusion
    Hyperventilation
    Subclavian steal
    Basilar artery migraine
    Narcolepsy
Neurocardiogenic (vasovagal; **most common etiology**)
    Emotional disturbance
    Pain
    Situational
    Carotid sinus hypersensitivity
    Reflex related
        Valsalva
        Micturition/defecation
        Cough, sneeze, vomiting
Orthostatic hypotension
    Volume depletion
    Anemia
    Autonomic dysfunction
Medication related
    Cardiovascular medications
        1. Beta-blockers/digoxin/CCBs
        2. Vasodilators
        3. Diuretics
        4. Central acting (clonidine)
    Psychoactive medications
    Many others
Toxic/metabolic
    Endocrinopathy
    Illicit drug use
Psychogenic
    Anxiety/panic disorder
    Conversion/somatization disorder

- Cardiac electrophysiologic study
- Cardiac stress testing/catheterization
- Echocardiography
- MRI/MRA/EEG

Treatment

▶ Treatment depends on ability to identify cause, correct abnormalities (i.e., volume depletion), and remove exacerbating factors (i.e., medications).

Disposition

▶ Determined by risk stratification/likelihood of serious etiology after ED evaluation.

Home

▶ Symptoms are classic or very suggestive of benign cause.
▶ Low overall risk for life-threatening causes.
▶ Etiology is determined in ED, and outpatient management is appropriate.

Observation Unit or Admit

▶ Symptoms are suggestive of life-threatening causes.
▶ High risk for life-threatening causes (CAD, CHF, age > 45 years).
▶ Recurrent unexplained syncope not clearly of benign cause.
▶ Additional testing required and not possible as outpatient.

◑ **PEARLS AND PITFALLS**

• Syncope is a frequent but diagnostically challenging EM presentation. A diagnosis is not made in many cases.
  ○ Age > 45 years, history of CHF/ventricular arrhythmia, and abnormal ECG are the best predictors of arrhythmia or death.
  ○ Diagnostic testing should be selective (labs, cardiac markers, and CT are unnecessary when the presentation is very suggestive of benign cause).

CHAPTER 3

ACUTE CORONARY SYNDROMES

Jim Edward Weber and Thomas E. VanHecke

▶ ACS is a spectrum of disease ranging from USA and non–ST-elevation MI to ST-elevation MI (STEMI).

▶ Ischemic heart disease is the number one cause of death in the U.S.

▶ Of the approximately 1.6 million patients treated for ACS annually, 500,000 have STEMI.

▶ Minimizing time to treatment has the greatest potential to decrease morbidity and mortality.

PATHOPHYSIOLOGY

▶ USA results from inadequate O_2 supply relative to myocardial O_2 demand secondary to rupture of an unstable plaque typically located within coronary vessels.

▶ Unstable plaques have soft, lipid-rich contents, with a thin, often sclerotic, foam cell–infiltrated, fibrous cap. Release of the lipid-rich atherogenic core causes adhesion, activation, and aggregation of platelets and initiates the coagulation cascade. A superimposed thrombus forms, occluding coronary blood flow resulting in myocardial ischemia.

▶ The most common cause of non–ST-elevation MI is microvascular embolization of platelet aggregates from non-occlusive thrombus at the site of plaque rupture.

▶ The most common cause of STEMI is *occlusive* thrombus at the site of a ruptured or fissured atherosclerotic plaque.

▶ AMI results in injury to both the conduction system (ectopy and dysrhythmias) and ventricular pump function ($\uparrow$ filling pressures).

▶ The degree and duration of occlusion as well as reserve blood flow determine the extent of myocardial damage and necrosis in ACS.

CLINICAL PRESENTATION

▶ The typical patient presents as diaphoretic, anxious, and in pain. The pain is usually substernal and described as a pressure, squeeze, or discomfort. The pain often radiates to the jaw or arms.

▶ Atypical symptoms, such as weakness, dyspnea, and dizziness, are more common in women, diabetics, and the elderly.

▶ Up to 20% of infarcts go unrecognized by physician or patient ("silent").

▶ Bradycardia and hypotension are commonly seen in inferior wall MI.

▶ Tachycardia and HTN are associated with anterior wall MI.

▶ Patients may present with heart failure, arrhythmias, pericardial friction rub, or cardiogenic shock.

EMERGENCY DEPARTMENT MANAGEMENT
Presentation/Diagnosis

▶ Triggering events for plaque rupture include stress, cold, cocaine use, smoking, or assuming upright posture.

▶ Risk factors for CAD include FH (men < 55 years; women, 65 years), cigarette smoking, HTN, diabetes, and hyperlipidemia.

▶ Patients with ACS cannot be initially categorized as USA or AMI until ECG and biomarkers become available. These patients are initially grouped together, because their pathophysiology, presentation, and management are similar.

▶ USA is a clinical diagnosis and can present as *new onset, rest,* or *increasing* (threshold, frequency, or duration) chest pain, typically lasting < 30 minutes.

▶ Symptoms persisting > 30 minutes are frequently associated with elevated biomarkers and AMI.

▶ Non–ST-elevation MI: Patients who present without ST-segment elevation have either USA or non–ST-elevation MI, a distinction that is ultimately made on the presence or absence of serum cardiac markers in the blood (Table 3-1). Most patients presenting with non–ST-elevation MI ultimately develop an non–Q-wave MI (non-Q MI) on the ECG; a few may develop a Q-wave MI (QWMI).

▶ STEMI: Patients with ischemic discomfort who present with ST-segment elevation on the ECG (see below). Although biomark-

TABLE 3-1.
TIMING OF RELEASE AND UTILITY OF CARDIAC MARKERS IN AMI

Subset	Cardiac troponins	Myoglobin	CK-MB	CK-MB isoforms
MI < 4 hours	–	+	–	–
4–12 hours	+	+	+	+
< 2–10 days	±	–	–	–
Early reinfarct	–	±	+	+

Modified from Califf RM. *Acute coronary syndromes essentials*. Royal Oak, MI: Physicians Press Publishers, 2003.

ers are useful for confirmatory and prognostic purposes, they are not required for the diagnosis of STEMI and should not delay treatment.

► Most STEMI patients ultimately develop a QWMI, whereas a few develop a non-Q MI.

► ECG changes may be present or absent with USA, and cardiac markers are normal.

• Patients with *non–ST-elevation MI* may present with a relatively normal ECG, with non-specific ST- and T-wave changes, or with ischemic ST-segment and T-wave changes.

• *Classic* ECG findings of ischemia include horizontal or downsloping ST depression ≥ 0.5 mm and/or symmetrically inverted T waves > 2.0 mm.

• The ECG diagnosis of *STEMI* requires ST elevation of ≥ 1 mm in two or more contiguous leads, usually associated by location (Table 3-2).

TABLE 3-2.
ECG CHANGES BY AMI LOCATION

Anterior	V_2–V_4
Inferior	II, III, aVF, V_5, V_6
Anteroseptal	V_1–V_3
Lateral	I, aVL, V_4–V_6
Anterolateral	V_1–V_6
Right ventricular	V_{4R}–V_6
Posterior MI	Large R > 0.04 mm, R/S > 1, and V_1–V_2 ST depression

Hyperacute T waves	ST-Elevation	Inverted T waves as ST	Q-waves
Begins 15 min. post-MI and resolves rapidly	Develops if transmural ischemia is present	decreases, and can persist	Develop within hours of AMI and can persist indefinitely

FIGURE 3-1.
Progression of ECG in AMI.

- Repolarization abnormalities evolve in a relatively predictable manner (Figure 3-1). Patients with new LBBB are to be presumed positive for AMI if they present with a typical ischemic history and have at least one of three ECG criteria. These criteria consist of either ST elevation ≥ 0.1 mV in leads with a positive QRS, ST depression ≥ 0.1 mV in V_1 to V_3, or ST elevation ≥ 0.5 mV in leads with a negative QRS.

▶ Serial ECGs should be performed in patients with ongoing chest pain and normal or non-specific changes on initial ECG because complete coronary occlusion and ST-segment elevation may occur, and reperfusion therapy (medical or mechanical) may be necessary.

▶ Several biochemical markers of myocardial necrosis have both diagnostic and prognostic utility in AMI. Each cardiac marker has advantages and disadvantages; therefore, no single marker is ideal. Because cardiac markers may not turn positive immediately (hours), initial management should be based on clinical presentation and initial ECG.

- Myoglobin is the most sensitive marker and is therefore useful for detecting very early MI. However, myoglobin has a low sensitivity for detecting late MI and has a high rate of false-positivity in patients with trauma, CPR, and renal failure.

- Troponin is more specific than CK-MB or myoglobin and is the best marker with musculoskeletal injury, small MI, or late (> 2–3 days) MI.

- CK-MB takes up to 72 hours to return to normal and is therefore useful for the detection of early reinfarction. However, CK-MB has a low sensitivity in very early AMI and can be falsely positive in the setting of trauma, CPR, cardioversion, or cardiac surgery.

▶ CXR should be performed to determine the presence or absence of CHF and to exclude non-ischemic etiologies for chest pain.

Treatment

▶ All ACS patients should receive ASA, nitrates, anti-thrombin therapy, and beta-blockers in the absence of contraindications.

▶ Usual therapeutic regime consists of the following:

- ASA, 325 mg PO (unless contraindicated).
- NTG, 0.4 mg SL q5min ×3 (hold if BP < 90 or concern for RV infarct).
- Morphine sulfate, 5–10 mg IV, titrate to pain.
- Unfractionated heparin (60 mg/kg bolus followed by 12 mg/kg/hour infusion) or LMWH. Enoxaparin (1 mg/kg SC) specifically preferred unless CABG anticipated within 24 hours.
- Lopressor, 5 mg IV q5min ×3 (hold if HR < 60 or BP < 90).
- Glycoprotein IIb/IIIa inhibitor for ACS patients undergoing intervention and medically managed patients with high-risk features. Routine use in patients without high-risk triggers is not supported by evidence-based trials.

▶ Patients with non–ST-elevation MI should be triaged to an invasive (mechanical) or conservative (medical) strategy based on risk stratification.

▶ Early (< 24 hours) intervention should be considered in patients with non–ST-elevation MI and high-risk features: recurrent angina/ischemia at rest despite therapy, elevated troponin, new ST-segment depression, angina/ischemia with CHF symptoms, or worsening mitral regurgitation.

▶ Clopidogrel should be given in addition to ASA in patients for whom catheterization is not planned during the next 24–36 hours, and to patients ineligible for CABG.

▶ Patients with STEMI should receive reperfusion therapy (fibrinolytic within 30 minutes) or PCI within 90 minutes.

▶ PCI with stenting, if available, is preferred over fibrinolytics for STEMI.

▶ Definitive treatment of AMI with cardiogenic shock is PCI. IABP counterpulsation may be used to bridge such patients to PCI.

Disposition

▶ CCU for patients with ACS and ongoing chest pain, ECG changes, dysrhythmias, or hemodynamic compromise.

▶ Monitored beds for patients with resolved chest pain, normal or non-specific ECG changes, and no complications.

▶ Chest pain observation unit for patients with low likelihood of MI. Serial ECG monitoring and enzyme analysis should be monitored (see Tables 3-1 and 3-2; Figure 3-1).

◑ **PEARLS AND PITFALLS**
   - Delay in diagnosis and initiation of reperfusion therapy worsen outcomes.
   - Failure to diagnose AMI in the absence of chest pain.
   - It is not uncommon for patients with ACS to have chest wall tenderness.
   - Failure to perform right-sided ECG in inferior MI. Presence of ≥ 1 mm ST elevation in lead V_{4R} indicates right ventricular infarction. Diuretics and NTG may worsen hemodynamics by reducing preload. IV fluids, dobutamine, and dopamine help maintain preload and cardiac output.
   - Lab investigations should be performed on patients with STEMI; however, they should not delay fibrinolysis or PCI.
   - Indications for rescue angioplasty or emergent CABG include continued hemodynamic instability and failed reperfusion after thrombolytics.
   - The ideal rapid triage is door to "balloon" within 90 minutes and door to "lytic" within 30 minutes for patients suitable for intervention.

CHAPTER 4

CONGESTIVE HEART FAILURE

David E. Newcomb

▶ Clinical syndrome caused by the inability of the heart to meet the circulatory demands of the body.
▶ 5 million cases nationwide and 0.5 million new cases every year.
▶ 1 million admissions for CHF annually.

PATHOPHYSIOLOGY

▶ Systolic dysfunction (60–80%)—reduced cardiac output.
  • Two-thirds of LV failures are caused by CAD.
  • Other causes include HTN, valvular heart disease, myocarditis, and idiopathic causes.
▶ Diastolic dysfunction (20–40%)—inadequate filling due to impaired relaxation.
  • Causes include restrictive cardiomyopathy, obstructive cardiomyopathy, ischemia, HTN, and idiopathic causes.
▶ Other causes: AF with RVR, thyrotoxicosis, severe anemia, alcoholism, cocaine, infiltrative diseases, peripartum cardiomyopathy, severe HTN, valvular disease.
▶ Pulmonary edema is caused by an increase in lung fluid secondary to leakage from pulmonary capillaries into the interstitium and alveoli.
▶ Common causes of CHF exacerbations include cardiac ischemia, arrhythmias, dietary indiscretion, medical non-compliance, infection, and anemia.

CLINICAL PRESENTATION
History

▶ Classically, patient presents with progressive fatigue, weakness, and exertional dyspnea.

TABLE 4-1.
CLINICAL PRESENTATION OF CHF

Symptom	Sensitivity (%)	Specificity (%)
Exertional dyspnea	100	17
Paroxysmal nocturnal dyspnea	39	80
Orthopnea	22	74
Peripheral edema	49	47

▶ Patients may complain of orthopnea, paroxysmal nocturnal dyspnea, progressive weight gain, or peripheral edema.

▶ Non-productive cough is common; patient may have pink frothy sputum in frank pulmonary edema (Table 4-1).

Examination

▶ Patient with pulmonary edema presents as anxious, diaphoretic, and often sitting upright. Hypoxic, tachycardic, and tachypneic. BP may be high, normal, or low.

▶ Auscultation reveals either rales or, occasionally, wheezing.

▶ S_3 or S_4 gallop.

▶ Hepatojugular reflex and increased JVD.

▶ Bilateral lower extremity edema.

▶ Patients with mild to moderate exacerbation have a less dramatic presentation but may still have many of the above exam findings.

EMERGENCY DEPARTMENT MANAGEMENT
Diagnosis

▶ The diagnosis of CHF is based on history and exam findings. Lab tests and the CXR may assist with decision-making.

Lab Tests

▶ Serum electrolytes, BUN/creatine: useful to document before initiation of diuretics.

▶ Cardiac enzymes: to assess for cardiac ischemia.

▶ BNP: produced by heart secondary to wall stress and used as a marker of heart failure. Most useful when trying to differentiate between CHF and COPD or asthma in a patient without a history of CHF.

- • Serum levels of BNP of < 100 pg/ml are unlikely to be from CHF.
- • Levels of 100–500 pg/ml may be caused by CHF. However, other conditions such as PE, primary pulmonary HTN, end-stage renal failure, cirrhosis, and hormone replacement therapy may also cause elevated BNP levels in this range.
- • BNP levels of > 500 pg/ml are most consistent with CHF.
- ▶ CBC: look for anemia or leukocytosis.
- ▶ LFTs: elevation may signify congestive hepatopathy.
- ▶ Digoxin level if indicated.

Other Studies

- ▶ ECG: evaluate role for ischemia or arrhythmia, may show LVH.
- ▶ CXR: cardiomegaly most commonly observed abnormality; findings may be delayed.
  - • Stage 1: pulmonary vascular redistribution "cephalization."
  - • Stage 2: interstitial edema with Kerley B lines.
  - • Stage 3: alveolar edema leading to classic butterfly appearance.
- ▶ Echocardiography: limited availability in ED but may help identify regional wall motion abnormalities, cardiac tamponade, and valvular heart disease.

Treatment

- ▶ Sitting position.
- ▶ IV access, cardiac monitor, and pulse oximetry.
- ▶ Supplemental O_2 to maintain saturation > 90%. For patients in pulmonary edema, this is usually 100% O_2 delivered via face mask.
- ▶ Consider need for non-invasive positive pressure ventilation. It can prevent intubation if initiated early in treatment.
- ▶ If patient is tiring or in obvious respiratory failure, secure airway and mechanically ventilate.
- ▶ Foley catheter may assist in a more accurate assessment of response to diuretics, particularly in elderly patients with decreased mobility.
- ▶ Initial pharmacologic treatment depends on BP:
  - • Hemodynamically stable patients:
    - ○ Diuretics: venodilation and reduced fluid overload. IV furosemide is most widely used. Peak effect is in 30 min-

utes. If no effect, may double dose. Start with IV dose equal to patient's oral daily dose.
- Furosemide, 40–80 mg IV.
○ Nitrates: vasodilatation. Begin with SL NTG or NTG paste, use IV NTG or nitroprusside for more severe cases.
- NTG, 0.4 mg SL q5min (unless BP < 100 mmHg).
- NTG infusion can be initiated once IV is established. Start at 10–20 mcg/minute and rapidly titrate up if BP tolerates.
○ Morphine: vasodilatation, decreased anxiety, sympathetic outflow.
- Morphine sulphate, 2–5 mg IV.
• Hypotensive patients:
○ Usually cannot tolerate diuretics, morphine, and nitrates. May be able to diurese cautiously once BP improves through use of inotropes. Most commonly used inotrope is dobutamine.
- Dobutamine: increases cardiac output and decreases wedge pressure.
- Started at 2 mcg/kg/minute IV.
- Perform invasive hemodynamic monitoring when inotropes are started.

Disposition

▶ Majority of patients are admitted to monitored bed for diuresis and to rule out cardiac ischemia as a cause for CHF exacerbation. Patients on inotropic support should be admitted to the ICU.
▶ Outpatient treatment may be considered if
- Mild CHF exacerbation with good response to ED interventions
- Normal vital signs
- Established diagnosis of CHF and a known or suspected cause for exacerbation that can be addressed, such as dietary indiscretion or medical non-compliance
- Assured compliance and close follow-up with primary care physician

CHAPTER 5

AORTIC DISSECTION

Christopher R. H. Newton

▶ Most common catastrophic event involving the aorta.
▶ Male to female ratio, 2:1.
▶ Patients are usually aged 60–70 years and have HTN.

PATHOPHYSIOLOGY

▶ Begins with a tear in the intima allowing blood to dissect into the media separating intima from adventia.
▶ 70% involve the ascending aorta.
▶ Atheromatous plaque limits extent of dissection—patients aged < 40 years have diffuse dissection; patients aged > 65 years tend to have localized dissection.
▶ HTN present in 70%. Other risk factors include congenital abnormalities of the aorta such as Marfan's disease (most common cause in patients aged < 40 years), pregnancy (most common cause in women aged < 40 years), trauma, cocaine, and syphilis.
▶ Stanford classification: type A involves ascending aorta and type B involves descending aorta only. Used for prognosis and to make management decisions.

CLINICAL PRESENTATION

▶ Classically sudden onset (85%) of pain (95%) usually located in the anterior chest (73%). The pain is often described as ripping or tearing (51%) and radiates to the back (53%). Localization of dissection can be inferred from the site of the pain; however, this estimate is often inaccurate.
▶ Dyspnea from aortic insufficiency caused by a proximal dissection. Diastolic murmur of aortic insufficiency (25%).
▶ Other signs and symptoms are seen in approximately one-third of cases and are related to obstruction of branch arteries. They include syncope (12%), focal neurologic signs/symptoms (18–

30%) including acute CVA (up to 5%), and, more rarely, GI hemorrhage, hematuria, or oliguria.

▶ Patient usually has HTN but can be hypotensive if dissected proximally into pericardial sac.

▶ Upper-extremity pulse/BP differences present in 30% of patients (also found in approximately 10% of general population).

EMERGENCY DEPARTMENT MANAGEMENT

Diagnosis

▶ Missed in up to 38% of patients on initial presentation; therefore, must maintain a high index of suspicion for the disease.

▶ ECG used primarily to exclude AMI. Most common finding is LVH.

▶ CXR should be done upright. Abnormal in 80%. Classically, there is mediastinal widening > 8 cm at T4 level. Other signs include left pleural effusion, indistinct aortic knob, extension of aortic shadow beyond calcified intima (> 1 cm), and deviation of trachea or mainstem bronchi.

▶ CT scan (sensitivity 83–94%, specificity 87–100%): rapid, non-invasive study that is often used as a first-line imaging modality in the ED. May also demonstrate other causes of symptoms. Disadvantages: difficulty imaging origin of intimal flap, involvement of branch vessels, and the aortic valve function. It also requires contrast.

▶ TEE (sensitivity 35–88%, specificity 39–96%): non-invasive, requires no contrast, and can be performed at the bedside, making it useful for hemodynamically unstable patients. Disadvantages: operator dependent and is also limited by institutional availability.

▶ Aortography (sensitivity 86–88%, specificity 75–94%): demonstrates anatomy and therefore is often preferred by cardiothoracic surgeons before surgery. Disadvantage: morbidity associated with a large contrast load.

▶ MRI (sensitivity and specificity 95–100%): lack of availability and long study times make this a poor choice for the ED work-up of suspected dissection (Figure 5-1).

Treatment

▶ Most important aspect of ED care is the control of arterial BP. The goal is to reduce rise of aortic pulse pressure (dP/dt) and

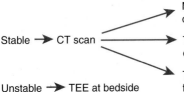

FIGURE 5-1.
ED work-up of suspected aortic dissection.

contractility of the LV. BP control should begin before definitive diagnosis if suspicion is high.

▶ BP control medications should be administered IV, with consideration of invasive BP monitoring.

• First choice is IV esmolol (beta-blocker), which has a very short half-life and allows rapid titration of effect. Decreases contractility and wall stress.

• IV nitroprusside is often used in combination with esmolol. Fenoldopam is also used at some centers to help control BP.

• Goal for BP control is systolic pressure of approximately 120 mmHg.

▶ Type A dissections are usually managed operatively. Surgery is contraindicated in patients with complications such as stroke. Operative mortality is 5–10% with a total in-hospital mortality for all proximal dissections of 30%.

▶ Type B dissections are managed medically with BP control.

▶ Endovascular stents are being studied in unstable proximal dissections and distal dissections complicated by organ or limb ischemia. The preliminary data are good, and they may play a role in the future management of both types of dissection.

Disposition

▶ Cardiothoracic surgeon should be consulted early, often before definitive diagnosis if suspicion is high. Patients who do not go directly to the OR are admitted to the ICU.

◐ **PEARLS AND PITFALLS**

• Most common mistake is to not consider the diagnosis.

• Consult cardiothoracic surgeon early.

• Imperative to have tight BP control.

CHAPTER 6

ATRIAL FIBRILLATION

Jeremy L. Cooke

▶ Atrial fibrillation (AF) is the most frequently managed arrhythmia in the ED.
▶ Both incidence and prevalence of AF rise with increasing age:
- 0.5–2% in patients aged 50–59 years
- 2–5% in patients aged 60–70 years
- 8.8% in patients aged > 80 years
▶ AF is associated with significant morbidity, including decreased exercise tolerance, embolic strokes, cardiomyopathy, and CHF.
▶ Mortality rates are doubled in patients with chronic AF compared with controls.

PATHOPHYSIOLOGY

▶ Multiple chaotic re-entrant impulses of various sizes are discharged throughout the atria, creating continuous electrical activity.
▶ Impulses arrive at the AV node and are propagated in an irregular fashion.
▶ Loss of organized atrial contraction ("atrial kick") and irregularity of ventricular response result in decreased cardiac output.
▶ The physiologic effects of a rapid ventricular response are broad and can range from asymptomatic to severe, life-threatening symptoms such as CHF, syncope, and angina.
▶ Rapid ventricular response rate increases O_2 demand and decreases diastolic filling time, which may cause ischemia in patients with underlying CAD.
▶ Stasis of atrial blood can produce cardiac clots and subsequent embolization, resulting in stroke and other embolic phenomena.

ETIOLOGY

▶ Immediate and life-threatening causes such as cardiac ischemia, CHF, and PE should be considered first (Table 6-1).

TABLE 6-1.
CAUSES OF AF

Cardiac	Non-cardiac
Ischemic heart disease	PE
HTN	Medication non-compliance
CHF	Thyroid disease
Pericarditis	Holiday heart syndrome
Valvular disease	Idiopathic
Sick sinus syndrome	Hypokalemia
Cardiomyopathy	Hypomagnesemia
Myocarditis	Medication use
Cardiac surgery	Electrocution
Congenital heart disease	Hypothermia
Infiltrative heart disease	Chest trauma

▶ Idiopathic and cardiac causes account for the largest percentage of AF.

▶ Obstructive sleep apnea may be an important risk factor.

▶ AF occurs in up to 20% of patients who present with AMI.

CLINICAL PRESENTATION

History

▶ Palpitations are the most common presenting symptom.

▶ Many elderly patients complain of vague symptoms, weakness, or dizziness.

▶ Chest pain, fatigue, dyspnea, and lightheadedness are also common and may indicate associated myocardial ischemia.

▶ Pleuritic chest pain may be seen with pericarditis or PE.

▶ Syncope is less common but may be a sign of a more severe disease process, such as aortic stenosis, sinus node dysfunction, cerebrovascular disease, hypertrophic cardiomyopathy, or an accessory pathway.

Physical Exam

▶ HRs may be normal but are usually tachycardic.

▶ Heart sounds and pulse are irregularly irregular.

▶ If HR is exceedingly high (> 160 bpm), consider thyrotoxicosis, fever, CHF, PE, dehydration, or acute blood loss.

▶ If HR is low, consider underlying conduction abnormalities or medications that may mask tachycardia.

TABLE 6-2.
DIFFERENTIAL DIAGNOSIS OF AF

Atrial flutter
Multifocal atrial tachycardia
PSVT
Sinus tachycardia
Pre-excitation syndromes:
   WPW
   Lown-Ganong-Levine syndrome

▶ BP measurements can be falsely reassuring. Mental status is a useful clinical indication of adequate cerebral blood flow.
▶ Respiratory compromise can indicate PE, CHF, or pneumonia.
▶ Fever can indicate sepsis, PE, endocarditis, or thyroid storm.
▶ Focal neurologic deficits may indicate a cerebral embolic event.

DIFFERENTIAL DIAGNOSIS OF ATRIAL FIBRILLATION (NARROW-COMPLEX TACHYCARDIAS)

▶ Consideration of the differential diagnosis in patients with suspected AF is very important, as the treatments for AF can have catastrophic consequences for patients with other cardiac arrhythmias (Table 6-2).

EMERGENCY DEPARTMENT MANAGEMENT

▶ Consider need for airway control or emergent cardioversion (i.e., ABCs).
▶ Brief, focused history and physical exam should occur simultaneously with the initial interventions, which include IV access, supplemental O_2, and cardiac monitoring.
▶ Obtain an ECG and a CXR. Further testing should be based on patient presentation and risk factors for other underlying disease.

Diagnosis

▶ ECG is the gold standard.
   • Irregularly irregular R-R intervals (use of calipers is helpful).
   • Absence of P waves.
   • Irregular fibrillatory wave forms (best seen in V_1).
▶ **Note:** An irregular, wide-complex tachycardia (WCT) suggests an SVT with aberrant conduction, which includes AF or multifo-

cal atrial tachycardia with underlying BBB and/or WPW syndrome. **Medications that slow AV conduction given to patients with WPW can induce VF arrest.** Consider early electrical cardioversion in rapid, wide-complex rhythms. Pre-excitation syndromes are typically found in younger patients whose ECGs usually demonstrate shortened PR intervals and a slurred upstroke of the QRS complex (delta wave).

▶ CXR: clues for cardiac or pulmonary disease.

▶ Lab studies: thyroid tests, CBC, chemistries, cardiac markers, drug levels, digoxin, theophylline.

Treatment

▶ The first treatment decision in rapid AF is determining whether the patient is stable.
  • Signs and symptoms of instability in rapid AF include chest pain, SOB, altered mental status, and symptomatic hypotension.

▶ Emergent DC cardioversion (synchronized) with at least 200 J is indicated in unstable patients despite known risk of thromboembolism (conversion rate success: 67–94%).

▶ Ventricular rate control improves the patient's overall hemodynamic status despite initial hypotension.

▶ CCBs: diltiazem, 10–20 mg IV, or verapamil, 5–10 mg.
  • First-line agents for rate control in narrow-complex rapid AF.
  • Risk of hypotension can be minimized by pre-treatment with IV calcium, 1–2 g.

▶ Beta-blockers: metoprolol, 5 mg IV, and/or esmolol infusion.
  • Benefit to using as first-line agent in clinical situations associated with high adrenergic tone such as thyrotoxicosis, acute hypertensive crisis, and MI.
  • Contraindicated in patients with severe bronchospasm or CHF.

▶ Digoxin: not indicated for emergency rate control.

▶ Chemical cardioversion agents such as ibutilide, amiodarone, and procainamide should be used in direct consultation with a cardiologist.

▶ Anticoagulation
  • AF duration of 48 hours or more
    ○ Literature supports anticoagulation before cardioversion.
    ○ Includes patients whose AF time is unknown or unclear.

- Role of anticoagulation in patients with AF duration of < 48 hours is less clear. There are three options:
  ○ In patients at low risk for thromboembolism and no known structural heart disease, perform cardioversion without TEE.
  ○ Perform a TEE:
    ■ If negative, cardiovert without anticoagulation.
    ■ If positive, anticoagulate for 3 weeks with follow-up TEE.
  ○ Anticoagulate all patients regardless of risk.
- Discussion of options with patient's primary care physician or cardiologist may be helpful.

Disposition

▶ In the U.S., patients with new-onset AF were often admitted for treatment, evaluation, and anticoagulation. This practice has been recently challenged in the literature.
▶ Suggested criteria for truly low-risk patients who might be discharged home safely include the following:
  - Younger patients (< 60 years)
  - Patients without significant comorbid disease
  - Patients in whom there is no clinical suspicion of PE or MI
  - Patients in whom AF converts in ED or rate is controlled
  - Patients for whom prompt follow-up is ensured
▶ In certain cases, patients may benefit from a brief work-up, which includes cardiac enzymes and TEE for risk stratification in an observational setting.

CHAPTER 7

TACHYDYSRHYTHMIAS AND CARDIOVERSION

Matthew J. Greenberg

▶ In adults, a tachydysrhythmia is defined as HR > 100 beats/minute.
▶ Patients may present with a variety of symptoms including palpitations, weakness, fatigue, nausea, dyspnea, pre-syncope, syncope, or symptoms of frank heart failure.
▶ Patients may also be asymptomatic and the dysrhythmia an incidental finding.

PATHOPHYSIOLOGY

▶ Normal electrical conduction in the heart:
  • The impulse is initiated in the SA node, travels to the AV node, slows, and proceeds through the His bundles terminating in the Purkinje fibers of the ventricles.
▶ Tachydysrhythmias are created via increased automaticity or re-entrant pathways.
  • Increased automaticity:
    ○ May occur at SA node or ectopic focus.
  • Re-entrant pathway:
    ○ Occurs with two electrical pathways of differing conduction speed and refractory period.
    ○ Often triggered by a PAC that induces a continuous circuit between the two pathways.
    ○ Activation in this manner can be either anterograde or retrograde.
    ○ WPW syndrome represents one example of a re-entrant tachycardia secondary to an accessory pathway.

IDENTIFICATION OF THE RHYTHM

▶ Narrow or wide
▶ Rate

▶ Are P waves present?
  • If so, in what relationship to the QRS?
  • Before or after the QRS?

TREATMENT

▶ If the patient is unstable, emergently cardiovert.
▶ If the patient is stable, consider pharmacologic treatment as determined by the underlying rhythm.
▶ Evaluate for underlying etiology and treat as appropriate.

Sinus Tachycardia

▶ Narrow-complex tachycardia.
▶ Rate 100–160.
▶ P wave precedes each QRS in a 1:1 ratio.
▶ Differential diagnosis includes dehydration, high adrenergic states, fevers, shock, heat stroke, hyperthyroidism, PE, sympathomimetics, withdrawal from alcohol or benzodiazepines, decreased vagal tone, anemia, hypoxia, and pain.
▶ Treat the underlying cause.

Supraventricular Tachycardia

▶ Narrow-complex tachycardia
▶ Rate typically 140–200
▶ Associated with ectopic focus and re-entrant pathway
▶ May have retrograde p waves after QRS
▶ Treatment
  • Vagal maneuvers: Valsalva, carotid sinus massage (if no carotid disease), ice water to face
  • Adenosine
    ○ Slows conduction through AV node to break rhythm and restore a sinus rhythm.
    ○ Half life < 10 seconds.
    ○ Dosing scheme: Initial bolus of 6 mg; if unsuccessful, may repeat with 12 mg twice.
    ○ Always give very rapid IV push with immediate flush.
    ○ Warn the patient of side effects, including nausea, feeling of anxiety, chest pain, dyspnea, vertigo, and syncope.
  • If adenosine is unsuccessful, consider LV function:

- ○ Normal LV function: beta-blocker, CCB, or digoxin may be used.
- ○ Decreased LV function: digoxin, amiodarone, diltiazem.
- • DC cardioversion can also be used (see below).
▸ SVT with WPW
- • These patients may present with rates > 200 beats/minute.
- • Treat these arrhythmias with caution.
- • As always, cardiovert the unstable patient.
- • Procainamide, 17 mg/kg IV infusion over 30 minutes, not to exceed 50 mg/minute, then 1- to 6-mg/minute drip hold for hypotension or 50% QRS widening.

Atrial Fibrillation/Atrial Flutter

▸ See Chap. 6.

Multifocal Atrial Tachycardia

▸ Narrow-complex tachycardia.
▸ Rate 100–180 beats/minute.
▸ Multiple foci with variable p wave morphology (at least three different morphologies required to constitute multifocal atrial tachycardia).
▸ Often associated with decompensated chronic lung disease or theophylline toxicity.
▸ Treat underlying condition—often resolves with O_2.

Junctional Tachycardia

▸ Narrow-complex tachycardia.
▸ Rate > 100 beats/minute.
▸ Absence of p waves, or retrograde p waves may be present.
▸ Associated with digoxin, catecholamine, and theophylline toxicities.
▸ Treat underlying cause; if none found, treat with same algorithm as SVT.

Ventricular Tachycardia

▸ See Chap. 17.

Unspecified Wide-Complex Tachycardia

▸ Rate > 100 beats/minute, and QRS > 0.12 seconds.

▶ May represent VT, SVT with aberrancy (such as an RBBB or LBBB), or pre-excitation.
- Pre-excitation represents a re-entrant tachycardia with ventricular activation through an accessory pathway.

▶ Differentiation of wide-complex tachycardia (WCT):
- BBB may be persistent and seen on previous ECG or may be rate dependent.
- AV dissociation and fusion beats are more consistent with VT.
- Extreme right or leftward axis is more consistent with VT.
- Concordance of the precordial QRS complexes is more consistent with VT.
- Irregularity, especially with a rate > 200 beats/minute, is most often representative of AF with aberrancy.

▶ If patient is hemodynamically unstable, cardiovert immediately; otherwise, attempt to determine SVT vs. VT and treat accordingly.
- Avoid the use of verapamil in undifferentiated WCT.
- Adenosine, amiodarone, lidocaine, procainamide, and cardioversion are considered safe in undifferentiated WCT.

DIRECT CURRENT CARDIOVERSION

▶ Used as first-line therapy in the unstable patient or if pharmacologic therapy is unsuccessful in a stable patient.

▶ Appropriate sedation should be attempted in all but the most unstable patients.
- Suitable agents include etomidate, methohexital, and midazolam.

▶ If discernible R waves are present, use in synchronized mode.
- This aligns the electrical charge so that it does not fall during repolarization.
- If VF is suspected or if T waves are more prominent than R waves, do not use synchronized mode.

▶ Paddles or "hands-off" pads can be positioned either antero-lateral or AP.
- Do not place directly over implantable defibrillators.

▶ Energy required for cardioversion is variable depending on the underlying rhythm.
- The AHA recommends a sequence of 100 J, 200 J, 300 J, 360 J; however, VT may convert with as few as 10–20 J in 80% of patients. Therefore, several authors recommend starting at 50 J.

EMERGENCY DEPARTMENT DISPOSITION

▶ Patients who are unstable at any point in time, have underlying abnormalities such as electrolyte disturbances, hypoxia, or overdose, or have ongoing arrhythmia require admission.

▶ Patients with easily converted SVT and no underlying abnormalities may be discharged after an observation period.

- Appropriate discharge instructions should include avoidance of possible precipitants, instruction in Valsalva, and appropriate follow-up.

CHAPTER 8

INFECTIVE ENDOCARDITIS

Stacey K. Noel

- ▶ Localized infection of the endocardium and valvular structures
- ▶ Occurs most commonly in individuals with predisposing risk factors
  - Congenital anatomic abnormalities (including MVP with regurgitation)
  - Prosthetic valves
  - Indwelling vascular lines or devices
  - History of IV drug abuse (usually right-sided disease)
  - Degenerative valve disease (i.e., aortic calcific stenosis)
- ▶ Epidemiology
  - Nearly two times more common in men
  - Aortic > mitral > tricuspid > pulmonic valve involvement
  - IV drug abuse mortality < 10%; 40% recurrence rate
  - Prosthetic valve recipients 3–7% occurrence, greatest risk in first 6 months postop, no difference mechanical vs. prosthetic prosthesis

PATHOPHYSIOLOGY

- ▶ Endothelial damage from blood turbulence, pressure gradient, injected.
  - Particulate matter, ischemia, or systemic inflammation.
- ▶ Deposition of platelets and fibrin at site of damage = sterile vegetation.
  - May also form due to hypercoagulability.
- ▶ Transient bacteremia (< 30 minutes) leads to colonization of sterile vegetations.
  - Highly invasive organisms may cause disease without pre-existing sterile vegetations.
  - *Staphylococcus aureus* is the most common cause of fulminant disease in native valves.

- *S. viridans* most common in prosthetic valves, but many others are possible.
- *Streptococcus* spp. may cause indolent disease.
- *S. aureus* most common in IV drug abuse patients.

▶ Organisms cause more platelet and fibrin deposition, leading to walled-off nidus of infection protected from usual cellular immune response.

▶ Vegetation fragments may embolize, leading to ongoing bacteremia and septic emboli.

▶ Valve destruction, myocardial abscess, conduction defects, and pericarditis may occur subsequently.

CLINICAL PRESENTATION

▶ History tends to be non-specific—intermittent fever, chills/rigors, malaise, fatigue, weight loss, exertional dyspnea.

▶ Exam findings include the following:
- Fever (90%)
- Murmur (80%)
- Embolic phenomena (> 50%):
    - Splinter hemorrhages
    - Osler's nodes: painful nodules on the fingertips
    - Janeway lesions: non-tender erythematous macules on hands and feet
    - Petechiae
    - Roth's spots (< 10%): retinal hemorrhages with central clearing
    - Distal abscesses
- Vital signs are often non-specific: BP may be lower owing to systolic dysfunction in fulminant cases.
- May also present with focal neurologic deficits.

EMERGENCY DEPARTMENT MANAGEMENT
Diagnosis

▶ Must have high index of suspicion—fever, new murmur, circulatory decompensation.

▶ Persistently positive blood cultures are gold standard—three sets from three different sites.

▶ TEE may reveal evidence of vegetations, abscess formation, or valvular incompetence. A negative exam does not exclude the diagnosis, however.
▶ Evidence of disparate septic emboli or CNS septic emboli.

Treatment

▶ Empiric antibiotics started based on clinical suspicion.
  • Native valve: nafcillin, 2 g IV + ampicillin, 2 g IV + gentamicin, 1 mg/kg IV
  • IV drug user, congenital heart defect, indwelling line, or hospital-acquired: nafcillin, 2 g IV + gentamicin, 1 mg/kg IV + vancomycin, 15 mg/kg IV
  • Prosthetic valve: vancomycin, 15 mg/kg IV + gentamicin, 1 mg/kg IV + rifampin, 600 mg PO
▶ Anticoagulation does not reduce risk of embolization and is potentially dangerous if patient has unrecognized septic emboli to brain or spinal cord.
▶ Consider cardiothoracic surgery consultation for patients with prosthetic valves or severe valvular incompetence.

Disposition

▶ Telemetry vs. ICU admission
▶ Prompt cardiology and infectious disease consultation
▶ Early surgical treatment indicated for
  • Increasing CHF
  • Inability to control infection with medical management
  • Valve dysfunction
▶ Mortality correlated with
  • Severity of CHF on presentation
  • Fulminant course
  • Age and comorbidity
  • CNS emboli

CHAPTER 9

ACUTE MYOCARDITIS AND ACUTE PERICARDITIS

Stacey K. Noel

MYOCARDITIS

▶ Inflammation of the myocardium with myocellular necrosis.
▶ Infiltrating cells include lymphocytes, plasma cells, histiocytes, and rarely, giant cells.
▶ Results in damage and malfunction of myocardial cells, systolic dysfunction.

Pathophysiology

▶ Caused by direct viral destruction or inflammatory damage to myocytes.
▶ Damaged myocytes release mediators activating humoral and cellular immune response → further inflammation.
▶ Many viruses have been implicated [e.g., coxsackievirus, echovirus, influenza, parainfluenza, EBV, hepatitis B virus (HBV), and HIV].

Clinical Presentation

▶ Chest pain/discomfort, usually not positional or reproducible
▶ Fever, myalgias, headache, malaise
▶ Progressive findings consistent with systolic depression and CHF—lower-extremity edema, hepatomegaly, exertional dyspnea, or pain
▶ Most common cause of sudden onset of CHF in a previously healthy young patient

Emergency Department Management

Diagnosis
▶ Usually based on combination of clinical presentation and echocardiographic findings.

▶ CXR may be normal or have cardiomegaly with pulmonary edema.
▶ ECG shows non-specific ST/T wave changes and/or variable AV blocks.
▶ Cardiac enzymes may be elevated (usually troponin I) during the first few weeks of symptoms.
▶ Echocardiography: dilated chambers and diffuse hypokinesis.

Treatment
▶ Supportive.
▶ Consider steroids but no conclusive data to support use.
▶ Antibiotics if a bacterial cause suspected.
▶ Symptomatic heart failure treatment: diuretics, pressors.
▶ Consider anticoagulation for suspected EF < 15–20%.

Disposition
▶ Telemetry vs. ICU admission

PERICARDITIS
▶ Infection or inflammation of pericardial linings
▶ Usually results in increase in pericardial fluid volume
▶ Spectrum of symptoms from pain alone to hemodynamic compromise

Pathophysiology
▶ Etiology
  • Idiopathic
  • Secondary infections (e.g., coxsackievirus, HIV)
  • Contiguous or sanguineous spread (e.g., TB, *Streptococcus*, *Staphylococcus*, *Histoplasma*)
  • Malignancy (leukemia, lymphoma, breast, lung, melanoma)
  • Pharmacologic (e.g., procainamide, hydralazine)
  • Post-pericardiotomy: 30% 2–4 weeks post-op
  • Post-radiation
  • Post-AMI (Dressler's syndrome)
  • Uremia
  • Myxedema

Clinical Presentation

History
► Sharp, stabbing, left-sided chest pain.
► Classically, pain increases with inspiration and lying supine, and decreases with leaning forward.
► Low-grade fever.
► May have dyspnea or dysphagia.

Exam Findings
► Vital signs usually normal.
► Abnormal vital signs (tachycardia, hypotension) with JVD; dyspnea may be sign of impending tamponade.
► Presence of a friction rub often changing with patient positioning.

Emergency Department Management

Diagnosis
► ECG changes:
  • Stage 1: diffuse ST elevations with upward concavity from sub-epicardial inflammation, PR depression
  • Stage 2: ST isoelectric, decreased T-wave amplitude
  • Stage 3: T-wave inversion
  • Stage 4: normalization of ECG
► Large effusion causes electrical alternans and/or low QRS amplitude.
► CXR usually normal to "waterbottle-shaped" cardiac silhouette.
► Echocardiogram is the gold standard.
  • Size of effusion may be difficult to determine.
  • Evaluate for evidence of tamponade.
► Cardiac markers may be elevated with marked myocardial involvement.

Treatment
► NSAIDs (usually Indocin).
► Treat underlying cause: e.g., dialysis for uremic, antibiotics for infective, and so forth.
► Steroids if systemic inflammation suspected or known.
► Ensure no myocarditis component (myopericarditis).
► Immediate ultrasound- or ECG-guided pericardiocentesis for clinical evidence of tamponade.

Disposition
▶ Consider discharge if no evidence of tamponade.

PERICARDIAL TAMPONADE

▶ Accumulated pericardial fluid rises to pressures greater than RV diastolic pressure.
▶ Results in loss of RV filling in diastole and hemodynamic collapse.
▶ Tamponade depends on rate of fluid accumulation, pericardial compliance, and end-diastolic RV pressure.
▶ Causes include malignancy, uremia, post-surgical, post-radiation, infectious, aortic dissection, or trauma.

Clinical Presentation

▶ Dyspnea is common.
▶ Tachycardia is early sign.
▶ Beck's triad of hypotension, JVD, and muffled heart sounds— late finding often pre-arrest.
▶ Narrow pulse pressure and pulsus paradoxus.

Emergency Department Management

Diagnosis
▶ Based on clinical presentation and confirmed by either bedside ultrasound or, if time permits, echocardiography
▶ ECG: low QRS voltage, electrical alternans

Treatment
▶ Treatment consists of pericardiocentesis. Timing of this is based on clinical stability. Patients with unstable vital signs should have this performed in the ED.
▶ Procedure:
  • Introduce cardiac or spinal needle just below xiphoid, aiming at the left shoulder; aspirate syringe plunger until blood or fluid is obtained.
  • ECG guided: attach ECG lead to needle.
  • Ultrasound guided: subxiphoid view of heart to "watch" needle position.
  • Fluid can be sent for cell counts, culture, and cytology.

► Large or recurring effusions may require placement of a pigtail drain via Seldinger technique.
► Most common complication is PTX.
► Rare but severe complication is cardiac or coronary laceration.
► Pericardiocentesis should always be followed by treatment for underlying cause of tamponade (e.g., antibiotics, dialysis, surgery).

Disposition
► Usually to the ICU for close monitoring for reaccumulation

CHAPTER 10

HYPERTENSIVE EMERGENCIES

Thomas G. Greidanus and
Christopher R. H. Newton

▶ There are 60 million people in the U.S. with HTN; approximately 1% develop hypertensive emergencies.
▶ Most commonly affects African-American males aged 40–60 years.
▶ HTN defined as BP > 160/95 mmHg.
▶ Hypertensive emergency is defined as elevated BP with evidence of acute end-organ dysfunction.
▶ Hypertensive urgency is best regarded as elevated BP (diastolic > 115 mmHg) with known target organ disease but without active compromise.

PATHOPHYSIOLOGY

▶ HTN most commonly affects the CNS, kidneys, and cardiovascular system.
▶ Malignant HTN: elevated BP associated with funduscopic changes including papilledema and evidence of encephalopathy or nephropathy.
▶ Hypertensive encephalopathy: elevated BP leading to cerebral dysregulation. Initially presents with headache, nausea/vomiting, and blurred vision that progresses to drowsiness, confusion, seizures, and coma if untreated.
▶ Usually rapid unexplained rise in BP in a patient with essential HTN, but must always consider other potential precipitants.
▶ Other causes of HTN in the ED that require careful monitoring and drug therapy include
  • Intracranial events (SAH)
  • Aortic dissection
  • Acute pulmonary edema

- Eclampsia
- Drug intoxication (e.g., cocaine, ecstasy)
- Drug withdrawal (e.g., clonidine, beta-blockers)
- Pheochromocytoma

CLINICAL PRESENTATION

History

▶ CNS symptoms include headache (85%), nausea/vomiting, blurred vision (60%), weakness, confusion, and seizures.

▶ Cardiovascular symptoms include chest pain, back pain, and dyspnea.

▶ Renal involvement is suggested by new onset of hematuria or oliguria.

▶ Ask about history of HTN, compliance with or recently stopping medications, and illicit drug use.

Exam

▶ Check BP in both extremities.

▶ Evaluate for altered mental status, focal neurologic findings, papilledema, and pulmonary edema.

EMERGENCY DEPARTMENT MANAGEMENT

Diagnosis

▶ Measure BP with an appropriately sized cuff.

▶ Asymptomatic patients with elevated BP do not need lab work or other studies in the ED.

▶ Lab studies for hypertensive emergencies include
- Electrolytes, BUN, and creatinine
- CBC
- UA to assess for hematuria or proteinuria

▶ Other studies
- CXR for cardiomegaly, evidence of pulmonary edema
- ECG to assess for LVH or ischemia
- Head CT if indicated for decreased mental status or concern about intracranial hemorrhage

Treatment

Hypertensive Emergency

▶ Goal is to stop progression of end-organ damage while preserving perfusion to vital organs. This requires rapid reduction of BP (approximately 25–30%).

▶ Invasive hemodynamic monitoring (intra-arterial catheter) should be performed in all patients with a hypertensive emergency requiring IV therapy.

▶ Specific therapy depends on the clinical situation, but the following are commonly used drug regimes:

- Hypertensive encephalopathy: IV nitroprusside or esmolol.
- ACS: IV beta-blocker in combination with NTG and morphine.
- Acute pulmonary edema: IV NTG in combination with loop diuretics.
- Aortic dissection: IV esmolol and fenoldopam.
- Pre-eclampsia: IV magnesium sulfate, hydralazine, and definitive treatment with delivery of the baby.
- Cocaine intoxication: IV benzodiazepines and phentolamine.
- Acute stroke BP treatment is potentially harmful and should only be considered if BP is very elevated (> 220/120 mmHg).

▶ Nitroprusside: rapid acting, relaxes smooth muscle, potential for cyanide toxicity at higher doses

- 0.25–10 mcg/kg/minute IV

▶ Esmolol: rapidly acting beta-blocker (duration 10 minutes)

- Load: 500 mcg/kg IV over 1 minute
- Infusion: 50–200 mcg/kg/minute

▶ Fenoldopam: dopamine receptor agonist that increases renal blood flow

- Infusion started at 0.1 mcg/kg/minute and is titrated q15min up to 1.7 mcg/kg/minute

▶ NTG

- Infusion: 10–20 mcg/minute and can rapidly increase this to desired effect

▶ Labetalol: non-selective beta-blocker with short duration of action that can be used for bolus therapy to reduce BP

- Start at 20 mg IV (can double this dose and repeat q20min up to 300 mg maximum)

Hypertensive Urgency
- ▶ Patients with hypertensive urgency can usually be managed with oral antihypertensives in the ED.
- ▶ Options include
  - • Labetalol, 200 mg PO
  - • Clonidine, 0.1–0.2 mg PO
- ▶ Patients being discharged should **not** be given IV antihypertensive medications.
- ▶ Unless immediate reduction in BP is warranted, antihypertensive medications are best initiated by the primary care physician. The exception to this is the patient with known HTN who has run out of medications and has appropriate follow-up.

Disposition

- ▶ Hypertensive emergencies should be admitted to the ICU for invasive hemodynamic monitoring.
- ▶ Hypertensive urgency with severely elevated BP may require admission to help reduce BP gradually and initiate therapeutic regime. However, the majority can be discharged to home if they have appropriate follow-up.
- ▶ All patients with documented HTN on ED visit need to have follow-up and BP recheck.

CHAPTER 11

ABDOMINAL AORTIC ANEURYSM

Brad J. Uren and Christopher R. H. Newton

- ▶ Common life-threatening emergency with a wide spectrum of clinical presentation.
- ▶ Typical patient is an elderly male with manifestations of atherosclerosis. Genetic predisposition. Other risk factors include smoking and HTN.
- ▶ Incidence is 2–4% of adult population.
- ▶ 50% Pre-hospital mortality.
- ▶ 50% Mortality for rupture that survive to ED.
- ▶ Initial misdiagnosis rate is 25–40%. The most frequent wrong diagnosis is renal colic.

CLINICAL PRESENTATION
History

- ▶ AAAs are usually asymptomatic until they expand or rupture.
- ▶ Patients with slow or contained leaks may present with abdominal or back pain.
- ▶ Classic presentation is sudden-onset, severe abdominal or back pain that radiates to the groin and is associated with a syncopal episode.
- ▶ Dissecting aneurysms have a variety of presentations, including mesenteric ischemia and/or limb ischemia if the dissection blocks flow to the individual branches of the aorta.

Physical Exam

- ▶ Vital signs variable. Normal vitals do not exclude AAA. Tachycardia and hypotension strongly suggest that the AAA is leaking or has ruptured.
- ▶ Pulsatile mass is present in 77% that have ruptured but is less frequently found if unruptured. Limited by obesity.

▶ Asymmetric or absent pulses to the lower extremities suggest thromboembolic event or dissection. The lower extremities can also show signs of ischemia from prolonged or severe interruption of blood flow.

EMERGENCY DEPARTMENT MANAGEMENT
Diagnosis

▶ Based on a high index of clinical suspicion in elderly patients who present with abdominal or back pain, especially if associated with syncope or hypotension. These symptoms alone may be sufficient evidence to call surgery and take them to the OR.

▶ Most patients require confirmatory studies:
  • Plain radiography: both insensitive and non-specific. Should not be used in the diagnostic work-up of suspected AAA. May see aortic wall calcification.
  • Ultrasonography: non-invasive, sensitive test (nearly 100%) that can be performed at the bedside. Used to measure aortic caliber and can detect free peritoneal blood. Limitations: no information about retroperitoneum or branch vessels. Unable to visualize aorta in 5–10% of patients secondary to bowel gas.
  • CT scan: also has a sensitivity of around 100% but is more accurate at detecting rupture, visceral artery involvement, and retroperitoneum. Limitations: contrast dye load, study time (patient must often be sent out of the ED), and cost.

Treatment

▶ Immediate surgical consultation should be initiated for any patient with either suspected or known AAA and unstable vital signs.

▶ Send CBC; type and cross six units PRBCs.

▶ IV access: two 16-G peripheral IVs.

▶ Supplemental O_2.

▶ Monitor, pulse oximetry.

▶ Unstable patients should receive aggressive resuscitation with crystalloid and blood products when available (consider O negative).

▶ Correct coagulation abnormalities if present.

▶ Minimally invasive endovascular surgery is now being performed on approximately 40% of AAAs.

Disposition

▶ Unstable patients should go directly to the OR.

▶ Surgical consultation should be obtained in hemodynamically stable patients with AAA > 5 cm, rapid interval enlargement in known AAA, or symptomatic AAA.

▶ All patients with AAA > 3 cm should have follow-up in the vascular surgery clinic.

CHAPTER 12

ACUTE ARTERIAL OCCLUSION

David E. Newcomb

▶ Abrupt interruption of blood flow to extremity resulting in inability to meet normal metabolic demands of tissues

PATHOPHYSIOLOGY

▶ Embolic occlusion (most common): from heart (80%) or aneurysmal thrombus.
▶ Thrombus formation: usually in the presence of pre-existing atherosclerosis and rupture of plaque causing acute local thrombosis.
▶ Direct injury to vessel, such as dissection from direct trauma or iatrogenic trauma from vessel catheterization.
▶ Emboli have highest morbidity because extremities do not have well-developed collateral circulation.
▶ Risk factors for PVD and acute arterial occlusion include smoking, hyperlipidemia, and diabetes.
▶ Limb salvage decreased at 4–6 hours after occlusion.

CLINICAL PRESENTATION

▶ Intermittent claudication may be the only manifestation of early PVD. Pain is precipitated by walking and relieved by rest.
▶ Acute arterial occlusion classically presents with some combination of the six Ps.
  • Pain: abrupt onset of severe pain. Local vessel thrombosis in the setting of atherosclerosis can be more insidious and is usually in the setting of pre-existing claudication pain. Patients with long-standing disease may have extensive development of collateral vessels; thus, complete occlusion may present less dramatically than acute embolic disease. The improvement of pain symptoms may indicate progres-

sion to a non-viable extremity rather than improvement in circulation.

- Poikilothermia: skin of the affected extremity is cool compared with the other side.
- Pallor.
- Pulselessness: examine both extremities for presence of pulse. Handheld Doppler is often required. If pulses can be observed using Doppler, the waveform may be monophasic or diminished. Absent or diminished pulses in the contralateral extremity suggest the presence of chronic PVD.
- Paralysis and paresthesias: represent underlying nerve damage from inadequate blood flow. Presence of sensory or motor deficits suggest limb-threatening ischemia.

▶ Skin over extremity may be atrophic and shiny.

▶ Auscultate for heart murmurs.

▶ The natural progression of symptoms usually is pain then paresthesias followed by paralysis.

DIFFERENTIAL DIAGNOSIS

▶ Trauma

▶ DVT

▶ Sciatica

▶ Peripheral neuropathy

▶ Raynaud's phenomenon

EMERGENCY DEPARTMENT MANAGEMENT
Diagnosis

▶ Diagnosis is usually clinical and based on prior history, presentation of current symptoms, and physical exam.

▶ Doppler ultrasonography and measurement of ABI should be included in the initial evaluation. These tests, however, should not delay vascular surgery consultation if an acute occlusion is suspected.

▶ ABI: ankle systolic pressure/brachial systolic pressure. Normal > 1.0, claudication 0.4–1.0, impending tissue damage or presence of rest pain < 0.4.

▶ Lab tests include CBC, chem 7, CK, type and screen, and PT/PTT.

▶ ECG: to evaluate for arrhythmia.

Imaging

▶ Duplex imaging: non-invasive, inexpensive study. Somewhat operator dependent and can be time-consuming. May be able to localize lesion and identify stenosis vs. occlusion.

▶ Angiography: regarded as gold-standard study; however, is invasive and has potential to cause nephrotoxicity. Helpful in discriminating embolic vs. thrombotic disease.

Treatment

▶ Once diagnosis is suspected, consult vascular surgeon immediately or, if unavailable, transfer patient to nearest hospital with vascular surgeon on call.

▶ Patient should be anticoagulated unless contraindicated and also given ASA.

▶ Definitive treatment for acute arterial occlusion entails revascularization in the form of intra-arterial thrombolytics, thrombectomy, or surgical bypass.

▶ If limb is non-viable, amputation may be required.

▶ There is **no** role for IV thrombolytics in the ED.

Disposition

▶ Patients with evidence of acute arterial occlusion are admitted to hospital for definitive care.

▶ Consider discharge for patients with
  • Known PVD and stable ABIs
  • No signs of limb-threatening ischemia and stable ABIs
  • Close follow-up with vascular surgery

CHAPTER 13

DEEP VENOUS THROMBOSIS

Diamond Vrocher III and Stephanie Hollingsworth

▶ 600,000 cases in the U.S. per year.
▶ Incidence: 1–2 events per 1000 people in the general population.
▶ Complications: PE, post-phlebitic syndrome, venous ulceration, venous insufficiency, chylothorax, and SVC syndrome.
▶ **Risk factors** are related to Virchow's triad of venous stasis, hypercoagulability, and endothelial injury (Table 13-1).

CLINICAL PRESENTATION

▶ Classic presentation is unilateral leg pain (50%), swelling (80%), and tenderness (75%).
▶ May also be erythema and edema or have palpable cord.
▶ Homans' sign (pain on passive dorsiflexion of the foot) is neither sensitive nor specific.
▶ Clinical signs and symptoms of PE: primary presentation of 10% of patients with confirmed DVT.
▶ Fever: patients may have a fever, usually low grade. High fever is usually indicative of an infectious process such as cellulitis or lymphangitis.

DIFFERENTIAL DIAGNOSIS

▶ Cellulitis: fever
▶ Venous insufficiency: burning, leg fatigue, swelling, throbbing, cramping, edema, calor, rubor, local tenderness, skin discoloration, stasis dermatitis, chronic non-healing leg ulceration, improved by walking
▶ Phlegmasia dolens (massive ileofemoral venous obstruction): edema, pain, and blanching (alba) → edema, agonizing pain, and cyanosis (cerulea) with possible bleb and bullae formation

TABLE 13-1.
RISK FACTORS FOR DVT

Previous DVT
Age
Immobilization (> 3 days)
Pregnancy/post-partum
Major surgery (previous 4 weeks)
Long plane or car trips (> 4 hours) in previous 4 weeks
Cancer
IBD
Multiple trauma
Lower-extremity fractures
Inherited disorders of coagulation/fibrinolysis
Estrogen therapy

    → gangrene → possible circulatory shock (in one-third) and/or arterial insufficiency

► Superficial thrombophlebitis: palpable, indurated, cordlike, tender subcutaneous venous segment

► Baker's cyst: often difficult to differentiate before ultrasound exam

► Asymmetric peripheral edema secondary to CHF, liver disease, renal failure, or nephrotic syndrome

► Lymphangitis or lymphedema

► Extrinsic venous compression (tumor, hematoma, or abscess)

► Hematoma or soft tissue injury

EMERGENCY DEPARTMENT MANAGEMENT

Diagnosis

► DVT should be suspected from patient's symptoms and physical exam findings. However, even in a classic presentation, the clinical diagnosis of DVT is unreliable.

► The combined use of a pre-test probability score, D dimer, and ultrasonography has been well studied. A simplified management scheme is suggested by (1) generating the pre-test probability using Wells clinical score for DVT and (2) following the algorithm in Figure 13-1.

► D dimer is a fibrin degradation product that is elevated in patients with DVT and PE.

► There are numerous rapid D dimer assays with generally high sensitivity but low specificity. Thus, the D dimer test is used to

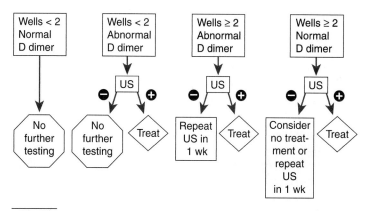

FIGURE 13-1.
Combined clinical score and D dimer for diagnosis of DVT in the ED.

rule out PE. To make clinical decisions based on D dimer, each physician must be familiar with his or her hospital's assay type. The Wells criteria are based on the SimpliRED D-dimer (Table 13-2).

▶ Duplex ultrasonography is a non-invasive test with sensitivity of 93% and specificity of 98%. Also can identify other causes of leg pain.

▶ Other imaging modalities: MRI, impedance plethysmography, contrast venography, and CT.

TABLE 13-2.
WELLS CLINICAL SCORE FOR DVT

Clinical parameter	Score
Active cancer (treatment ongoing or within 6 months or palliative)	+1
Paralysis, paresis, or recent plaster immobilization of the lower extremities	+1
Recently bedridden for > 3 days or major surgery < 4 weeks	+1
Localized tenderness along the distribution of the deep venous system	+1
Entire leg swollen	+1
Calf swelling > 3 cm compared to the asymptomatic leg (measured 10 cm below tibial tuberosity)	+1
Pitting edema (greater in the symptomatic leg)	+1
Collateral superficial veins (non-varicose)	+1
Alternative diagnosis (as likely or greater than that of DVT)	–2

High probability ≥ 3; moderate probability 1 or 2; low probability ≤ 0.

Treatment

- ▶ **Anticoagulation:** mainstay of therapy. Begin anticoagulation with heparin or LMWH (usually 5–7 days) followed by warfarin for 3–6 months.
  - • **Heparin:** 80 U/kg IV bolus followed by 18 U/kg/hour maintenance infusion. Monitor aPTT and titrate maintenance dose to effect (aPTT of 1.5–2.5 times control).
  - • **Enoxaparin (Lovenox):** 1 mg/kg SC bid (or 1.5 mg/kg SC qd). Currently, the only LMWH approved for outpatient DVT therapy. It is at least as effective as unfractionated heparin, requires no lab monitoring, can be given SC as outpatient, and has fewer bleeding side effects.
  - • **Warfarin (Coumadin):** adult: 2–10 mg/day; pediatric: 0.05–0.34 mg/kg/day; adjust according to desired INR of 2–3. Contraindicated in pregnancy.
- ▶ **IVC filter:** consider if anticoagulation is contraindicated or ineffective.
- ▶ **Compression hose:** routinely recommended.
- ▶ **Thrombolysis:** indicated for massive ileofemoral thrombosis or upper-extremity DVT. Administered with heparin. Decreased post-phlebitic syndrome but markedly increased risk of bleeding complications.
- ▶ **Thrombectomy:** typically reserved for patients with massive ileofemoral thrombosis.

Disposition

- ▶ Outpatient treatment with LMWH is rapidly becoming the treatment of choice if no contraindication exists (suspected concomitant PE, extensive ileofemoral DVT, morbid obesity, renal failure, significant comorbidities, or poor follow-up).
- ▶ For patients beginning on warfarin, arrange for close monitoring of INR until therapeutic goal is attained.
- ▶ Most patients require 3 months of oral anticoagulation. Those with certain risk factors require longer therapy.

- ◑ **PEARLS AND PITFALLS**
  - • Consider occult malignancy; in patients with no other identifiable risk factor, cancer is newly diagnosed within 2 years in up to 25% of patients with DVT.

- PE is the primary non-traumatic cause of mat⟨
  during pregnancy and post-partum. Bed rest du⟨
  nancy increases the risk 20-fold.
- Never begin warfarin therapy without prior heparinization,
  because warfarin can produce a hypercoagulable state in
  the first 5 days.

CHAPTER 14

APPROACH TO AIRWAY MANAGEMENT

Eugene Kenny and Michael Lutes

INDICATIONS

▶ Airway protection: altered mental status, increased risk of aspiration
▶ Ventilation: respiratory failure that leads to inadequate gas exchange
▶ Oxygenation: inability to maintain adequate O_2 levels (e.g., CHF, asthma, ARDS, pneumonia)
▶ Patency: mass, edema, or hematoma that threatens closing the airway
▶ Drug administration: patients with inadequate IV access or cardiac arrest. Drugs that can be given endotracheally: Narcan, epinephrine, lidocaine, and atropine   (typical doses are 2–2.5 times the IV dose)

AIRWAY ASSESSMENT

▶ No single anatomic feature can reliably predict difficult intubations; however, various predictors have been found to be suggestive.
▶ **Worrisome characteristics include**
  • Thyromental distance: less than three finger breadths
  • Mallampati class greater than II
  • Inability to open mouth greater than three finger breadths
  • Neck mobility at atlanto-occipital less than 35 degrees
  • Evidence of obstruction: stridor, hematoma, hoarseness, or subcutaneous air

PREPARATION

▶ Adequate preparation is the most important step in successful intubations.

Equipment

▶ Laryngoscope: curved (Macintosh) or straight (Miller). Always check light and have alternate handle available.
▶ Bag valve mask with O_2 reservoir.
▶ ETTs: always have several sizes, check balloon, and lubricate.
▶ Suction: with Yankauer tip attached, make sure suction connected and on.
▶ Stylet: recommended for emergency intubations to increase success.
▶ IV: one functioning IV is essential.
▶ Monitors: pulse oximetry, ECG leads, BP, and end-tidal CO_2.
▶ Rescue airways: see below.

Patient Preparation

▶ See Airway Assessment above.
▶ Obtain ample history, respiratory/cardiac status, and information about diseases that affect C-spine stability (RA, ankylosing spondylitis) if time permits.
▶ Positioning: The bed should be at midchest of intubator, and patient should be in the "sniffing position" (head extended and neck flexed) if possible. In trauma patients in whom C-spine precautions need to be maintained, an assistant should stabilize the head when the cervical collar is removed, and neck movement should be considered.

Preoxygenation

▶ Patients should be preoxygenated with 100% O_2 via face mask for 3 minutes to minimize O_2 desaturation during intubation.
▶ Alternatively, four maximal breaths of 100% O_2 provides adequate oxygenation if time does not permit.
▶ Cricoid pressure (Sellick maneuver) must be maintained if ventilations are needed.
▶ Consider an oropharyngeal airway in an obtunded patient.

Premedication

▶ Lidocaine: consider in elevated ICP; however, no proven benefit in humans and requires 3–5 minutes before intubation.
▶ Opiates: consider fentanyl for analgesia in awake patients and to blunt sympathetic response to intubation in patients with aortic dissection, ischemic heart disease, and elevated ICP.

▶ Atropine: indicated for children aged < 5 years to prevent bradycardia and excessive secretions.

RAPID SEQUENCE INTUBATION

▶ Safest and most effective for the majority of ED intubations.
▶ Assumes that the patient has a full stomach and that a definitive airway can be obtained, even if initial intubation attempts are unsuccessful.
▶ Paralytics should be administered immediately after sedative. Wait 45–60 seconds for optimal intubating conditions.
▶ Do not give positive pressure ventilation after paralysis unless intubation attempts are unsuccessful and the patient becomes hypoxic.
▶ Maintain cricoid pressure after sedation to minimize aspiration.

Medications

▶ These drugs provide optimal intubating conditions and minimize side effects for the patient; however, they also create an apneic patient without an airway. The characteristics of the individual medications must always be considered (Tables 14-1 and 14-2).

Endotracheal Tube Placement

▶ Laryngoscope should be held in left hand and the mouth opened with right thumb and index finger.
▶ Laryngoscope blade is inserted in the right side of the mouth and tongue is swept to the left, being careful to avoid the teeth and lips.
▶ A curved blade is advanced into the vallecula between the epiglottis and base of the tongue; up and outward pressure elevates the epiglottis allowing a view of the larynx.
▶ A straight blade is advanced until the tip is under the epiglottis and gently lifted to expose the vocal cords.
▶ ETT is placed through the vocal cords with the right hand, under direct visualization.
▶ The BURP maneuver (an assistant provides backward, upward, and rightward pressure against the larynx) has been shown to increase success.
▶ After the tube has been placed, the stylet is withdrawn, cuff is inflated, and bag valve mask is attached.

TABLE 14-1.
SEDATIVES USED IN AIRWAY MANAGEMENT

Medication	RSI dose	Typical 70-kg dose	Onset	Duration	Cautions/notes
Etomidate	0.3 mg/kg	20 mg	30 seconds	3–5 minutes	Little hemodynamic effect
Midazolam (Versed)	0.3 mg/kg	20 mg	2 minutes	1 hour	Hypotension Amnesia
Fentanyl	1–2 mcg/kg	100 mcg	1 minute	30–60 minutes	Chest wall rigidity
Ketamine	1–2 mg/kg	100 mg	30–60 seconds	5–15 minutes	Bronchodilation Emergence phenomenon HTN

TABLE 14-2.
PARALYTICS USED IN AIRWAY MANAGEMENT

Medication	RSI dose (mg/kg)	Typical 70-kg dose (mg)	Maintenance dose (mg/kg)	Onset	Duration (minutes)	Cautions/notes
Succinylcholine	1–2	100	—	30–60 seconds	5–10	Depolarizing[a]
Vecuronium	0.15–0.30	10	0.1	2–5 minutes	30–60	—
Rocuronium	0.6–1.2	70	0.6	2 minutes	30	—
Atracurium	0.5	35	0.4	3–5 minutes	20–40	—

[a]**Succinylcholine** can cause hyperkalemia in patients with crush injuries, burns, or denervating injuries more than 3 days old. Also, it can cause increased IOP and ICP.

▶ Common pitfalls include standing too close to the patient (which limits view), levering the blade on the upper teeth, and hurrying to intubate a patient without adequate preparation of the patient, equipment, and yourself!

Placement Confirmation

▶ Visualize the tube pass through the cords.
▶ Listen over the epigastrium for gurgling sounds, which would indicate esophageal placement.
▶ Symmetric chest rise and bilateral breath sounds.
▶ End-tidal CO_2 detector (colorimetric detector should turn yellow) now considered standard of care in the ED. Color change does not occur in patients with cardiac arrest.
▶ CXR to confirm location.
▶ Secure the tube with a collar or tape.

DIFFICULT AIRWAYS

▶ Multiple difficult airway algorithms exist. Avoiding bad outcomes requires always having a backup plan and being familiar with various rescue airway techniques.

NASOTRACHEAL INTUBATION

▶ **Indications:** when it is difficult or impossible to access the mouth (patient with a wired jaw, obstruction, or severe tongue swelling). The patient should be breathing spontaneously if nasotracheal intubation is attempted.
▶ **Contraindications:** suspected basilar skull fracture, nasal fracture, or coagulopathy. Usually is more time-consuming than other methods.
▶ **Procedure:** Use topical vasoconstrictors/anesthetics (phenylephrine, lidocaine, or cocaine) in the nose to prevent bleeding and discomfort. Insert a lubricated tube perpendicularly to the face and advance gently cephalad. In the spontaneously breathing patient, air movement can be auscultated through the tube. Advance the tube during inspiration toward the sound of the breath sounds. Most common problem is placing the tube in the esophagus, which can be corrected by extending the neck, directing the tube anteriorly.

COMBITUBE

▶ **Indications:** patients who cannot be intubated or ventilated, to avoid a surgical airway.

▶ **Contraindications:** children < 4 feet tall, intact gag reflex, esophageal pathology, or caustic ingestions. Combitubes do not provide a definitive airway.

▶ **Procedure:** Check balloons and preoxygenate the patient. Lift the patient's tongue and jaw and insert Combitube with the curve of the pharynx. The two balloons should be inflated, and the patient ventilates through the blue (longer) lumen. In most cases, the tip of the Combitube lies in the esophagus, and ventilating through the blue (pharyngeal) port forces air from the fenestrations in the tube into the trachea. If no breath sounds are heard or if there is no end-tidal CO_2 present, then the Combitube was placed in the trachea, and the patient should be ventilated through the tracheal lumen. Tube placement should be confirmed by auscultation and end-tidal CO_2.

LARYNGEAL MASK AIRWAY

▶ **Indications:** patients who cannot be intubated or ventilated, to avoid a surgical airway.

▶ **Disadvantages and contraindications:** incomplete protection of the airway and increased risk of gastric insufflation, inability to provide high pressures in asthmatic patients, epiglottitis, FB in upper airway or larynx.

▶ **Advantages:** blind technique, which does not require visualization of the larynx or paralytics; success is independent of abnormal anatomy that may make intubation difficult.

▶ **Procedure:** LMA is a semi-rigid tube and inflatable mask, which is placed blindly in the hypopharynx. The cuff is deflated and lubricated, and the LMA is pressed against the hard palate and advanced into the posterior pharynx.

▶ **Intubating LMAs (ILMAs)** are available that allow placement of an ETT through the LMA after it is in place.

NEEDLE CRICOTHYROTOMY/TRANSTRACHEAL JET VENTILATION

▶ **Indications:** failed non-surgical technique in the "cannot intubate, cannot ventilate" patient or significant trauma that does not allow orotracheal intubation; primarily used in children aged < 8 years.

▶ **Contraindications:** significant laryngeal trauma or total obstruction at the level of the larynx.

▶ **Procedure:** The cricothyroid membrane is identified and punctured with a 12- to 16-ga catheter-over-needle. The catheter is attached to a syringe with saline, and the catheter is advanced when air is aspirated. The catheter is attached to a pressurized O_2 source (50 psi for adults; 20–30 psi for children aged > 5 years, and a bag should be used for children under 5). 1 second of inflation and 2–3 seconds of exhalation give the proper ventilation rate.

SURGICAL CRICOTHYROTOMY

▶ **Indications:** failed non-surgical technique in the "cannot intubate, cannot ventilate" patient or significant trauma that does not allow orotracheal intubation.

▶ **Contraindications:** significant laryngeal trauma, age < 10 years, or expanding neck hematoma.

▶ **Procedure:** Oxygenate the patient while prepping the neck. A vertical incision is made in the midline through the skin inferior to the thyroid cartilage over the cricoid membrane, and then a horizontal incision is made through the cricothyroid membrane. The hole must be immediately controlled with a hemostat, blade handle. A tracheal hook should be used to retract the tracheal cartilage and a 6.0 ETT or tracheal tube is inserted into the trachea and secured.

PERCUTANEOUS CRICOTHYROTOMY

▶ The same **indications** and **contraindications** as surgical cricothyrotomy.

▶ **Procedure:** Many kits are available and are based on the Seldinger technique. A catheter-over-needle is inserted through the cricothyroid membrane, and air is aspirated to confirm location. A guidewire is placed through the catheter and the catheter withdrawn. A tracheal tube with a dilator is placed into the airway over the wire. Tube placement is confirmed in the usual manner.

SPECIAL POPULATIONS
Pediatric Patients

▶ Anatomic differences:
  - Larger occiput causes neck flexion when supine. Placing a towel under the neck can facilitate the correct sniffing position.
  - The more anterior opening of the larynx, the larger tongue, and floppy epiglottis favor the use of a laryngoscope with a straight blade in children.
  - ETTs without cuffs are used in children under age 8, as the narrowest portion of the airway is at the cricoid ring.
▶ Equipment
  - The equipment needed for pediatric RSI is essentially the same as that in adults, but care must be taken to ensure that the devices are all of the proper size. Weight- or length-based references, such as the Broselow emergency tape, are useful for selecting the proper size equipment.
  - ETT size: estimated with formula: $(16 + \text{age in years})/4$.
  - ETT insertion depth: tube diameter $\times 3$.
  - Use uncuffed tubes in children under age 8.
  - Straight blade preferred in children under age 8.
▶ Medications
  - Atropine, 0.02 mg/kg IV, should be given to all patients aged ≤ 5 years to prevent vagal-induced bradycardia during intubation and to help minimize secretions.
  - Sedating agents: etomidate, 0.2–0.3 mg/kg IV; midazolam, 0.1–0.2 mg/kg IV; or ketamine, 1–2 mg/kg IV.
  - Paralytic agents: succinylcholine, 1.5–2.0 mg/kg IV; rocuronium, 1.0–1.2 mg/kg IV.
▶ Rescue devices
  - Bag valve mask ventilation
  - LMA
  - Needle cricothyrotomy with jet insufflation is the preferred emergency surgical airway in children under age 8; standard surgical cricothyrotomy may be performed in children 8 years and older.

Obstetric Patients

▶ Several anatomic and physiologic changes make RSI more challenging in obstetric patients.

▶ Progesterone-induced increases in total body water lead to vascular engorgement and edema of important respiratory tract structures including the oro- and nasopharynx, larynx, and trachea. Bleeding with instrumentation is more likely. Tissue edema of the airway structures may necessitate the use of smaller-than-predicted ETTs.

▶ Decreased functional residual capacity (FRC) owing to diaphragmatic elevation and increased O_2 consumption contributes to more rapid O_2 desaturation during RSI.

▶ Relaxation of the lower esophageal sphincter increases risk of aspiration.

▶ The supine position should be avoided, as the gravid uterus can compress the IVC, ultimately leading to decreased cardiac output.

CHAPTER 15

APPROACH TO SHOCK

Holly Weymouth and Laura Roff Hopson

▶ Reduction in tissue perfusion resulting in decreased tissue O_2 delivery.

▶ Treatment of underlying disorder in addition to adequate resuscitation is crucial to survival.

PATHOPHYSIOLOGY

▶ **Hypovolemic:** decreased preload. Caused by hemorrhage or fluid loss.

▶ **Cardiogenic:** pump failure. Leading cause is AMI. Also caused by cardiomyopathies, dysrhythmias, mechanical abnormalities (papillary muscle rupture, ventricular septal rupture), and obstructive disorders (e.g., cardiac tamponade, massive PE). Spiral of decreased perfusion resulting in decreased pump function resulting in decreased perfusion, and so on.

▶ **Vasodilatory:** severe decrease in SVR and maldistribution of blood volume. Caused by sepsis, anaphylaxis, neurogenic shock, toxins, burns, pancreatitis, myxedema, and ischemia reperfusion syndrome due to prolonged shock of any cause.

CLINICAL PRESENTATION

▶ Hypoperfusion of end organs. Clinical signs include altered mental status, oliguria, metabolic (lactic) acidosis, and hypotension.

▶ **Hypovolemic:**
  • Hypoperfusion. Cool, mottled extremities. Narrow pulse pressure, poor capillary refill, low JVP.
  • Suggested by findings of trauma, blood loss, or dehydration.

▶ **Cardiogenic:**
  • Hypoperfusion, narrow pulse pressure, increased JVP, pulmonary edema (most but not all patients), gallop rhythm, ECG

changes (ST elevation or non-specific). 75% of patients have LV failure. RV failure classically presents with hypotension with distended neck veins and no evidence of pulmonary edema.

- 90% of patients develop after hospital admission but generally (75%) within 24 hours of onset of cardiac ischemia (mean time to onset 5–7 hours).
- Risk factors include increasing age, diabetes, and prior MI.

▶ **Vasodilatory:**
- Hypoperfusion, but in contrast to hypovolemic and cardiogenic shock, patients typically have increased cardiac output and signs of peripheral vasodilation. Early signs include hyperemic extremities, bounding pulses, brisk capillary refill, hyperdynamic heart sounds, and wide pulse pressure.

DIAGNOSIS

▶ **Cardiogenic:**
- ECG, CXR, cardiac enzymes, echocardiography (determine EF, wall motion abnormalities, valvular dysfunction, tamponade), CT scan (rule out PE if clinical suspicion). Typical hemodynamic profile includes wedge pressure > 15 mmHg with a CI < 2.2 L/minute/m^2.

▶ **Hypovolemic:**
- History and physical exam to identify source of volume loss. Consider sources of occult blood loss (aortic dissection, ruptured ectopic pregnancy). Consider causes of impaired venous return (tension PTX, status asthmaticus, mechanical ventilation, restrictive cardiac disease).

▶ **Vasodilatory:**
- Fever, leukocytosis, or leukopenia.
- Evaluate for an infectious source (consider TSS in a menstruating woman). Blood cultures may not help ED management but should be obtained from two or three separate sites (no organism identified in one-third of cases).

▶ **Miscellaneous causes:**
- Consider if more common causes not apparent or in patients unresponsive to treatment.
- In adrenal insufficiency, baseline cortisol < 25 mg/dl is useful diagnostic threshold or if cortisol response to corticotropin stimulation test is < 9 mg/dl regardless of baseline.

- Evaluate for other causes with detailed history and lab tests such as thyroid function, catecholamine levels, and toxicology screens.

TREATMENT

▶ Goal for all types of shock: Restore normal tissue perfusion quickly to prevent multiple organ system failure.

▶ **Airway/breathing**
  - Early ET intubation if respiratory failure, hypoxemia, significant hemodynamic instability, or depressed mental status.
  - Mechanical ventilation and paralytics decrease O_2 demand of respiratory muscles and optimize oxygenation.

▶ **Circulation**
  - *Volume resuscitation.* Crystalloid or blood products if hemorrhagic/hypovolemic shock. Titrate to desired clinical endpoints [increased BP, CVP, urinary output (UOP), decreased HR] and watch for signs of fluid overload if large volume infusions or concern for cardiogenic shock. Use warmed fluids to avoid hypothermia. Small (250-cc) boluses if suspect cardiogenic shock.
  - *Vasoactive therapy.* Determine if low or high cardiac output state. For low cardiac output (e.g., cardiogenic shock), consider dobutamine if SBP > 80 mmHg, or dopamine if SBP < 80 mmHg. Some suggest that a combination of both may be preferred. Amrinone or milrinone can be added in refractory hypotension. For high cardiac output state (e.g., septic shock), phenylephrine or norepinephrine is preferred. Dopamine also produces vasoconstriction at doses > 10 mg/kg/minute. Vasopressin is not first-line therapy but may be added and eliminates need for catecholamines. Epinephrine (1–10 mg/kg/minute) may be used in severe shock and has both alpha- and beta-adrenergic effects.
  - Early goal-directed therapy in septic shock is shown to improve mortality (30.5% in-hospital mortality vs. 46.5% for standard therapy).
    - Maintain CVP 8–12, MAP > 65 mmHg, UOP > 0.5 ml/kg/hour, and central venous or mixed venous O_2 saturation > 70%.
    - Accomplish this with fluids to keep CVP 8–12 and pressors to achieve MAP > 65 mmHg. Transfuse PRBCs for

$SvO_2 < 0\%$ until HCT is $> 30\%$. If SvO_2 remains low, use inotropes.
- No evidence of mortality benefit for $NaHCO_3$, even in severe acidosis.

▶ **Treat underlying cause**
- **Hypovolemic.** Stop hemorrhage/fluid loss.
- **Cardiogenic.** Improved survival with early revascularization with PCI or CABG in patients aged < 75 years recommended based on results of SHOCK trial. Aggressive medical therapy (thrombolytics + vasopressors + IABP) if transfer is needed for revascularization. Elderly patients aged > 75 years may also benefit from early revascularization. Optimize all other parameters, such as electrolytes. Correct dysrhythmias.
- **Septic.** Treat with early administration of broad-spectrum antibiotics and debridement of necrotic/infected tissues if present. Early goal-directed volume resuscitation improves outcome. Low-dose corticosteroids (hydrocortisone, 200–300 mg/day) may improve hemodynamics if there is relative adrenal insufficiency. Activated protein C may be indicated in severe sepsis with end-organ failure or APACHE II score > 25 and no bleeding risks.
- **Adrenal insufficiency.** Suspect if refractory hypotension despite vasopressors or if a history of exogenous steroid administration. Stress dose replacement steroid is hydrocortisone, 100 mg q8h. Dexamethasone can also be used and does not interfere with subsequent corticotrophin stimulation testing.

CHAPTER 16

ANAPHYLAXIS

Scott A. Kelley and Laura Roff Hopson

▸ Largely underreported, but estimated incidence 1–3% in the U.S.
▸ Wide range of severity from minor to life-threatening.
▸ An estimated 30,000 anaphylactic reactions to foods are treated in EDs and 150–200 fatalities occur each year in the U.S.

PATHOPHYSIOLOGY

▸ Exposure to antigenic stimulus that binds to IgE on mast cells and basophils, leading to the sudden systemic release of chemical mediators (including histamine, tryptase, chymase, nitric oxide, and heparin). Prior exposure to antigen is necessary for full-blown anaphylaxis to occur.
▸ Anaphylactoid reaction is similar but does not require prior exposure to antigen and is not IgE mediated.
▸ Death most commonly results from cardiopulmonary effects such as laryngeal edema, respiratory failure, and circulatory collapse.
▸ Common causes of IgE-mediated anaphylaxis are insect stings, medications (e.g., penicillin and sulfa), latex, peanuts, and shellfish.

CLINICAL PRESENTATION

▸ Initially present with nasal itching or lump in throat that can rapidly progress to systemic manifestations of disease.
▸ Urticaria and angioedema are the most common manifestations (92%) and generally arise within 5–30 minutes of exposure to an antigenic stimulus. Reactions to some agents (e.g., ASA) may not develop for several hours. Rarely, reactions are biphasic, with recurrent symptoms manifesting again up to 38 hours (mean of 10 hours) after the initial attack.

▶ Cardiorespiratory: chest pain, SOB, cough, hoarseness, wheezing, syncope, and laryngeal edema.

▶ Other cutaneous: generalized pruritus, flushing, morbilliform rash, and pilar erecti.

▶ GI: dysphagia, heartburn, abdominal cramps, diarrhea, nausea, and vomiting.

▶ Close attention to vitals for hypotension, tachycardia, and tachypnea.

▶ Full-blown anaphylaxis leads to progressive upper airway swelling and obstruction, hypotension, and tachycardia that must be managed aggressively to avoid cardiovascular collapse.

DIFFERENTIAL DIAGNOSIS

▶ Other forms of shock (hemorrhagic/hypovolemic, cardiogenic, septic)

▶ Flush syndromes (carcinoid, pheochromocytoma, postmenopausal, oral hypoglycemic agents with alcohol)

▶ Syndromes of acute respiratory failure (status asthmaticus, FB aspiration, PE, epiglottitis)

▶ "Restaurant" syndromes (monosodium glutamate, sulfites, scombroidosis)

▶ Excess endogenous production of histamine (systemic mastocytosis, basophilic leukemia, acute promyelocytic leukemia, hydatid cyst)

▶ Non-organic diseases (panic attacks, globus hystericus)

▶ Other conditions: hereditary angioedema, serum sickness

EMERGENCY DEPARTMENT MANAGEMENT
Diagnosis

▶ Primarily based on history and physical exam (presence of urticaria, angioedema, and other associated signs in the context of exposure to known antigenic stimulus).

▶ Consider ECG to rule out primary cardiogenic cause of hemodynamic collapse.

▶ Consider CXR to exclude cardiopulmonary causes of hypotension and/or SOB, such as tension PTX and cardiac tamponade.

▶ Labs and work-up are usually regarded as otherwise unhelpful in the acute setting unless patient has significant comorbidities.

Treatment

▶ Assessment and maintenance of ABCs are necessary before proceeding to other management steps.

▶ Whether anaphylactic (IgE mediated) or anaphylactoid (IgE independent), treatment is the same.

▶ **Epinephrine** (0.1–0.5 mg aqueous 1:1000 dilution) SC.

▶ May administer IV epinephrine 1:1000 (0.1 ml in 10 ml of NS) as a last resort if hypotension is refractory to multiple doses of SC epinephrine (risk for lethal arrhythmias with IV administration). May require multiple epinephrine doses before response.

▶ Maintain a low threshold for intubation (cricothyrotomy may be required). Administer supplemental O_2.

▶ Place patient in Trendelenburg position to maximize perfusion of vital organs.

▶ Eliminate any ongoing exposure to inciting stimulus, such as stopping IV infusions or removing topicals.

▶ Volume resuscitation with crystalloid. Vasodilation and leaky capillaries may require large volumes to treat hypotension.

▶ Adjunctive pharmacologic therapy:

- **H_1-receptor antagonists** (e.g., diphenhydramine, 25–50 mg for adults and 1 mg/kg for children) diminish urticaria, angioedema, or pruritus.

- **H_2-receptor antagonists** (e.g., ranitidine and cimetidine) have an additive benefit with H_1 blockers.

- **Corticosteroids** may prevent persistent or biphasic anaphylaxis (e.g., methylprednisolone, 1–2 mg/kg/day IV q6h) but require several hours to take effect.

- **Inhaled beta-2 agonists** (e.g., albuterol) combat bronchoconstriction.

- **Glucagon** (e.g., 1–5 mg IV push followed by infusion) may reverse hypotension and bronchoconstriction, especially in patients on beta-blockers.

- **Vasopressors** (e.g., dopamine, norepinephrine) for refractory hypotension.

Disposition

▶ Patients with hypotension and/or significant upper airway compromise should be admitted to the ICU setting even if responsive to therapy. With complete resolution of symptoms, a monitored bed may be appropriate.

► Patients who are on beta-blockers, have significant comorbidities, and are elderly have a higher likelihood of delayed reactions and should be admitted for observation unless symptoms are minor.

► Patients without hypotension or upper airway compromise who have a complete response to therapy may be considered for discharge after a 4- to 6-hour observation period. Discharged patients should be given a 3- to 5-day course of oral steroids and also antihistamines.

► Individuals at high risk for severe anaphylaxis should be advised to carry self-injectable epinephrine (e.g., EpiPen) at all times and wear a MedicAlert bracelet.

► Prevention relies on identification of the causative agent, and referral to an allergist for skin testing is indicated.

CHAPTER 17

ADVANCED CARDIAC LIFE SUPPORT

Matthew J. Greenberg

▶ ACLS as indicated by the AHA involves the skills necessary to recognize and treat the patient presenting in cardiopulmonary arrest or in the peri-arrest period.

▶ These skills involve the initial assessment, airway management, artificial ventilation, ECG interpretation, and electrical and pharmacologic treatment of the underlying rhythms and their possible etiologies.

AIRWAY

▶ Establishment of an appropriate airway in persons unable to protect their airway.
  • ET intubation is generally considered the gold standard.
  • Alternatives such as Combitubes and LMA may be considered.

BREATHING

▶ Provide adequate ventilatory support.
  • An appropriate rate, approximately 10–12 breaths/minute.
  • An appropriate volume, 10–15 ml/kg.
    ○ Some recent data suggest 6–7 ml/kg may have fewer adverse events.
  • Supplemental O_2 at 100% FiO_2 is appropriate in the immediate resuscitation period.

CIRCULATION

▶ Adequate monitoring of the circulatory state for HR, BP, and ECG rhythm.

▶ Provide appropriate circulatory support including CPR, fluid therapy, and vasoactive support as needed.

▶ Appropriately recognize and treat electrical abnormalities of the heart with pharmacologic and/or electrical therapy.
▶ Provide acute intervention for ACS in the form of thrombolytics or PCI.

ASSESS THE CARDIAC RHYTHM

▶ Per AHA guidelines, therapies are directed at individual dysrhythmias with a concurrent goal of correcting any underlying pathology.

Ventricular Fibrillation and Pulseless Ventricular Tachycardia

▶ Electrical therapy has been shown to be most effective the earlier it is initiated.
  • Standard monophasic regimen of three stacked shocks: 200 J, 300 J, and 360 J followed by pharmacotherapy.
  • All subsequent shocks at 360 J.
  • Goal is to defibrillate within 4 minutes of onset of VF/pulseless VT.
  • Repeat defibrillation as needed after pharmacologic treatments for continued VF/pulseless VT.
  • An equivalent biphasic regimen may alternatively be used.
  • Do not shock directly over implantable automatic defibrillators.
▶ If no defibrillator present and witnessed arrest, consider precordial thump.
  • A firm thump by a closed fist from a height of 12–15 inches can generate approximately 5 J.
▶ **Pharmacotherapy:**
  • Vasopressin, 40 units IV × 1 (half-life 20 minutes), or
  • Epinephrine, 1 mg IV q3–5min
    ○ Escalating- or "high-" dose epinephrine has not been shown to have any mortality benefit.
▶ For ongoing VF or pulseless VT, consider antiarrhythmics:
  • Amiodarone, 300 mg IV, may repeat 150 mg IV
  • Lidocaine, 1.0–1.5 mg/kg IV q3–5min, to a maximum dose of 3 mg/kg
  • Procainamide, 50 mg/minute, to a maximum infusion of 17 mg/kg
▶ VT with an appearance of torsades de pointes
  • Magnesium, 1–2 g IV

TABLE 17-1.
POSSIBLE REVERSIBLE ETIOLOGIES OF PEA AND ASYSTOLE

Hypovolemia
Hypokalemia
Hyperkalemia
Hypothermia
Overdose (TCA, ASA, beta-blocker, CCB, digoxin)
Hypoxia
PE
MI
Pericardial tamponade
Tension PTX
Acidosis

Pulseless Electrical Activity

▶ See Table 17-1.
▶ Attempt to correct any of the above etiologies (Table 17-1).
▶ Ultrasound may be of some benefit in identifying cardiac motion without palpable pulse vs. electrical activity with cardiac standstill.
▶ Pharmacology:
   • Epinephrine, 1 mg IV q3–5min, or
   • Vasopressin, 40 units IV × 1 (half-life 20 minutes)
   • Atropine, 1 mg IV repeated q3–5min, with a maximum dose of 0.04 mg/kg (if HR < 60)

Asystole

▶ Asystole indicates a complete absence of electrical cardiac activity, which can be either primary or secondary in the setting of deterioration of VT or VF.
▶ Mortality for patients presenting in asystole is high.
▶ Always verify asystole in two leads 90 degrees from each other.
▶ Transcutaneous pacing:
   • Initiate early.
   • Use in conjunction with pharmacologic agents.
   • For asystole, start at highest output and titrate down to maintain capture, then add 2 mA as a safety margin.
▶ Pharmacotherapy:
   • Epinephrine, 1 mg IV q3–5min, or
   • Vasopressin, 40 units IV × 1
   • Atropine, 1 mg IV repeated q3–5min with a maximum dose of 0.04 mg/kg

POST-ARREST CARE

► Diligent monitoring is essential.
  • Invasive monitoring such as CVP, IA BP, and Swan-Ganz catheters may be warranted.
► BP augmentation may be needed with vasopressors (see Chap. 15).
  • Dopamine, 5–20 mcg/kg/minute IV
  • Norepinephrine, 0.5–30.0 mcg/minute IV
  • Dobutamine, 2.5–15.0 mcg/kg/minute IV
► Ongoing antiarrhythmic therapies:
  • Consider antiarrhythmic infusion of agent that was used during resuscitation.
  • Lidocaine, 1–4 mg/minute IV.
  • Amiodarone, 0.5 mg/minute IV.
  • Procainamide, 20 mg/minute to a maximum dose of 17 mg/kg IV.

SPECIAL CONSIDERATION: PATIENT WITH HEART TRANSPLANT

► Atropine is ineffective in the denervated heart.
► Consider rejection as an etiology.
  • If patient survives initial arrest, methylprednisolone, 1 g IV.
  • Consult transplant surgeon.

ENDING RESUSCITATIVE MEASURES

► Look for and honor DNR orders.
► Do not initiate resuscitation in the setting of unrecoverable injury (e.g., exposed brain matter, rigor mortis).
► Resuscitation may be ended if appropriate DNR orders are found even after resuscitation is initiated.
► End resuscitation after a reasonable effort has been attempted and further intervention is futile.

FAMILY PRESENCE DURING RESUSCITATION

► Several recent studies have shown that family presence during resuscitative efforts can help the grief process and improve survivor satisfaction in the patient's care.

▶ A trained liaison, such as a social worker educated in resuscitation, can greatly facilitate this practice.

◑ **PEARLS AND PITFALLS**
  - If no IV access, consider alternatives such as IO.
  - Lidocaine, epinephrine, and atropine can be given at twice the normal dose via an ETT, followed by an NS flush.

CHAPTER 18

APPROACH TO DEATH IN THE EMERGENCY DEPARTMENT

Constance J. Doyle and Kirsten G. Engel

SUDDEN DEATH NOTIFICATION AND THE ACUTE GRIEF RESPONSE

▶ As providers of emergency care, we are faced more frequently with unexpected death than clinicians in most other fields.

▶ The opportunity to care not only for victims of sudden death but also for the survivors represents one of the greatest challenges in our profession.

▶ We often fail to recognize the vital role that we play in these settings and the great opportunity that we have to positively influence the lives of a patient's family and friends.

DISTINGUISHING FEATURES OF SUDDEN DEATH

▶ Unexpected, no preparation/anticipation

▶ Often affects young, healthy individuals

▶ No prior relationship between family and ED staff, with no basis for mutual respect and trust

▶ Time constraints

▶ Uncertainty about cause of death (frustrating to staff, upsetting and disconcerting to family)

▶ Other issues (e.g., cultural/language differences)

▶ Anger that the decedent caused other injuries or deaths

▶ Lifestyle issues or illegal activity that becomes apparent in context of death

▶ Our own personal experiences and emotional responses to death

▶ Failure to resuscitate as a personal failure as a doctor

▶ Conflicts of needing to care for other live patients who are waiting vs. caring for grieving family members

THE ACUTE GRIEF RESPONSE

▶ The inherent features of sudden death make grieving more complex within the context of the grief response.

▶ Sudden death precipitates an abrupt transition with the unexpected loss of significant relationships.

▶ Survivors are at increased risk for pathologic/atypical reactions (absent, distorted, exaggerated responses). High frequency of subsequent depression, suicidality, substance abuse. New onset or exacerbation of illness.

▶ Basis of healthy grief response is established in the initial interactions with ED staff; any interference with or disruption of this process can lead to pathologic reactions/increased morbidity and mortality.

SIX PHASES OF SUDDEN DEATH NOTIFICATION

Initial Contact

▶ Notifying next-of-kin—social worker, RN, MD, hospital security

▶ Phone calls

- Identify yourself, the institution, patient's name, and person spoken with.
- Avoid notification over the phone unless directly questioned.
- Emphasize the gravity of the patient's condition by using the words *seriously ill* or *injured and unconscious.*

Arrival of Family

▶ Arrival of family should be anticipated; ED staff should greet them and provide any available information.

▶ Family should be escorted to a private conference room.

▶ Information updates should be provided every 10–15 minutes with warnings of impending death.

▶ Consider family presence during resuscitation if possible; family members should be screened and accompanied at all times by trained support staff that are not part of the resuscitation team.

Notification of Death

▶ Give yourself a brief period of time to transition from the intensity and stress of the resuscitation and prepare to speak to the family with empathy and sensitivity.

▶ Introduce yourself, make good eye contact, and identify all family members in the room.

▶ Provide a brief summary of the resuscitation effort and reassure the family that everything possible was done to help their loved one.

▶ Use clear unambiguous language: *dead, death,* or *died.*

▶ If possible, reassure the family that the patient did not suffer.

▶ Allow time for reflection/response and encourage the family to speak with you about their feelings.

The Grief Response

▶ Early stages
  • Anticipatory anxiety
  • Shock/disbelief with associated physical (choking, SOB, throat tightness, and intestinal upset) and emotional symptoms (numbness, bewilderment, a sense of unreality, and a blunted affect)
  • Denial, which serves as a defense mechanism and helps to give the mind time to deal with the sudden tragedy

▶ Later stages
  • Anger mixed with guilt
  • Ultimate acceptance and reorganization

Viewing the Body

▶ Whenever possible, provide the family with the opportunity to view the deceased and, if ambivalent, provide gentle encouragement.

▶ Use the patient's name and never refer to "the body."

▶ Prepare the deceased for viewing.

▶ Family members should be accompanied by a social worker or other ED staff so that appropriate support and information can be provided.

▶ If the death was in the context of a crime or homicide, family may not be able to touch the deceased.

▶ In medical examiner's cases, tubes and lines need to remain in place during the viewing.

Concluding Process

▶ Complete appropriate paperwork (e.g., autopsy, organ donation).

▶ Be sure to allow family members the opportunity to ask questions and provide them with your contact information for any future questions.

▶ Threats of suicide or other violence must be taken very seriously and addressed with appropriate support/evaluation.

▶ Ensure that no family member leaves the ED alone.

▶ Whenever possible, follow up with surviving family members within 1–2 weeks after the event or designate staff such as pastoral care.

▶ Sympathy cards to the family are usually appreciated.

CHAPTER 19

APPROACH TO DYSPNEA

Keith E. Kocher

▶ Subjective feeling of unpleasant or uncomfortable respiratory sensations.

▶ Objectively interpreted as respirations that are labored, difficult, or stressful.

▶ Sensation is thought to result from a mismatch between central respiratory motor activity and incoming afferent information from receptors in the airways, lungs, and chest wall—when feedback from the peripheral receptors indicates that work of breathing is greater than would be expected by the patient's level of activity.

▶ Broad differential—two-thirds of patients presenting to the ED have cardiac or respiratory cause.

▶ May have normal physical exam.

▶ May also have the following associated findings:
  • Tachypnea: rapid breathing
  • Orthopnea: dyspnea in recumbent position
  • Paroxysmal nocturnal dyspnea: orthopnea that awakens patient at night

DIFFERENTIAL DIAGNOSIS

▶ See Table 19-1.

CLINICAL PRESENTATION

▶ History: Inquire about onset, severity, associated symptoms, past medical history, current medications/compliance/recent changes, and occupational exposures.

▶ Abrupt onset → CHF, PE, ACS, PTX.

▶ Air hunger, need to breathe, urge to breathe → CHF, PE, asthma, COPD.

▶ Increased work or effort of breathing → COPD, asthma, myopathy.

TABLE 19-1.
DIFFERENTIAL DIAGNOSIS OF ACUTE DYSPNEA

Cardiovascular	Respiratory	Other
Ischemic heart disease	Asthma, COPD	Psychogenic
CHF	PE	Anemia
Pericardial effusion/ tamponade	PTX	Sepsis
Cardiac arrhythmia	Pneumonia	
	Upper airway obstruction (FB, anaphylaxis/angioedema, hemorrhage)	

► Chest tightness with wheeze → asthma, COPD, and must consider CHF.

► Rapid, shallow breathing → interstitial fibrosis, psychogenic.

► Suffocating, smothering → pulmonary edema.

► Heavy breathing, breathing more → metabolic acidosis, deconditioning, psychogenic.

► Cough, fever, and focal lung findings → pneumonia.

► Absence of lung findings, tachycardia, and hypoxia → PE.

► Abrupt onset in setting of MI with loud murmur → acute valvular insufficiency.

► Known exposure, facial swelling, rash → anaphylaxis or angioedema.

DIAGNOSIS

► Given the subjective nature of dyspnea and its wide differential, careful history is important and is an initial guide; physical exam should further define work-up.

► **Oxygenation/ventilation**

• Pulse oximetry (gross measurement of oxygenation but no information regarding $PaCO_2$).

• ABG (shows hypercapnia, also metabolic acidosis as cause of hyperventilation).

• Bedside assessment of work of breathing (may have normal ABG despite respiratory distress)—can consider doing walking pulse oximetry to give additional information regarding disposition.

• Peak expiratory flow before/after bronchodilators.

▶ **CXR:** look for infiltrate, pulmonary edema, effusion, PTX, and cardiomegaly (pericardial effusion vs. cardiomyopathy).

▶ **ECG:** look for arrhythmia, myocardial ischemia, or signs of PE.

▶ **Labs**

- **CBC:** anemia, chronic (= MCV low, RDW high) vs. acute.
- **CIPs:** if concerned about cardiac ischemia as cause.
- **BNP:** can potentially help differentiate between respiratory and cardiogenic causes of dyspnea.
- **D dimer:** can be used to exclude PE in low-risk population.

▶ **Nasopharyngeal scope:** may be used to evaluate upper airway if concerned about FB.

TREATMENT

▶ ABCs: ensure adequate airway first, then assess breathing.

▶ Supplemental O_2: to maintain O_2 saturation > 90%.

▶ Definitive management of acute dyspnea: establishment of the airway (intubation) followed by adequate oxygenation and ventilation (mechanical ventilation).

▶ Consider non-invasive positive pressure ventilation early (CPAP, BiPAP) as patient must be conscious and able to cooperate—may prevent intubation in CHF and some COPD patients.

▶ In general, goal is adequate oxygenation/avoiding hypoxia (PaO_2 > 60 mmHg, SaO_2 > 90%) and adequate ventilation/avoiding hypercapnia ($PaCO_2$ < 45 mmHg).

▶ Often early in ED care, there is a need to treat aggressively before having made a specific diagnosis—e.g., initiate diuresis with NMTs and steroids in elderly with history of CHF and COPD and non-specific exam findings.

DISPOSITION

▶ Admission criteria vary with underlying disease; however, consider for those with abnormal vital signs or where underlying process has not been sufficiently reversed.

▶ Certain diagnoses have EBM-tested criteria or national guidelines for determining admission—e.g., NIH asthma guidelines. However, these do not supplant sound clinical judgment.

CHAPTER 20

APPROACH TO HEMOPTYSIS

Erich C. Kickland and James Mattimore

▶ Hemoptysis is defined as expectorated blood originating from a source below the vocal cords.

▶ Massive hemoptysis: > 600 ml of expectorated blood in a 24-hour period. Treat as life-threatening emergency.

▶ Most commonly minor and treatable or self-limiting and can be worked up as an outpatient.

▶ True hemoptysis must be differentiated from pseudohemoptysis and hematemesis.

▶ Pseudohemoptysis occurs when blood originates from a source above the vocal cords, usually the naso- or oropharynx.

▶ Most common cause worldwide is TB.

ETIOLOGIES

▶ See Table 20-1.

CLINICAL PRESENTATION

▶ True hemoptysis is usually bright red, foamy, and associated with coughing. It does not contain food particles and has an alkaline pH.

▶ Differentiate from hematemesis by presence of GI symptoms, but note that high-volume hemoptysis can result in swallowed blood that mimics hematemesis.

▶ May be able to visualize directly the source of pseudohemoptysis on exam.

▶ Chronic cough, recurrent blood in sputum → bronchiectasis.

▶ Smoker > age 40, hemoptysis duration > 1 wk, history of weight loss → lung cancer.

▶ Acute cough, wheeze → bronchitis.

▶ Pleuritic chest pain, SOB, leg swelling → PE.

TABLE 20-1.
ETIOLOGIES OF HEMOPTYSIS

Bronchiectasis (~20%) Lung cancer (~20%) Bronchitis (~20%) Infection (~15%)	Unknown (termed cryptogenic or idio- pathic hemoptysis: 15–30%) Coagulopathy (< 5%) CHF (< 5%) Other (including trauma: ~10%)

▶ Fever, purulent sputum → pneumonia.

▶ Fever, night sweats, weight loss → TB, aspergilloma, lung abscess.

▶ Recent travel to Asia, South America, Middle East → schistosomiasis.

▶ Associated hematuria → Goodpasture syndrome.

▶ History of AIDS/immunosuppression → TB, Kaposi's sarcoma.

▶ History of recent Swan-Ganz catheterization, lung biopsy, or
bronchoscopy → iatrogenic.

▶ History of crack cocaine use → diffuse alveolar hemorrhage.

▶ Female, recurrent hemoptysis concurrent with menses → cata-
menial hemoptysis.

▶ Rales, peripheral edema, murmur → CHF, mitral stenosis.

▶ Pediatric considerations → cystic fibrosis, FB aspiration, vascular anomalies, bronchial adenoma.

▶ Multiple patients or uncommon age distribution for common
pathology → consider bioterrorism (plague, tularemia, T2
mycotoxin, among others).

DIAGNOSIS

Lab Tests

▶ CBC (assess magnitude and duration of bleeding)

▶ PT, PTT (assess for coagulopathy)

▶ UA, serum chemistries (if pulmonary-renal syndrome suspected, or if fluid resuscitation required)

▶ T&S (moderate hemoptysis) or type and cross (if hemodynamically unstable or coagulopathy suspected)

▶ Sputum exam utility based on clinical suspicion: Gram's and
acid-fast bacterial stains; cultures, including fungal; cytology if
malignancy suspected (adequate sample > 25 PMNs and < 10
epithelial cells)

Imaging

▶ CXR: essential in all. May reveal predisposing condition (cancer, cavitary lesions, infiltrates) or help localize blood.

▶ High-resolution CT: study of choice for stable ED patients with normal CXR. Obtain study with contrast when possible. Not as sensitive as bronchoscopy for detection of mucosal lesions. May be obtained as outpatient in patients with minor hemoptysis and normal CXR.

▶ Fiberoptic bronchoscopy: in the ED, mainly indicated in unstable patients. Allows direct visualization and potential treatment of bleeding source.

▶ Other studies, such as V/Q scan or pulmonary arteriography, should be used only in selected cases as guided by the clinical scenario.

MANAGEMENT/DISPOSITION
Massive Hemoptysis

▶ Hemoptysis with hemodynamic or respiratory instability indicates risk of death.

▶ IV (two large bore), O_2, monitor, suction.

▶ ET intubation to protect airway. Use ≥ 8-mm inner diameter tube when possible to facilitate bronchoscopy.

▶ Place affected side in dependent position.

▶ Send labs: CBC, coagulation studies, type and cross.

▶ Transfuse PRBCs, FFP for continuous heavy bleeding with hemodynamic compromise.

▶ Obtain pulmonary, thoracic surgery consults early.

▶ Consider interventional radiology for embolization of bleeding source.

▶ Admit to ICU or transfer via ACLS if appropriate services are unavailable.

Moderate, Active Hemoptysis

▶ Bleeding < 600 ml/24 hours with stable vital signs.

▶ IV (two large bore), O_2, monitor.

▶ Provide suction, IVF as indicated.

▶ Send labs: CBC, coagulation studies, T&S.

▶ Send sputum studies as directed by differential.

▶ Obtain CXR.
▶ Usually admitted for further work-up and/or treatment of underlying cause.

Minor Hemoptysis or Hemoptysis by History

▶ Minimal bleeding observed in ED or by history.
▶ CXR in all, labs if indicated.
▶ Usually infectious etiology requiring antibiotics ± cough suppressants.
▶ If CXR is negative and history and exam do not warrant further inpatient management, contact primary care provider regarding continuation of work-up as outpatient.
▶ Discharge with clear instructions to return if worse.

CHAPTER 21

ASTHMA

Jeffrey Callard

▶ Asthma affects approximately 5% of the U.S. population.
▶ Accounts for 2 million annual ED visits in the U.S.

PATHOPHYSIOLOGY

▶ Reversible airflow obstruction caused by smooth muscle contraction, vascular congestion, bronchial wall edema, and thick mucous secretions.
▶ Triggers that can initiate an asthma exacerbation include allergies, viral URI (most common), exercise, medications, GERD, cold exposure, and inhaled irritants.

CLINICAL PRESENTATION

▶ Classic presentation is recurrent bouts of wheezing, cough, and dyspnea. Chest tightness. Symptoms often occur at night.
▶ Inquire about duration of attack, current medications, previous hospitalization, and intubation.
▶ Vital signs may be variable and do not necessarily reflect the severity of obstruction. Classic exam findings of tachycardia, tachypnea, and wheezing may normalize in worsening obstruction.
▶ Severe airway obstruction indicated by ability to speak only a few words, poor air movement or silent chest, use of accessory muscles, HR > 120, RR > 30, and mental status changes.

DIFFERENTIAL DIAGNOSIS

▶ See Chap. 19.

EMERGENCY DEPARTMENT MANAGEMENT
Diagnosis

▶ The diagnosis of asthma is usually based on history and physical exam.

▶ In most asthma exacerbations, diagnostic studies are of little value. Studies are more helpful in ruling out alternative diagnoses.

▶ CXR shows evidence of hyperinflation. It is not routinely indicated, but may be indicated in fever, focal exam findings, failure to respond to treatment, or first episode of wheezing.

▶ Pulse oximetry is also used as an indicator of severity of disease.

▶ Measuring PEFR before and after treatment can provide an objective measurement of airflow obstruction. It is an unreliable predictor of need for admission. PEFR < 100 L/min initially or < 30–50% predicted baseline suggests severe disease.

▶ ABGs are useful in patients with impending respiratory failure, including fatigue, altered mental status, worsening after treatment, or pulse oximetry < 90%.

▶ Lab studies are not routinely indicated.

Treatment

▶ The goal for the treatment of asthma is to reverse airflow obstruction, reduce inflammation, and provide adequate oxygenation. Beta-adrenergic agonists, anticholinergics, and corticosteroids are the mainstays of the emergent treatment of asthma.

▶ $Beta_2$-adrenergic agonists increase cAMP, which results in bronchodilation.

▶ Inhaled agents are administered via nebulizer.

▶ **Albuterol,** 0.5% solution, 2.5 mg in 2- to 3-cc NS q20min × 3 is the usual regime. Continuous nebulization for 1 hour with albuterol has been used in severe asthmatics.

▶ Anticholinergics promote bronchodilation by decreasing cGMP. The primary effect is in the large airways. Ipratropium bromide (Atrovent) is the most widely used agent.

▶ **Atrovent,** 500 mg in 2 cc of NS q20–30min for three doses and then q4–6h.

▶ Corticosteroids decrease airway inflammation. They should be given to all except those responding immediately to a single nebulized treatment. Oral and IV routes are equally efficacious, the IV route being chosen when concerns regarding airway or absorption are an issue.

▶ Methylprednisolone, 125 mg IV.

▶ Prednisone, 60 mg PO. Discharged patients should be given 4–5 days of prednisone, longer may require tapering.

▶ Magnesium sulfate should be considered for severe asthmatics. There may be some benefit in preventing intubation in these patients, but studies are conflicting.

▶ Magnesium sulfate, 2 mg IV over 5 minutes.

▶ Heliox (helium and O_2) decreases airway resistance and respiratory work. It is used in some centers and may have some benefit.

▶ Fortunately, intubation is rarely necessary. The decision is usually made on clinical exam and findings and not on lab tests. Some of the indicators include exhaustion, deterioration despite aggressive therapy, or change in mental status. Use a large-bore tube; consider ketamine, 1–2 mg, for induction because of bronchodilator effect. If intubated, allow permissive hypercapnia to prevent barotrauma. Tidal volume 8–10 cc/kg, RR of 10–12.

▶ Methylxanthines, formerly a mainstay in ED treatment, are no longer recommended.

▶ Antibiotics should not be prescribed routinely in asthma.

Disposition

▶ Depends on the patient's response to therapy, improvement of wheezing, dyspnea, and air exchange. Other factors to consider include previous history of exacerbations, admissions, and social situation.

▶ Consider admission if patient fails to improve or deteriorates in the ED, has hypoxia or tachycardia after treatment, or is already on maximal treatment as an outpatient.

▶ If discharged, patients should be advised to use inhaler with spacer device, 2 puffs q4h, and given prednisone, 40–60 mg PO daily for 5 days. They may need refills on inhalers.

▶ All asthmatics need follow-up in 2–5 days and education on proper inhaler and spacer use.

CHAPTER 22

CHRONIC OBSTRUCTIVE PULMONARY DISEASE

Elke G. Marksteiner

- ▶ 1 in 4 adults affected and is the fourth leading cause of death in the U.S.
- ▶ Male > females, elderly.
- ▶ Majority directly related to smoking.
- ▶ Chronic irreversible disease that has a less than dramatic response to therapy.
- ▶ Three components of disease include emphysema (destruction of lung parenchyma), bronchitis (airway inflammation), and asthma (airway hyperreactivity).

PATHOPHYSIOLOGY

- ▶ Causes: cigarette smoking, passive smoke exposure, air pollution, and occupational exposures as well as genetic risk factors such as alpha-1-antitrypsin deficiency, cystic fibrosis.
- ▶ Chronic smoking triggers production of elastase, which results in destruction of alveolar septi.
- ▶ Bronchial wall inflammation, wall thickening by smooth muscle hyperplasia, and damage to endothelium → impaired mucociliary response.
- ▶ V/Q mismatch can ultimately result in cor pulmonale and polycythemia.
- ▶ Airway obstruction by bronchoconstriction and mucus plugging.
- ▶ Exacerbations caused by PTX, PE, atelectasis pneumonia, and viral infection.

CLINICAL PRESENTATION

- ▶ Dyspnea or worsening dyspnea with exertion
- ▶ Productive cough, chronic sputum production
- ▶ Inability to speak in full sentences

▸ Tachycardia and tachypnea
▸ Lip pursing, accessory muscle use, and diaphoresis
▸ Decreased breath sounds, rhonchi, and wheezing
▸ Decreased mental status suggests CO_2 narcosis
▸ Pulsus paradoxus, distant heart sounds, loud P_2
▸ Signs of right-sided heart failure (distended neck veins, enlarged liver)

DIFFERENTIAL DIAGNOSIS
▸ See Chap. 19.

EMERGENCY DEPARTMENT MANAGEMENT
Diagnosis
▸ Based primarily on clinical presentation; however, the following tests may aid diagnosis:
- Pulse oximetry: < 90% indicates severe hypoxia. Many with severe disease live around 88–90% so must correlate with symptoms, HR, and RR.
- ABG: not required for diagnosis but may be useful to compare to prior results. Hypoxia is usually present but increases with severity of exacerbation. Respiratory failure suggested by PaO_2 < 60, $PaCO_2$ > 60, or pH < 7.30.
- CXR: hyperinflated lungs, increased retrosternal airspace, flattened diaphragms, and bullae. Used to exclude coexisting disease processes (e.g., pneumonia, PTX, and CHF).
- ECG: to detect ischemia or dysrhythmias. Signs of COPD include P pulmonale (peaked P in II, III, and AVF), low voltage, right axis deviation, and poor R-wave progression. RV hypertrophy and multifocal atrial tachycardia.
- Pulmonary function tests: less useful than in asthma because patients do not have significant reversible component.
- Labs do not assist clinical decisions but are usually obtained in admitted patients:
  ○ CBC: polycythemia or elevated WBC
  ○ Electrolytes, because bronchodilator and diuretic therapy can cause hypokalemia
  ○ Theophylline level

Treatment

► O_2: goal to maintain O_2 saturation > 90% (monitor for apnea owing to removal of hypoxic drive to breathe).
► Bronchodilators: mainstay of therapy, most rapid response.
  • Beta$_2$-agonist: Albuterol, 2.5–5.0 mg (0.5–1.0 ml of 0.5% solution) nebulizer treatment q20min × 3, then hourly. If patient is able, MDI with spacer has equal efficacy with adequate dosage.
  • Anticholinergics: ipratropium bromide nebulization, 0.5 mg q4h. Onset of action up to 20 minutes. Synergistic with albuterol.
► Corticosteroids: indicated in all acute exacerbations, but less compelling evidence that they work in COPD.
  • Prednisone, 60 mg PO daily, or
  • Methylprednisolone, 125 mg IV, if cannot tolerate PO route.
  • Patients discharged to home should have 7- to 10-day course of prednisone.
► Antibiotics: recent meta-analysis supports antibiotics for exacerbations of COPD. A macrolide or respiratory fluoroquinolone is ideal monotherapy for patients being discharged. Admitted patients should follow guidelines for inpatient pneumonia.
► Decision to intubate is made clinically. It is based on patient's mental status, respiratory distress, and response to therapy. If patient arrives in extremis, then should consider non-invasive ventilation with CPAP or BiPAP early on, as this may decrease need for intubation.

Disposition

► Admit patient if no significant clinical improvement despite initial treatment, presence of significant comorbidities or inciting factors, failure of previous outpatient treatment, old age, insufficient home support.
► Walking pulse oximetry may help predict who can be discharged in borderline patients.
► Discharge patient with close outpatient follow-up, home O_2 if needed, bronchodilator treatment, and 7- to 10-day course of steroids.

CHAPTER 23

PNEUMONIA

Amer Z. Aldeen and Rahul K. Khare

▶ Pneumonia is defined as infection of the pulmonary alveolar tissue and is generally divided into two groups according to setting: community-acquired and nosocomial (in hospitals and nursing homes).

▶ Pneumonia is the number one cause of death due to infection in the U.S., and the sixth leading cause of death overall.

▶ Four million cases occur each year; 25% of patients are hospitalized.

▶ While overall mortality is < 1%, hospitalized patients with pneumonia have up to 25% mortality.

▶ Bacteria are the most common cause, followed by viruses, parasites, and fungi.

PATHOPHYSIOLOGY

▶ Bacteria from upper airways migrate down to lung parenchyma, which is normally a sterile environment.

▶ Immune-compromised states (cancer, chemotherapy, HIV), extremes of age, and impairment in normal defenses (altered mental status, smoking, COPD) all contribute to increased risk of severe pneumonia requiring hospitalization.

▶ Aspiration is an important mechanism for developing both community-acquired and nosocomial pneumonia.

▶ Co-infection between viruses and bacteria is now recognized as extremely common.

▶ The most likely causative agents are
  • Bacterial (Table 23-1)
  • Viral
    ○ Influenza (RSV in infants)
    ○ Parainfluenza
  • Fungal → *Cryptococcus, Aspergillus, Blastomyces, Histoplasma,* coccidioidomycosis

TABLE 23-1.
BACTERIAL CAUSES OF PNEUMONIA

Community-acquired	Nosocomial
Streptococcus pneumoniae *Haemophilus influenzae* *Mycoplasma pneumoniae* *Legionella pneumophila*	Gram-negative bacilli (including *Pseudomonas aeruginosa*) *Staphylococcus aureus* Anaerobes

- Other
  - *Chlamydia pneumoniae*
  - *Pneumocystis carinii*

CLINICAL PRESENTATION

▶ Fever (80%), cough, dyspnea, and pleuritic chest pain are the cardinal symptoms of pneumonia, although no constellation of signs and symptoms is 100% predictive.

▶ Sudden onset of severe symptoms is more likely to represent a bacterial cause.

▶ Accurate measurement of RR and temperature (rectal) is essential.

▶ Rales, egophony, and dullness to percussion are often seen in pneumonia; however, wheezes, rhonchi, or decreased breath sounds may be the only findings present.

▶ RR is considered the "lost vital sign"; tachypnea is often the only clinical sign of pneumonia in the elderly.

▶ A thorough history may help elicit the most likely infectious agent responsible (Table 23-2).

DIFFERENTIAL DIAGNOSIS

▶ See Chap. 19.

EMERGENCY DEPARTMENT MANAGEMENT
Diagnosis

▶ CXR is the mainstay of diagnosis and differentiates between pneumonia and bronchitis.

▶ Up to 10% of patients who have pneumonia may have negative initial CXRs—if history and physical exam are strongly indicative of pneumonia, treatment is warranted.

TABLE 23-2.
PATIENT HISTORY FOR PNEUMONIA

History	Likely pathogen(s)
COPD, smokers, alcoholics	*Klebsiella, Haemophilus influenzae, Legionella, Moraxella*
Bloody sputum	Pneumococcus, TB
Currant-jelly sputum	*Klebsiella*, pneumococcus
GI symptoms	*Legionella*
IV drug abuse	*Staphylococcus aureus*
Post-influenza	Pneumococcus, *S. aureus*
HIV	*Pneumocystis carinii, Cryptococcus*
Transplant patient	CMV, *Aspergillus*, pneumococcus, opportunistic agents
Travel	Midwest → *Blastomyces, Histoplasma*
	Southwest → coccidioidomycosis
	International → TB
Animal exposure	Cats/cattle → *Coxiella burnetii*
	Birds → *Chlamydia psittaci*

▶ Obtain two sets of blood cultures before antibiotic therapy in patients who are being hospitalized.

▶ Urinary antigen testing has good accuracy for detecting pneumococcus and excellent accuracy for detecting *Legionella*, although not routinely done in the ED.

▶ Pleural effusions associated with pneumonia should be sampled to check for presence of empyema, which requires urgent tube thoracostomy drainage.

Treatment

▶ Antibiotics are the mainstay of treatment—a 10- to 14-day course is generally given, depending on the severity (Table 23-3).

▶ Drug-resistant pneumococcus and MRSA are becoming more prevalent in the community setting.

Disposition

▶ Admit all patients who are hypoxic (SpO$_2$ < 92%), severely tachypneic (RR > 25), at extremes of age, or who have serious comorbid conditions.

▶ A prospectively validated pneumonia severity score exists to aid clinical decision-making in the disposition of pneumonia patients, but in unclear cases, sound clinical judgment should prevail.

TABLE 23-3.
TREATMENT OF PNEUMONIA

Patient	Disposition	Treatment	Alternative	Alternative
CAP: < 60 years and non-smoker	Outpatient	Azithromycin, 500 mg PO ×1, 250 mg PO qd	Fluoroquinolone PO[a]	Doxycycline, 100 mg PO bid
CAP: > 60 years healthy or smoker	Outpatient	Azithromycin PO + 2° cephalosporin[b]	Fluoroquinolone PO[a]	Doxycycline PO
CAP: > 60 years with comorbidity or smoker	Inpatient	Azithromycin, 500 mg IV qd + 3° cephalosporin[c]	Fluoroquinolone IV[a]	—
Nosocomial	Inpatient	APA[d,e,f,g] (double cover)	—	—
Pneumocystis carinii (add prednisone if PO_2 <70)	Both (21 days total)	SMX-TMP, 5 mg/kg IV or 2 DS tabs PO q8h	Clindamycin[b] + primaquine, 30 mg PO qd	Pentamidine, 4 mg/kg IV qd
Influenza	Both	Oseltamivir, 75 mg PO bid × 5 days	Zanamivir, 10 mg inhaled bid × 5 days	—
Fungal	Both	Fluconazole,[h,i] 400 mg PO/IV qd	Amphotericin B, 1 mg/kg IV qd	—

[a] Fluoroquinolone (all PO/IV qd) → gatifloxacin, 400 mg; levofloxacin, 500 mg; moxifloxacin, 400 mg.
[b] 2° cephalosporin (all PO q12h) → cefdinir, 300 mg; cefpodoxime proxetil, 200 mg; cefprozil, 500 mg; cefuroxime axetil, 500 mg.
[c] 3° cephalosporin → cefotaxime, 2 g IV q4–8h; ceftriaxone, 1–2 g IV qd.
[d] Add vancomycin, 1 g IV q12h, if suspicion is high for MRSA.
[e] Add linezolid, 600 mg PO/IV q12h, if suspicion is high for VRE.
[f] Add metronidazole, 500 mg IV tid, or clindamycin, 600 mg IV q6h, for aspiration if other antibiotics have poor anaerobic coverage.
[g] Anti-pseudomonal antibiotics (APAs) include piperacillin/tazobactam, 3.375 g IV q6h; ticarcillin/clavulanate, 3.1 g IV q6h; imipenem-cilastatin, 500 mg IV q6h; meropenem, 1 g IV q8h; ceftazidime, 2 g IV q8h; cefepime, 2 g IV q12h; fluoroquinolones; tobramycin, 5 mg/kg IV qd; amikacin, 15 mg/kg IV qd.
[h] voriconazole, 400 mg IV/PO qd, may be necessary for Aspergillus species.

CHAPTER 24

PNEUMOTHORAX

Ann Hess

- ▶ PTX is defined as air or gas in the pleural cavity.
- ▶ Primary spontaneous PTX—most common in tall, young males with no underlying lung disease.
  - • Patients are usually in their twenties, M:F ratio is 6:1, recurrence rate is 28%.
- ▶ Secondary spontaneous PTX is observed in elderly with underlying parenchymal disease—e.g., COPD.
  - • Patients are usually in their sixties, M:F ratio is 3:1, recurrence rate is 43%.
- ▶ Smoking is major risk factor for both primary and secondary PTX.
- ▶ Traumatic PTX (most common cause) results from injury often secondary to medical intervention.
- ▶ Tension PTX caused by creation of one-way valve and air trapping that can lead to cardiovascular collapse and death.

PATHOPHYSIOLOGY

- ▶ PTX arises when air enters the potential space between the visceral and parietal pleura.
- ▶ Alveolar pressure exceeds the pressure in the lung interstitium → alveolar rupture.
- ▶ Air moves into the interstitium and the hilum, resulting in pneumomediastinum. From the mediastinum, air enters the pleural space.

CLINICAL PRESENTATION
History

- ▶ Symptoms are related to size and rate of development.

▶ Primary PTX usually occurs at rest, and virtually all patients have ipsilateral pleuritic chest pain or acute dyspnea.
  • Symptoms often resolve within 24 hours even if the PTX is untreated.
▶ In secondary PTX, the most common complaint is dyspnea, usually severe even in the setting of a small PTX, and most patients also complain of ipsilateral chest pain.
  • Symptoms do not resolve spontaneously.

Exam

▶ Tachypnea, tachycardia (most common finding), hypoxia.
▶ If small (< 15% volume of hemithorax), the exam may be normal.
▶ Larger PTXs have classic findings of hyperresonant percussion, decreased chest wall movement, decreased tactile fremitus, and distant/absent breath sounds.
▶ In the setting of trauma, patient may have subcutaneous emphysema.
▶ In tension PTX, patients develop severe hypoxemia, increased JVD, and hypotension before cardiovascular collapse.

EMERGENCY DEPARTMENT MANAGEMENT
Diagnosis

▶ By history and confirmed by an upright PA CXR, which reveals a thin, visceral pleural line (< 1 mm width) displaced from the chest wall.
▶ Expiratory CXR may be helpful to identify small apical PTX; however, the routine use of expiratory film does not improve the diagnostic yield.
▶ The exact size of PTX is often difficult to determine from CXR.
▶ It is important to differentiate PTX from large bulla. If the diagnosis is unclear, may consider obtaining a chest CT.
▶ ABG may reveal an increased A-a gradient and a respiratory alkalosis.

Treatment

▶ The goals are to evacuate air and prevent recurrences.
▶ In the ED, emphasis is placed on eliminating the intrapleural air. This can be accomplished by a number of methods includ-

ing observation, supplemental O_2, catheter aspiration, mini catheter placement, and standard thoracostomy.

► **Supplemental O_2:** often overlooked as a valuable tool. The rate of pleural air absorption is 1.25%/day. O_2 increases this rate 3–4 times by creating a pressure gradient between the pleural space and the tissue capillaries, enhancing absorption of pleural nitrogen first, as well as other gases.

► **Observation** may be used if the patient is not dyspneic and the PTX is < 15%. Approximately 23% of these patients go on to require a chest tube for progression of symptoms.

► **Aspiration** aims to evacuate pleural air and re-expand the collapsed lung. This is accomplished by placing a small catheter (can be an IV catheter) between the fourth and fifth intercostal space in the anterior axillary line using the Seldinger technique and attaching a three-way stopcock and large syringe for aspiration.

► **Heimlich valve:** involves placement of a catheter with a one-way valve, which can be left in place until lung expansion occurs, or it can be converted to a small-bore chest tube if air leak persists.

► **Chest tube:** is recommended for primary PTX failing aspiration and is advocated for most secondary PTX. Small-bore tubes (7–14 F) can be safely used if patient is not undergoing mechanical ventilation or has risk of occlusion from pleural effusion.

► Guidelines:
  • Small primary PTX (< 15% of the hemithorax): Treat with supplemental O_2. Most physicians hospitalize these patients for observation; however, if the patient is young and otherwise healthy, may consider discharge to home after a 6-hour ED observation and repeat CXR. These patients must have follow-up at 24 hours.
  • Moderate-sized primary PTX: Simple aspiration is successful for 70%. If aspiration fails, attach catheter to a one-way Heimlich valve or water seal device and use the apparatus as a chest tube.
  • Secondary PTX: 20–28 F chest tube to water seal, and hospitalize secondary to risk of respiratory compromise, reserving the use of suction for ongoing air leaks.

► PTX in the setting of trauma should have 36 F chest tube placed.

► Tension PTX is an emergency. It should be treated by inserting a 14–16 F catheter into the second or third intercostal space in the midclavicular line. This should result in an immediate rush of air and rapid clinical improvement. The catheter is left in place until a chest tube is secured in position.

Disposition

► Patient may be discharged after observation if PTX is small and patient is asymptomatic; however, most patients are admitted for treatment and observation as outlined above.

► Referral to pulmonologist and/or thoracic surgeon is indicated for recurrent primary PTX and all secondary PTX.

CHAPTER 25

PULMONARY EMBOLISM

Christopher R. H. Newton

▶ Third leading cause of death in the U.S.
▶ Majority caused by lower-extremity DVT.
▶ Requires high index of suspicion to make this often difficult diagnosis.

PATHOPHYSIOLOGY

▶ Thrombus forms in the deep venous system in the lower extremities and propagates distally, lodging in pulmonary vasculature.
▶ Risk of embolization highest in first 2 weeks after thrombus formation.
▶ Virchow's triad includes venous stasis, hypercoagulability, and endothelial damage and predisposes to development of DVT.
▶ Major risk factors include prolonged immobilization, recent surgery, prior DVT/PE, obesity, malignancy, and other hypercoagulable states.

CLINICAL PRESENTATION

▶ There is no typical presentation of PE. Rather, a collection of non-specific historical and exam findings, together with risk factors, should raise the suspicion for PE.

History

▶ Classic triad of dyspnea, hemoptysis, and pleuritic chest pain present in < 20%.
▶ History of chest pain (especially pleuritic) or dyspnea (> 80%) with risk factors for DVT should raise suspicion for PE.
▶ Can present with syncope (10–15%) or feeling of anxiety (≤ 50%).

Examination

▶ Tachypnea (RR > 16) is the most commonly observed abnormal vital sign. Tachycardia and hypoxia should also raise suspicion for PE.

▶ Cyanosis is rarely present and indicates massive PE.

▶ Focal lung findings (wheeze, rales, and pleural friction rub) may also be present but are uncommon and non-specific.

DIAGNOSIS

▶ Gold standard test is a pulmonary angiogram. However, because of the risks associated with the procedure, it is done infrequently.

▶ Diagnosis is usually based on combination of clinical presentation, risk factors, and interpretation of non-invasive tests.

▶ **ECG** is most useful for excluding other diagnoses, such as pericarditis and MI. Sinus tachycardia is the most common abnormality. May have non-specific ST changes, new RBBB, P-pulmonale, or S1Q3T3 pattern.

▶ **CXR** is most commonly normal on presentation. Hampton's hump: wedge-shaped pleural infiltrate. Westermark sign: relative oligemia distal to engorged pulmonary arteries in massive PE. Again, similar to the ECG, it is most helpful in excluding other causes of the patient's complaint.

▶ **Clinical probability** estimation is an important component of the evaluation of PE. While symptoms and signs are non-specific, it is possible to estimate the pre-test probability of PE using clinical expertise. In addition, two simple scoring rules have been derived and validated to classify patients as low, moderate, or high probability for PE.

▶ **D dimer** is a non-specific marker for thromboembolic disease formed when cross-linked fibrin is lysed by plasmin. The D dimer test has high sensitivity, but low specificity, for PE. It is most useful to rule out PE in low-probability patients. A variety of rapid D dimer assays are available.

▶ **ABGs** can demonstrate the degree of hypoxemia; however, a normal or grossly abnormal PaO_2 does not exclude or confirm the diagnosis.

▶ **V/Q scans** have been used as a primary modality for diagnosis of PE but are non-diagnostic in a large percentage of patients with suspected PE, especially in patients with effusion or infiltrate on CXR. Results are classified as normal, indeterminate, low, intermediate, or high probability for PE. Diagnostic use is dependent on the clinical probability of PE.

- A normal V/Q reliably excludes disease.
- High pre-test probability + high-probability V/Q → admit for anticoagulation.
- Low pre-test probability + low-probability V/Q → look for another cause of patient's symptoms.
- All other combinations of clinical suspicion and V/Q results usually require further testing.

▶ **Computed tomoangiography (CTA)** is rapidly replacing V/Q scans to evaluate patients with suspected PE. CTA is especially useful for PE in larger pulmonary vasculature, and improving technology is leading to better accuracy in sub-segmental pulmonary arteries. It may also demonstrate other pathology that explains the patient's symptoms.

▶ **Pulmonary angiography** remains the gold standard for inconclusive PE work-ups. It is associated with 4% morbidity and 0.5% mortality and thus is not performed in most patients.

TREATMENT

▶ Anticoagulation is essential to prevent thrombus progression and recurrent embolization.

▶ The standard regime consists of a heparin bolus of 80 U/kg (max 5000 U), then a continuous infusion of 18 U/kg (max 1280 U) after coagulation studies have been sent.

▶ LMWH has replaced unfractionated heparin in the treatment of DVT and is also being used more commonly in the treatment of PE. It has been proven to be as effective as unfractionated heparin, has a lower incidence of bleeding complications, and is easier to administer.

▶ Oral anticoagulation with Coumadin should be initiated as an inpatient and is continued for 3–6 months in most patients.

▶ Thrombolytic therapy should be considered for patients with massive PE and circulatory collapse.

▶ Patients should all be admitted to hospital for monitoring of anticoagulation.

CHAPTER 26

TUBERCULOSIS

Rahul Rastogi

- ▶ 10 million new cases per year worldwide.
- ▶ 3 million deaths annually accounting for 6% of deaths worldwide.
- ▶ Resurgence in the U.S. due to immigration, IV drug abuse, homelessness, HIV.
- ▶ TB is an AIDS-defining opportunistic infection.
- ▶ 60% mortality if untreated.

PATHOPHYSIOLOGY

- ▶ *Mycobacterium tuberculosis*, an acid-fast aerobic rod, accounts for the majority of infection.
- ▶ Transmission through inhaled aerosolized bacilli.
- ▶ Droplets may evaporate into "droplet nuclei" and remain suspended in the air and cause infection.
- ▶ Risk factors: malnutrition, elderly, HIV, ESRD, steroid use, IV drug abuse.
- ▶ Primary infection:
  - Bacilli replicate in the alveoli after being ingested by macrophages and may be taken to regional lymph nodes.
  - Granulomas or tubercles form locally in 2–6 weeks.
  - Ghon complex: peripheral lung lesion (granuloma) with calcified hilar lymph nodes.
  - Majority of patients are asymptomatic, and host immune system contains primary infection while bacilli remain dormant and viable.
  - Bacilli are typically not present in the sputum.
- ▶ Reactivation:
  - Most common form of disease, usually seen in elderly.
  - 10% of immunocompetent individuals will reactivate, with majority in the first 2 years of exposure.
  - Triggers for reactivation include systemic illnesses, immunocompromised states, and steroid use.

- Nearly 80% of reactivation manifests as pulmonary disease involving the apical posterior segments of the upper lobes or the superior segments of the lower lobes.

CLINICAL PRESENTATION

▶ Most common symptom is chronic cough. May also have hemoptysis.

▶ Other symptoms are non-specific and include weight loss, night sweats, and low-grade fevers.

▶ Chest exam often is unremarkable but may have focal lung findings.

▶ Extrapulmonary disease occurs through lymphatic or hematogenous dissemination. Symptoms are dependent on the organ system involved and severity of involvement.

▶ Miliary TB: hematogenous spread that can affect the entire body. May present with generalized symptoms but can also have a more fulminant course.

DIAGNOSIS

▶ Difficult diagnosis in the ED, but must consider in any patient with respiratory symptoms in high-risk group.

▶ **Skin testing** is the standard test for detecting TB.
  - PPD or Mantoux testing is a delayed type hypersensitivity using intradermal PPD.
  - Interpretation is 48–72 hours after placement on the dorsal side of the forearm.
  - Measure only the area of induration, not the area of erythema.
  - Positive test indicates presence of infection but not necessarily active disease.
  - 25% of active TB patients may have a negative test. False-positive reactions also occur.
  - Criteria for interpreting test as positive include
    - > 5 mm induration: known HIV, abnormal CXR, and close contact with TB patient
    - > 10 mm induration: resident or employee at long-term care facility, IV drug abusers, immigrants from endemic areas
    - > 15 mm: all persons

▶ **Sputum** should be sent for stain and culture.

- Acid-fast bacilli are detected with Ziehl-Neelsen or fluorescent stain. Positive smears have 98% specificity. All should be confirmed with culture.
- Sputum culture is the gold standard but takes 3–6 weeks to identify acid-fast bacilli. Faster DNA and PCR probes are now available but not widely used.
- Sputum should be obtained from the patient on 3 consecutive days to exclude the diagnosis.
▶ Labs tend to be non-specific.
  - CBC may reveal microcytic anemia with monocytosis.
  - Hyponatremia, thrombocytopenia, and leukopenia may be present in miliary TB.
  - Blood cultures should be drawn.
  - All patients not known to be HIV positive should be tested for HIV.
▶ **CXR** may have a variety of findings.
  - Infiltrate with unilateral hilar adenopathy
  - Classic upper-lobe infiltrates in reactivation TB
  - Fine nodules in all lung fields in miliary TB

TREATMENT

▶ If diagnosis is suspected, patient should wear mask and be placed in isolation room.
▶ Due to drug resistance and frequently changing susceptibilities, it is suggested that the CDC web site be reviewed for the most up to date antibiotic therapy.
▶ Currently, uncomplicated patients follow four-drug regime:
  - Isoniazid (INH), rifampin (RIF), pyrazinamide (PZA), and either ethambutol (EMB) or streptomycin for 8 weeks followed by INH and RIF for 16 weeks (this may be tailored based on susceptibility testing).
  - HIV-positive patients are treated with a similar regime for much longer duration.
  - Prior to initiating these drugs, baseline labs should include LFTs, CBC with platelet count, and BUN/creatinine. Also get serum uric acid if treating with PZA, and visual acuity if treating with EMB.
▶ Multi-drug resistance, defined by resistance to INH and RIF, is common and often related to non-compliance with standard therapeutic regime.

▶ Treatment should not wait on confirmatory testing in high-risk patients.

DISPOSITION

▶ All patients with suspected active TB should be admitted to the respiratory isolation room.

CHAPTER 27

APPROACH TO ABDOMINAL PAIN

John Kahler

HISTORY

▶ Ask about onset (sudden vs. gradual), severity, and aggravating vs. alleviating factors.
▶ Associated symptoms, recent travel, or antibiotic use.
▶ Past medical and surgical history.
▶ LMP in females of childbearing age.

PHYSICAL EXAM

▶ Observe
  • Patient is unable to get comfortable (kidney stone, ovarian torsion, gallstone).
▶ Inspect abdomen
  • Distended (obstruction)
  • Redness/swelling (incarcerated hernia, cellulitis, herpes zoster)
▶ Auscultate
  • Diminished bowel sounds (peritonitis)
  • Bruits (vascular pathology)
▶ Shake bed
  • Pain worsens or localizes (peritonitis, diverticulitis, appendicitis).
▶ Palpation
  • May require analgesia if too painful to examine (e.g., morphine, 2–4 mg IV)
  • Genital exam (hernias, testicular torsion)
  • Rectal exam for occult blood (positive in colitis, bowel infarction, PUD)

DIFFERENTIAL DIAGNOSIS

▶ See Table 27-1.

TABLE 27-1.
DIFFERENTIAL DIAGNOSIS OF ABDOMINAL PAIN

RUQ	**Back**
Biliary colic	AAA
Acute cholecystitis	Pancreatitis
Hepatitis	Acute cholecystitis
Pancreatitis	Kidney stone
Kidney stone	Retrocecal appendicitis
RLL pneumonia	Psoas abscess
Herpes zoster	**LUQ**
RLQ	Kidney stone
Appendicitis	PUD
Ovarian/testicular pathology	LLL pneumonia/PE
Kidney stone	Constipation
IBD	Splenic infarct/rupture
Herpes zoster	Herpes zoster
Epigastrium	**LLQ**
PUD	Diverticulitis/abscess
Acute cholecystitis	Kidney stone
Hiatal hernia	Ovarian/testicular pathology
AMI	Constipation
Pancreatitis	Incarcerated hernia
	Herpes zoster

MANAGEMENT

▶ Pain management:
- Analgesia should not be withheld and may actually improve physical exam in some studies.
- Morphine, 2–5 mg IV, or Dilaudid, 0.5–1.0 mg IV. Titrate to level of discomfort.

▶ Immediate surgical consultation if the following suspected:
- Appendicitis
- AAA
- Ectopic pregnancy
- Peritonitis

DIAGNOSTIC TESTING

▶ Pregnancy test in females of childbearing age (must rule out ectopic).
▶ CBC is non-specific, but elevated WBC can suggest acute inflammatory process or infection.

▶ UA to rule out urinary infection and stones and determine hydration status.

▶ Acute abdominal series (plain films) is only indicated if obstruction, free air, or FB suspected.
  • Low threshold in immunosuppressed patients or elderly

▶ Electrolytes if comorbidities present for renal disease, patient is elderly or critically ill, or IV contrast dye is needed.

▶ Amylase/lipase to exclude pancreatitis.

▶ LFTs if RUQ pain present.

▶ Ultrasound:
  • Testicular: rule out torsion.
  • Pelvic: rule out ovarian pathology, ectopic pregnancy, or undifferentiated lower abdominal pain in females.
  • Aortic: rule out AAA.
  • RUQ: rule out biliary obstruction, acute cholecystitis.
  • Renal: kidney transplant patients, evaluate for kidney stones in pregnant patients.

▶ CT scan:
  • Non-contrast: study of choice for kidney stone evaluation
  • IV/oral contrast good to evaluate for
    ○ Appendicitis
    ○ Diverticulitis, IBD
    ○ Intra-abdominal abscess

◗ **PEARLS AND PITFALLS**
  • Pain out of proportion to the physical exam in the elderly suggests bowel infarction/ischemia.
  • AAA commonly missed and mistaken for musculoskeletal back pain.
  • Do not misdiagnose. If etiology is unknown, the diagnosis is "abdominal pain of unclear etiology" and patient will require re-examination in 12–24 hours.
  • If surgical emergencies (appendicitis, AAA, torsion, perforation) are suspected, consult prior to definitive testing.

APPROACH TO DIARRHEA

John Kahler and Matthew K. Hysell

- ▶ Remains a leading cause of death worldwide.
- ▶ Mortality is mostly related to dehydration.
- ▶ Vulnerable populations:
  - Travelers, elderly (mortality 3%), children, immunosuppressed patients, homosexual men, and HIV patients
- ▶ Definition: three or more loose or watery stools, or one or more bloody stools in 24-hour period (daily stool weight > 200 g).
  - Acute: < 14 days
  - Persistent: > 14 days
  - Chronic: > 1 month
- ▶ Epidemics (U.S.) caused by contaminated food, person-to-person contact, and contaminated water.

PATHOPHYSIOLOGY

- ▶ Increased intestinal secretion (*Vibrio cholerae*, *Escherichia coli*)
- ▶ Decreased intestinal absorption (*Salmonella*, *Campylobacter*, *Yersinia*, *Shigella*, *E. coli*, *Entamoeba histolytica*)
- ▶ Increased osmotic load (lactose intolerance, laxatives)
- ▶ Abnormal intestinal motility (IBS, hyperthyroidism)

DIFFERENTIAL DIAGNOSIS

- ▶ Infectious (most common)
  - Virus 50–70%
    - ○ Less severe, except in children
    - ○ Norwalk, *Rotavirus*, and *Enterovirus*
  - Bacteria 15–20%
    - ○ More severe
    - ○ *E. coli*, *V. cholerae*, *Campylobacter jejuni* (most common), *Salmonella*, *Clostridium difficile*, *Yersinia*

- Parasites 10–15%
  - *E. histolytica* (colon).
  - *Giardia lamblia*, *Isospora*, *Cyclospora*, *Microsporidium*, and *Cryptosporidium* all infect the small intestine.
- Unknown 5–10%
▶ IBD
- Ulcerative colitis
- Crohn's disease
▶ Medications
- Antibiotics, laxatives, antacids, colchicine, lithium, tube feeds
▶ Radiation
▶ Intestinal ischemia
▶ Endocrine: hyperthyroidism

DIAGNOSIS AND MANAGEMENT

▶ Heme positive/negative? (Hemoccult stool, fecal leukocytes)
- Helps differentiate the need for stool cultures and empiric antibiotics
▶ Lab tests
- Stool culture (*Salmonella, Shigella, Campylobacter*)
  - Obtain if invasive diarrhea (heme positive), toxic patients, children, immunosuppressed, diarrhea persists for more than 3–4 days, or patient is starting antibiotics.
- *C. difficile* assay if recent antibiotic use
- Electrolytes if dehydrated, toxic, or comorbidities
- CBC if hemorrhage is suspected or present
- Lactate if intestinal ischemia is suspected
- Ova and parasites if traveler or chronic diarrhea
- Rotazyme assay not necessary in majority of pediatric cases

TREATMENT

▶ Fluids
- IV: Ringer's lactate, 1–2 L NS or bolus
  - 20 cc/kg in children (NS)
- Oral rehydration recommended if possible (must contain sodium, potassium, and glucose).

- ○ WHO-recommended solution:
  - 1 L purified water, 20 g of glucose (40 g sucrose), 3.5 g of sodium chloride, 5 g of sodium bicarbonate, 1.5 g of potassium chloride
▶ Empiric antibiotics
  - Shorten the duration of symptoms in select populations.
  - Consider in the following patients if diarrhea appears invasive and infectious:
    - ○ Fever, bloody stool, and toxic appearing.
    - ○ Also consider in immunocompromised, elderly, significant comorbidities, health care workers, child care workers, patients with prosthetic joints, and travelers with significant symptoms.
  - Avoid if *C. difficile* is suspected (or start Flagyl, as below).
  - Adults: ciprofloxacin, 500 mg bid for 3–5 days.
    - ○ Alternative agents:
      - Bactrim, bid for 3–5 days
      - Flagyl, 500 mg tid, if *C. difficile* suspected (or await assay results)
      - Cipro, 1 g × one dose, if cholera suspected (high volume, non-invasive watery stools)
  - Children: Zithromax (standard dosing).
    - ○ May be less likely to induce hemolytic uremic syndrome in patients with *E. coli* 0157:H7.
▶ Diet
  - Avoid caffeine, milk, soda, and sports drinks (if high glucose load).
  - Recommend starches (rice, noodles, potatoes), cereal, salted crackers, bananas, soup, and boiled vegetables.
▶ Anti-diarrheal agents
  - Imodium (adults) is safe in non-invasive diarrhea and invasive infectious diarrhea when patient is non-toxic and on empiric quinolones.
  - Bismuth-subsalicylate (Pepto-Bismol) is used in prevention and treatment of traveler's diarrhea in adults.
    - ○ Treatment: 2 tabs (30 ml) q30min (max 8 doses/day)
    - ○ Prevention: 2 tabs (30 ml) 4× daily (meals and qhs)
    - ○ May cause black stools, tinnitus, and drug interactions
  - Kaopectate (may be used in older children) is safe in invasive diarrhea as it may bind toxins but does not affect intestinal motility.

◑ **PEARLS AND PITFALLS**

- Bloody diarrhea and pain out of proportion to the exam in the elderly suggest mesenteric ischemia.
- Seizures with diarrhea may suggest shigellosis.
- Dysentery with RLQ pain may suggest *Yersinia*.
- Avoid anti-diarrheal agents in patients with toxic dysentery.
- Maintain a low threshold for admitting the elderly with diarrhea.
- Viral gastroenteritis is a diagnosis of exclusion.

CHAPTER 29

APPROACH TO JAUNDICE

Steven Schmidt

- ▶ Jaundice is the clinical picture of yellow skin and sclera in conjunction with serum bilirubin > 2.0–2.5 mg/dl.
- ▶ Bilirubin comes from catabolism of RBCs (80%) or ineffective erythropoiesis plus breakdown of muscle myoglobin and cytochromes (20%). Hepatocytes conjugate the bilirubin and excrete it into bile.
- ▶ Pseudojaundice can occur with excessive ingestion of foods rich in beta-carotene (e.g., squash, melons, carrots). Unlike true jaundice, there is no scleral icterus or elevation of bilirubin level.

DIFFERENTIAL DIAGNOSIS

- ▶ See Table 29-1.

CLINICAL PRESENTATION

- ▶ Gradual-onset jaundice:
  - Ascites, pruritus, spider angiomata → cirrhosis
- ▶ Acute jaundice:
  - Fever, abdominal pain → hepatitis, acute cholecystitis
  - Asymptomatic or with back or joint pains → hemolytic anemia
- ▶ Recurrent mild jaundice in otherwise healthy patient:
  - Familial causes (e.g., Gilbert syndrome)
- ▶ Painless jaundice, weight loss in elderly patient:
  - Malignancy

DIAGNOSIS

- ▶ Lab tests

TABLE 29-1.
DIFFERENTIAL DIAGNOSIS OF JAUNDICE

Indirect (unconjugated) hyperbilirubinemia
    Overproduction:
        Spherocytosis
        Autoimmune disorders
        Erythropoietic disorders (sickle cell anemia, thalassemias, etc.)
        Excessive heme metabolism (large hematoma reabsorption)
    Decreased uptake:
        Gilbert syndrome
        Drug-related (rifampin [RIF], contrast agents)
    Decreased conjugation:
        Gilbert syndrome
        Crigler-Najjar syndrome
        Hepatocellular disease
        Drug inhibition (chloramphenicol)
Direct (conjugated) hyperbilirubinemia
    Intrahepatic cholestasis:
        Infection
          Viral hepatitis
          Infectious mononucleosis
          Leptospirosis
        Toxic
          Alcohol
          Acetaminophen
          Phenytoin
          Carbon tetrachloride
        Familial
          Rotor syndrome
          Dubin-Johnson syndrome
        Other
          Sarcoidosis
          Lymphoma
          Liver metastases
          Amyloidosis
          Cirrhosis
          Cholestatic jaundice of pregnancy
    Extrahepatic cholestasis:
        Intrinsic to the ductal system:
          Gallstones
          Strictures (surgical, congenital, primary sclerosing
            cholangitis)
          Infection (CMV, cryptosporidium, bacterial cholangitis)
          Malignancy (hepatic, cholangiocarcinoma)
        Extrinsic to the ductal system
          Pancreatitis
          Pancreatic adenocarcinoma

- Determine if direct/indirect bilirubin by obtaining serum bilirubin level with fractionation and UA (only conjugated bilirubin gets excreted as urobilinogens).
  - If unconjugated, look at CBC (with smear, looking for schistocytes and increased reticulocytes → hemolysis), consider Coombs' test and Hgb electrophoresis.
  - If conjugated, look at AST, ALT, alkaline phosphatase, gamma glutamyl transpeptidase (GGTP).
  - If normal, suggests non-hepatic cause (systemic infection, familial causes, pregnancy).
  - If abnormal, pattern suggests cause of disease.
    - Predominance of aminotransferase elevation suggests hepatocellular disease.
    - Marked elevations of alkaline phosphatase, GGTP suggest biliary obstruction.
- Imaging
  - Ultrasound: first line, most sensitive for imaging biliary stones (> 95% sensitivity).
  - CT scan can provide information on both liver and pancreatic parenchymal disease.
  - ERCP: imaging of ductal stones/strictures, can also be therapeutic (removal of intraductal stones, placement of stent across stricture).
  - Percutaneous transhepatic cholangiography (PTC): imaging ductal stones/strictures.
- Liver biopsy
  - Useful if serum and imaging studies do not lead to a firm diagnosis.

TREATMENT AND DISPOSITION

- Treatment and disposition depend on underlying etiology. Jaundice alone is not an indication for admission.
- If discharging a patient, make sure that he or she has proper follow-up.

CHAPTER 30

APPENDICITIS

Elke G. Marksteiner

- ► Most common cause of acute abdomen.
- ► 7% of the population will have appendicitis during their lifetime.
- ► Incidence is highest in the 10- to 19-year-old age group.

PATHOPHYSIOLOGY

- ► Obstruction of the appendiceal lumen by
  - Lymphoid hyperplasia in young patients
  - Food matter
  - Fecaliths or adhesions
  - Viral illness or bacterial infection
- ► Mucosal secretion continues despite obstruction, which leads to an increase in intraluminal pressure and subsequent thrombosis of small vessels as well as decreased lymphatic drainage causing the wall of the appendix to become necrotic.
- ► Bacterial overgrowth ensues with predominantly *Escherichia coli*, *Peptostreptococcus*, *Bacteroides fragilis*, and *Pseudomonas* species.
- ► Initial luminal distention triggers visceral afferent pain fibers.
  - Pain at this time is usually vague and poorly localized (first 24 hours).
  - Later, peritoneal inflammation involves somatic pain fibers, which localizes pain to the RLQ.

CLINICAL PRESENTATION
History

- ► Initially, non-specific abdominal pain in epigastric or periumbilical region that eventually localizes to RLQ (81% sensitive, 53% specific).
  - Anorexia (68% sensitive, 36% specific), nausea (58% sensitive, 37% specific), vomiting (51% sensitive, 45% specific).

- Low-grade fever and leukocytosis usually occur later in the course. Perforation is more likely in patients with higher WBC and fever exceeding 39.4° C (103° F).

Exam

▶ As illness progresses, localized tenderness in the RLQ over McBurney's point (one-third of distance along a line between the right superior iliac crest and the umbilicus).

▶ Pain in the RLQ with palpation of the LLQ (Rovsing sign).

▶ Pain with internal rotation of the right hip (obturator sign).

▶ Pain in the RLQ brought on by extension of the right hip (iliopsoas sign). Sensitivity 16%, specificity 95%.

▶ Location of pain, however, can be atypical depending on location of appendix.

▶ Rebound tenderness, voluntary and involuntary guarding, and tenderness on rectal exam may develop with progression of peritoneal irritation.

▶ Elderly and young children often have atypical presentation that can delay diagnosis.

DIFFERENTIAL DIAGNOSIS

▶ See Chap. 27.

EMERGENCY DEPARTMENT MANAGEMENT

Diagnosis

▶ Usually based on history and exam finding of focal RLQ tenderness.

▶ Women of childbearing age should have pelvic exam and pregnancy test to exclude gynecologic etiologies of pain.

▶ CBC, if WBC > 10,000/μl. Sensitivity is 70–90%. 30% of patients with acute appendicitis have normal WBC.

▶ UA to rule out a UTI.

- Abnormal UA found in 19–40% of patients, possibly related to extension of appendiceal inflammation to the ureter.

▶ Radiographic studies should be performed in patients in whom the diagnosis is unclear.

- CT of abdomen/pelvis with contrast is best radiographic study (96% sensitivity, 94% accuracy).

- Plain radiographs usually have limited diagnostic value; however, appendicolith, localized RLQ ileus, loss of psoas shadow, and free air on plain film can suggest appendicitis.
- Ultrasound is useful if abnormal. However, it is operator dependent, and study may be limited by body habitus, gas in bowel, or by a retrocecal appendix.
  - Often test of choice in young children

Treatment

▶ Surgery for acute appendicitis.
  - Patient needs to be NPO, adequately fluid resuscitated.
▶ If perforated appendicitis/abscess, cover anaerobic bacteria, enterococci, and gram-negatives.
  - Ampicillin/sulbactam, 3 g IV, or piperacillin/tazobactam, 3.375 g IV.

Disposition

▶ If appendicitis likely based on exam, get early surgical consultation.
▶ If appendicitis is suspected but diagnosis remains somewhat unclear, obtain additional studies, including imaging study.
▶ If diagnosis of appendicitis unlikely, patient should be observed in ED for a period of time and discharged with clear and explicit instructions on which worrisome symptoms should prompt their return to the ED.
▶ Discharged patients should have re-examination performed at 12–24 hours by either their primary care physician or in ED if follow-up cannot be established.

CHAPTER 31

PANCREATITIS

Diann M. Krywko

- ▶ Inflammatory process in which pancreatic enzymes auto-digest the gland
- ▶ 80% mild, 20% severe acute pancreatitis
- ▶ Mortality rate: overall 5%, mild 1%, severe acute 10–25%
- ▶ Male predominance

PATHOPHYSIOLOGY

- ▶ Developed countries' etiologies: alcohol (40%), gallstones (35%), idiopathic (20%), ERCP, trauma, drug, hereditary, hypercalcemia, hypertriglyceridemia, and duct abnormalities causing ductal blockage.
- ▶ All pathways lead to cellular edema, vacuolization, and premature intracellular activation of trypsinogen and digestive enzymes resulting in auto-digestive injury.
- ▶ Complications include pseudocyst, abscess, GI hemorrhage, pancreatic and extra-pancreatic malignancy, chronic pancreatitis with ensuing exocrine and endocrine dysfunction, and necrotizing pancreatitis, sterile or infected (40–70%).

CLINICAL PRESENTATION

- ▶ Severe epigastric abdominal pain radiating to back, nausea, vomiting, and dehydration.
- ▶ Tachycardia, tachypnea, hypotension, and fever.
- ▶ Grey Turner's sign (bluish discoloration of flanks) and Cullen's sign (bluish discoloration of periumbilical area) are both caused by retroperitoneal leak of blood in hemorrhagic pancreatitis (1–3%, appears in 48 hours, no additional mortality).

DIFFERENTIAL DIAGNOSIS

- ▶ See Chap. 27.

TABLE 31-1.
RANSON'S CRITERIA

At admission:
  Age > 55 years
  WBC > 16,000/mm^3
  Serum glucose > 200 mg/dl
  LDH > 350 or 2 times normal
  AST > 250 or 6 times normal
At 48 hours:
  HCT decrease > 10%
  BUN increase > 5 mg/dl
  Calcium < 8 mg/dl
  PaO$_2$ < 60 mmHg
  Base deficit > 4 mEq/L
  Fluid sequestration > 6 L

EMERGENCY DEPARTMENT MANAGEMENT
Diagnosis

▶ Lab: useful diagnostically, not prognostically. Serum amylase and/or lipase (> 3 times elevation) supports diagnosis.
  • Amylase rises within 2–12 hours, peaks within 48 hours, normalizes in 3–5 days.
    ○ Poor sensitivity: elevated by intra-abdominal, parotid, and submandibular gland inflammation; renal insufficiency (25% renal clearance); macroamylasemia; hypertriglyceridemia.
    ○ Specificity increased using cutoff of > 2 to 3 times normal limit.
  • Lipase rises within 4–8 hours, peaks at 24 hours, normalizes in 8–14 days.
    ○ Sensitivity affected by intra-abdominal and lingual gland inflammation, renal insufficiency, macromolecule.
    ○ More specific than amylase.
  • ALT > 150 IU/dl (3 times increase), PPV 95% of acute gallstone pancreatitis.
  • Triglyceride, calcium, CRP (sensitivity 83–100%, PPV of 37–77%, 150 mg/L) (Table 31-1).
▶ Mortality based on combination of admission and 48-hours criteria:
  • 0–2, < 5% mortality

- 3–4, 20% mortality
- 5–6, 40% mortality
- 7–8, 100% mortality
▶ Sensitivity/specificity 85%.
▶ Ranson's criteria are based on alcoholic pancreatitis.
▶ Note that amylase and lipase are not included in criteria.
▶ Radiology testing:
  - Ultrasound:
    ○ Detects gallstones, CBD dilation, sludge, mass, peripancreatic fluid.
    ○ Limited by bowel gas.
    ○ Gallstone pancreatitis detection sensitivity is 70%.
  - Contrast-enhanced CT differentiates pancreatitis from other hyperamylasemic intra-abdominal pathology, delineates complications with same specificity/sensitivity as Ranson's criteria.
    ○ CT indications:
      ■ Establish diagnosis
      ■ Assess severity
      ■ Diagnose complications
    ○ CT sensitivity/PPV near 100% for detecting pancreatic necrosis 4–10 days after symptom onset.
  - MRI is superior to CT for distinguishing uncomplicated pseudocyst vs. necrosis.
  - ERCP:
    ○ Procedure of choice for cholangitis, increasing pancreatitis severity, and if CBD stone present.
    ○ Diagnostic for papilla obstruction/ductography (tumors, strictures, diverticula, pancreas divisum, and annular pancreas), bile microscopy, and sphincter of Oddi manometry.
    ○ Therapeutic for stone removal, sphincterotomy, stricture dilation, and necrotomy.
    ○ It is invasive with complications (50% elevate enzymes, 7% mild, 1% severe acute pancreatitis, and 0.01% mortality rate).

Treatment

▶ Diagnostic and supportive.
▶ NPO.
▶ Aggressive fluid resuscitation, O_2, and analgesia.
▶ Antibiotics indicated only if > 30% necrosis diagnosed on CT.

► Prophylactic IV antibiotics that penetrate pancreatic tissue include imipenem (drug of choice), ciprofloxacin, metronidazole, and bacitracin.

► NG tube controversial as early trophic enteric feeding gaining favor.

Disposition

► Patients with a Ranson's score > 2 should be placed in the ICU for resuscitation and monitoring.

► Those with mild pancreatitis (Ranson's score 0–2) should be admitted for pain control, made NPO, given IV fluids, and monitored for progression of disease.

CHAPTER 32

CHOLELITHIASIS AND CHOLECYSTITIS

Scott Ferguson and Laura Roff Hopson

▶ Gallstone prevalence increases with age. By age 60, 20% of women and 10% of men are affected.

▶ Risk factors: age, female, high estrogen states (multiparity, pregnancy), prolonged fasting/bile stasis (TPN, critical illness), rapid weight loss, diabetes, obesity, FH.

▶ **Biliary colic:** transient obstruction of the cystic duct by a gallstone.

▶ **Acute cholecystitis:** prolonged cystic duct obstruction with subsequent gallbladder (GB) inflammation and superinfection.

▶ **Choledocholithiasis:** obstruction of the CBD by gallstone.

▶ **Cholangitis:** infection of the CBD with underlying anatomic abnormality such as choledocholithiasis, tumor, or stricture.

PATHOPHYSIOLOGY

▶ Obstruction at GB neck or cystic duct causes **biliary colic** by distention of GB.

▶ If obstruction is prolonged, then the increased pressure and PG synthesis cause localized GB wall ischemia/inflammation **(cholecystitis).**

CLINICAL PRESENTATION

▶ **Biliary colic:** misnomer as pain is not colicky
  • Typically, pain builds over several minutes to moderate/severe intensity.
  • Located in the RUQ or epigastrium.
  • May radiate to the right shoulder/scapula or interscapular area.

- Classically lasts 1–4 hours and resolves once the stone dislodges. Peak time of onset around midnight.
- Attacks classically occur after a fatty meal, but in one-third of patients, the pain is unrelated to eating.

▶ If symptoms persist for longer than 4–6 hours, progression to **acute cholecystitis** is likely (90% from prolonged cystic duct obstruction from stones, 10% acalculous). RUQ tenderness (73–81% sensitive). Murphy's sign: inspiratory arrest with palpation over the GB (58–71% sensitive and 85–89% specific).

▶ Consider atypical presentations of acute cholecystitis, particularly in elderly patients.

DIFFERENTIAL DIAGNOSIS

▶ See Chap. 27.

EMERGENCY DEPARTMENT MANAGEMENT
Diagnosis

▶ Biliary colic
- Physical exam shows RUQ or epigastric tenderness without peritoneal signs.
- Afebrile with labs, WBC, and LFTs being normal.

▶ Acute cholecystitis
- Physical exam reveals RUQ tenderness.
- Murphy's sign: inspiratory pause on palpation of RUQ.
- Fever present in 35%, leukocytosis in 63%, abnormal LFTs (any one of ALT, AST, or bilirubin) in 70%.

▶ Acalculous cholecystitis (10% of cases)
- Usually in patients with a prolonged critical illness such as major surgery or burns, or in those receiving prolonged TPN.
- GB distention and bile stasis result in functional obstruction.
- Many patients are not able to localize their pain and have only unexplained fever, leukocytosis, or sepsis.
- 20% have elevated transaminases and bilirubin.

▶ Imaging
- Plain films: 10% of stones are radio-opaque.
- Ultrasound is the initial imaging study of choice.
  - 88% sensitive and 80% specific for presence of cholelithiasis.

- ○ Able to detect signs of cholecystitis (sonographic Murphy's sign, GB wall thickening > 4–5 mm, pericholecystic fluid, increased blood flow by Doppler).
  - ○ If ≥ 3 signs present, PPV is 80–90% for acute cholecystitis.
  - ○ Consider choledocholithiasis if CBD dilated (> 10–12 mm).
- HIDA
  - ○ 97% sensitive and 90% specific for acute cholecystitis.
  - ○ False positives in ≤ 40% of critically ill patients.
  - ○ False-positive rate decreased by administration of morphine.
  - ○ Failure to visualize GB indicates cystic duct obstruction. Failure to visualize duodenum indicates CBD obstruction.
- CT
  - ○ 50% of stones visualized.
  - ○ May show other signs of cholecystitis.
  - ○ Best test to evaluate for other intra-abdominal pathology.

Treatment

▶ Once stones become symptomatic, consider surgical referral as the rate of recurrent biliary colic is high (70% in next 2 years), and 1–2% per year risk of complications (acute cholecystitis, pancreatitis).

▶ Symptomatic therapy in the ED: IVF, correct electrolytes, control of emesis via antiemetics or NGT if refractory.

▶ Pain control with NSAIDs (ketorolac, 30 mg IV) or opiates (Dilaudid, 1–2 mg IV).

▶ Cholecystectomy is the definitive treatment, but if major comorbidities preclude surgery, may treat with ursodiol to try to dissolve stones.

▶ IV antibiotics for acute cholecystitis to cover gram-negatives and anaerobic organisms.
- Some possibilities include ampicillin/sulbactam, piperacillin/tazobactam, cefotetan, and ampicillin/gentamicin/metronidazole.

▶ Critically ill or hemodynamically unstable patients may be managed with a percutaneous cholecystostomy and interval cholecystectomy once stable.

Disposition

▶ Outpatient surgical referral for biliary colic patients whose symptoms have resolved. Send home with prescriptions of ibuprofen and/or narcotics.

▶ Emergent surgical consultation and admission for patients with acute cholecystitis or refractory biliary colic symptoms.

▶ Consideration for ERCP if suspicion of choledocholithiasis.

▶ Timing of surgery in acute cholecystitis is controversial. Immediate surgery vs. "cooling off" with antibiotics for 48–72 hours.

CHAPTER 33

DIVERTICULITIS

Nathaniel S. Bowler

- ▶ Diverticulosis refers to the presence of small mucosal pockets in the wall of the colon.
- ▶ Diverticulitis refers to the presence of inflammation and infection in a diverticulum.
- ▶ Diverticulosis affects one-third of the population older than age 45 and up to two-thirds of the population older than age 80.
- ▶ Highest incidence is in the U.S., Europe, and Australia and is likely related to an overall deficiency of dietary fiber.
- ▶ ≤ 25% of patients with diverticulosis progress to have diverticulitis.

PATHOPHYSIOLOGY

- ▶ Diverticula are characterized structurally by mucosal herniation through the colonic wall.
- ▶ Diverticulitis results when a diverticulum becomes obstructed by impacted stool in its neck, leading to inflammation and eventual perforation if not treated.
- ▶ In Western societies, ≤ 90% of patients have involvement of the sigmoid colon.
- ▶ Cases may progress to perforation, abscess formation, intestinal obstruction, or diverticular fistula.

CLINICAL PRESENTATION

- ▶ 93–100% present with abdominal pain, primarily located in the LLQ, in the case of sigmoid diverticulitis.
- ▶ Other symptoms may include nausea, vomiting, constipation, diarrhea, dysuria, and urinary frequency.

▶ Fever is common, and other vital sign abnormalities may be present.
  • Tachycardia and hypotension should increase suspicion for perforation and signal a need for resuscitation.
▶ Physical exam usually demonstrates localized tenderness in the LLQ, except in the case of right-sided pathology.
▶ Localized guarding, localized rebound tenderness, or a palpable mass may be present.
▶ Rectal exam may reveal tenderness and should be tested for blood (gross bleeding is rare in diverticulitis).
▶ 25% of patients with diverticulitis are Hemoccult positive.

EMERGENCY DEPARTMENT MANAGEMENT
Diagnosis

▶ Initial studies should include a CBC, UA, and a flat and upright abdominal X-ray to screen for perforation or obstruction.
▶ In classic presentations of diverticulitis, in which other gynecologic or urologic pathology has been effectively ruled out, the diagnosis of diverticulitis can be made based on clinical criteria alone.
▶ In cases in which the diagnosis is in question, imaging modalities include CT scan, contrast enema, and ultrasound.
  • The imaging test of choice is CT scan, which has a sensitivity ≤ 97% and a specificity of 75–100%. This method has the added advantage of being able to localize pathology to other organ systems and, as a result, has become the diagnostic modality of choice in most EDs.

Treatment

▶ Treatment options are oral or parenteral antibiotics, and surgical or percutaneous drainage.
▶ Certain factors influence the approach.
  • Age: Acute diverticulitis is more virulent in the elderly.
  • Pain: Patients often need IV narcotics.
  • Health of the patient: Immunosuppressed patients, diabetics, steroid use, and renal failure patients may need IV antibiotics and re-assessment.
  • Location: Right-sided diverticulitis is more virulent than left.

- ▶ Antibiotic choice should cover gram-negative rods and anaerobes.
  - Appropriate IV regimens include
    - ○ Metronidazole or clindamycin **plus** an aminoglycoside, monobactam, or third-generation cephalosporin.
    - ○ Ampicillin/sulbactam, ticarcillin/clavulanate, and cefotetan are single antibiotic alternatives.
  - Appropriate oral regimens include
    - ○ SMX-TMP **plus** metronidazole
    - ○ Quinolone **plus** metronidazole
- ▶ Diverticular abscesses can be treated conservatively or aggressively.
  - Small pericolic abscesses may resolve with antibiotic therapy and bowel rest alone.
  - Large abscesses can be treated by percutaneous or surgical drainage.
  - Elective resection of the area of affected colon is often considered after two attacks of uncomplicated diverticulitis.

Disposition

- ▶ Uncomplicated diverticulitis in patients able to tolerate PO, who do not have systemic symptoms or peritoneal signs, and in whom pain can be controlled with oral pain medications can be considered for outpatient treatment.
  - Patients being discharged must be reliable enough to take medications and have follow-up with a primary care physician.
  - They should be discharged on a clear liquid diet, oral antibiotics, and appropriate pain medications.
- ▶ All others should be admitted to the hospital on bowel rest and IV antibiotics.

CHAPTER 34

BOWEL OBSTRUCTION

Carol H. Schultz

SMALL BOWEL OBSTRUCTION

▶ Etiology: adhesions (60%), malignant tumors (20%), hernia (10%), IBD (5%)

▶ Adhesions: 80% from pelvic surgery when small bowel is tethered at root of mesentery and mobile in pelvis

Pathophysiology

▶ Distention stimulates secretions and peristalsis leading to more distention.

▶ Severe distention increases intraluminal hydrostatic pressure and bowel wall edema.

▶ Third-spacing of fluid increases and massive dehydration may result in hypovolemic shock.

▶ Bacterial translocation occurs in 59% of cases and is the result of intestinal stasis, rapid proliferation of bacteria with transmural migration, and infection of mesenteric lymph nodes and organs.

▶ Bowel ischemia and necrosis may occur rapidly followed by perforation, peritonitis, and death from sepsis.

Clinical Presentation

▶ Abdominal pain, distention, nausea, vomiting, lack of bowel movement or lack of flatus, and history of abdominal surgery or cancer.

▶ Pain described as intermittent and crampy early, then constant and severe later.

▶ Abdominal tenderness ± peritonitis, heme-positive or bloody stools, and incarcerated hernia.

▶ Strangulation presents with constant pain, fever, tachycardia, peritonitis, painful mass, bloody stools, leukocytosis, and acidosis and has a 10–30% mortality rate.

Emergency Department Management

Diagnosis

▶ Plain radiographs
- Radiographs are 50–60% diagnostic and may show dilated loops of bowel and air-fluid levels.

▶ CT scanning
- CT scan shows proximal bowel filled with fluid and/or air with a transition zone and collapsed bowel distally, a beak-like narrowing at the point of obstruction from adhesions, masses, or IBD.
- CT scan signs of strangulation include bowel wall thickening, pneumatosis intestinalis, portal venous gas, mesenteric haziness, and non-enhancement of bowel wall after IV contrast (same findings as in ischemic bowel).
- One study reports sensitivity of 92% and specificity of 71%.
- Useful when plain films are negative despite high clinical suspicion.

Treatment

▶ Resuscitation with isotonic IV fluids.
▶ NPO.
▶ NG decompression provides symptomatic relief and decreases need for operative decompression.
▶ Monitor urinary output (UOP).
▶ 88% of patients with complete obstruction from adhesions had resolution following 2–3 days of conservative treatment without an increase in rate of strangulation or mortality, and those requiring surgery had no untoward effects with delayed surgery.
▶ Immediate surgical consultation when strangulation is suspected.
▶ Mortality rate is 3–5%.

Disposition

▶ Admission with conservative treatment.
▶ If signs of sepsis occur, surgery may need to be consulted in the ED.

LARGE BOWEL OBSTRUCTION

▶ Colorectal carcinoma is the leading cause (53%).

▶ Other etiologies include volvulus (17%), diverticular disease (12%), extrinsic compression (6%), stricture, hernia, fecal impaction, adhesions, and pseudo-obstruction.

Pathophysiology

▶ Same as in SBO.
▶ Distention is greater than in SBO, and the risk of ischemia and perforation is higher.
▶ There is an increased risk of perforation with a competent ileocecal valve and closed loop.

Clinical Presentation

▶ History of sudden distention suggests volvulus.
▶ Alteration in bowel habits over months suggests sigmoid carcinoma.
▶ Complaints of obstipation, abdominal pain, distention, and vomiting (feculent).
▶ Exam reveals distention, variable bowel sounds, and tenderness ± mass, peritoneal signs, dehydration, and hypovolemic shock.
▶ Pseudo-obstruction presents with pain, minimal tenderness, and absent bowel sounds.

Emergency Department Management

Diagnosis

▶ Acute abdominal series were found to be 84% sensitive and 72% specific, whereas the contrast (water-soluble) enema was 96% sensitive and 98% specific.
▶ Colonoscopy is useful in determining the etiology and may facilitate decompression.
▶ CT scanning is useful in diagnosing masses, diverticular abscess, and intussusception.

Treatment

▶ Immediate surgery for perforation or ischemia
▶ Percutaneous drainage and IV antibiotics for abscess
▶ Decompression for volvulus and pseudo-obstruction
▶ Supportive care including resuscitation with isotonic saline IV and NG decompression
▶ Surgery if medical management fails

SIGMOID VOLVULUS
Pathophysiology

▶ The axial twist of colon around its mesentery

Clinical Presentation

▶ Bimodal peaks: infants and elderly population
▶ Abdominal pain, distention, constipation, and vomiting
▶ History of previous large bowel obstruction in 40–60%

Management

▶ Sigmoid volvulus looks like a bent inner tube or inverted U-shaped sigmoid loop on abdominal radiographs.
▶ Confirmed by contrast enema, which may reveal "bird's beak" where contrast encounters obstruction.

Treatment

▶ Decompressed by colonoscopy
▶ Fluoroscopic or endoscopic rectal tube placement
▶ Surgery

CECAL VOLVULUS
Pathophysiology

▶ Torsion of the ascending colon just above the ileocecal valve.
▶ Incidence peaks at ages 20–40.

Clinical Presentation

▶ Similar to SBO

Management

▶ Cecal volvulus looks like a coffee bean on plain radiograph.
▶ CT scan has higher specificity than plain films; should be used when diagnosis is in question.

Treatment

▶ Barium enema can be attempted initially unless patient has peritonitis, sepsis, or free air.

▶ Emergent surgery to reduce the volvulus and ischemia as quickly as possible if barium enema was unsuccessful.

PSEUDO-OBSTRUCTION OR OGILVIE SYNDROME
Clinical Presentation
▶ Similar symptoms as SBO.
▶ Higher incidence in elderly with multiple medical pathologies.

Management
▶ Aggressively treat underlying medical conditions, fluid or electrolyte deficits.
▶ Risk of perforation correlates with the duration of distention more than the degree of distention; however, ≥ 10 cm must be treated aggressively.
▶ Treatment consists of supportive care, decompression, and pharmacologic manipulation.

CHAPTER 35

INFLAMMATORY BOWEL DISEASE

David E. Newcomb and Rahul K. Khare

▶ Two main entities: Crohn's disease and ulcerative colitis.
▶ Both have similarities in clinical presentation, complications, and treatments.
▶ Both disorders present in a pattern of exacerbations and quiescent periods with a bimodal age distribution, affecting patients in the teens to 30s, and again in the 60s.
- Crohn's disease
  ○ Transluminal inflammation (all layers) of bowel wall.
  ○ Gives mucosa cobblestone appearance.
  ○ Can involve any component of the GI tract from the mouth to perianal areas; primarily involves small bowel (80%).
  ○ Incontiguous areas of inflammation lead to "skip lesions" throughout GI tract.
- Ulcerative colitis
  ○ Mucosal inflammation primarily of the large bowel but rarely involves distal ileum in severe cases.
  ○ Submucosal inflammation in a continuous fashion throughout the entire large bowel (no skip lesions).
  ○ Almost always involves rectum, and inflammation is geographically continuous.
  ○ Peak incidence 20–30 years.

CLINICAL PRESENTATION
▶ Features common to both disorders
- Constitutional: fever, weight loss, fatigue
- GI: diarrhea, abdominal pain, sclerosing cholangitis, bloody stools
- Cutaneous: erythema nodosum, pyoderma gangrenosum
- Arthralgias/bone: ankylosing spondylitis, large joint peripheral arthritis, osteomalacia

TABLE 35-1.
DIFFERENTIAL DIAGNOSIS OF IBD

Infectious enteritis
Clostridium difficile colitis
Mesenteric ischemia
Lactose intolerance
Appendicitis
Diverticular disease
Malignancy
IBS

- Anemia
- ► Features unique to Crohn's disease
  - Malabsorption, osteomalacia, pernicious anemia
  - Fistulas to retroperitoneum, skin, bladder
  - Perianal skin tags, fissures, and abscesses
  - Relatively more bowel strictures and obstructions
- ► Features unique to ulcerative colitis
  - Most common complaint is bloody diarrhea with abdominal pain.
  - More likely to develop toxic megacolon.
  - More likely to develop colon cancer.

DIFFERENTIAL DIAGNOSIS
- ► See Table 35-1.

EMERGENCY DEPARTMENT MANAGEMENT
Diagnosis
- ► Diagnosis based on history, exam, biopsy, and exclusion of other disease entities.
- ► Positive FH helpful.
- ► Definitive diagnosis made by colonoscopy and biopsy.
- ► In patients with known disease, evaluation focused on ruling out common complications.
- ► Imaging
  - Plain abdominal X-rays to evaluate for evidence of perforation, obstruction, toxic megacolon, loss of normal bowel markings

- CT scan to evaluate for strictures, fistulas, abscess, and perforation
  - Also may aid in differentiating Crohn's disease from ulcerative colitis based on location of lesions
▶ Lab evaluation
  - CBC: WBC may be elevated, Hgb to determine degree of anemia.
  - Electrolytes, BUN/creatinine may be abnormal if diarrhea/dehydration severe.
  - PT/PTT if significant bleeding or severe malabsorption suspected.
  - CRP or ESR may help in determining severity of flare.

Treatment

▶ Steroids generally initiated with the discussion of accepting hospital team.
▶ Treatment must also focus on common complications such as electrolyte derangements, hypovolemia, anemia, dehydration, obstruction, fistulas, and toxic megacolon.
▶ Medical treatment:
  - Mesalamine (5-ASA), 1 g PO qid or 1 rectal suppository PR bid
    - May be used for exacerbations and long-term suppression
  - Topical (rectal) and oral steroids for more severe and/or refractory cases
    - Hydrocortisone enema, 60 mg
    - Prednisone, 40–60 mg PO qd
    - Solu-Medrol, 60–125 mg IV q6h
  - Role for selected antibiotics in Crohn's disease with colonic involvement, Flagyl, 500 mg PO tid.
  - For severe cases not responsive to above treatments, immuno-suppressive agents such as cyclosporine, azathioprine, methotrexate, and anti–tumor necrosis factor (TNF) antibodies may be necessary.
  - Anti-motility agents may reduce diarrhea but are contraindicated with toxic megacolon.
▶ Surgical treatment:
  - In cases unresponsive to medical therapy, surgical excision may be required.
  - Colectomy often curative in ulcerative colitis.
  - Crohn's disease has a relatively high rate of reoccurrence after surgical therapy.

Disposition

▶ Admission
- Patients with surgical complications, moderate to severe exacerbations, or those failing outpatient treatments
- Presence of complications that warrant admission such as dehydration, or anemia requiring transfusions

▶ Discharge
- Patients with mild to moderate exacerbations of known disease with absence of complications or features requiring hospitalization.
- Consultation with gastroenterologist/primary care physician while in ED or close follow-up must be arranged.

CHAPTER 36

ACUTE MESENTERIC ISCHEMIA

Andrew R. Barnosky

▶ Acute vascular compromise of the intestine threatening bowel viability and causing acute abdominal pain
▶ Patients generally older than age 50 (with median age of 70)
▶ Female to male distribution of 2:1
▶ Mortality > 50%

PATHOPHYSIOLOGY

▶ SMA occlusion most common site (50%) of acute mesenteric ischemia occlusion (SMA supplies distal duodenum to splenic flexure).
▶ Mesenteric arterial embolism most common mechanism.
▶ Source of emboli is generally the heart, from left atrial or ventricular thrombi that fragment during dysrhythmia, or embolization from valvular lesions.
▶ Risk factors include CHF, CAD, dysrhythmias (particularly AF), and valvular heart disease.
▶ Ischemic injury allows release of bacteria, toxins, and vasoactive peptides. May lead to septic shock, cardiac failure, and multisystem organ failure.
▶ Necrosis can occur within 10 hours of onset of symptoms.

CLINICAL PRESENTATION

▶ Classically, pain is out of proportion to clinical findings: severe abdominal pain without significant abdominal exam findings.
▶ Pain is initially visceral in nature and poorly localized.
▶ Patients generally > age 50, often experiencing sudden abdominal pain lasting > 2 hours, often refractory to narcotics.
▶ Severe, poorly localized, acute abdominal pain, with nausea, vomiting, and diarrhea.

▶ Subacute presentations may have less severe presentation with abdominal pain and distention and occult GIB.

▶ Physical findings often non-diagnostic early. Later, abdominal distention, diffuse abdominal tenderness, diminishing bowel sounds. Eventually, exquisite tenderness to palpation (late), heme-positive stool (late, in 25% of cases).

▶ Classic triad of SMA embolism: GI emptying, abdominal pain, and underlying cardiac disease.

DIFFERENTIAL DIAGNOSIS

▶ See Chap. 27.

EMERGENCY DEPARTMENT MANAGEMENT

Diagnosis

▶ Routine lab and X-rays often non-specific; waiting for abnormal results to develop prevents early diagnosis.

▶ Late presentation has increase in WBC (75% have > 15,000 cells/mm^3) and lactate with hemoconcentration, metabolic acidosis with base deficit, and hyperamylasemia.

▶ Plain radiographs early are normal or may show adynamic ileus, distended air-fluid loops, and bowel wall thickening. Later, may show pneumatosis and/or gas within the portal system.

▶ Abdominal CT may show indirect evidence of ischemia (edema of bowel wall or intramural gas).

▶ Angiography remains the gold standard (but contraindicated if shock or vasopressor therapy present).

Treatment

▶ O$_2$, cardiac monitoring, and two large-bore IVs.

▶ Must correct hypovolemia, hypotension, and metabolic abnormalities quickly with IV crystalloid solutions.

▶ IV administration of broad-spectrum antimicrobials.

▶ Notify vascular or general surgeon immediately if diagnosis is a possibility.

▶ Pre-operative angiogram improves laparotomy outcome.

▶ Prompt laparotomy necessary to resect necrotic bowel, remove embolus, or bypass arterial obstruction.

▶ Papaverine infusion into SMA diminishes mesenteric vasoconstriction (60 mg bolus followed by 30–60 mg/hour continuous
infusion).

▶ Percutaneous transluminal angioplasty and intra-arterial infusion of thrombolytic agents may be therapeutic while diagnostic study of angiogram is being done.

Disposition

▶ All patients should be seen by a surgeon and go to the OR or be
admitted to the ICU.

CHAPTER 37

GASTROINTESTINAL BLEEDING

Matthew K. Hysell

- ▶ Volume resuscitation is of paramount concern.
- ▶ An NGT is necessary in many cases.
  - Hematochezia usually, but not always, represents lower GI pathology.
  - Melena frequently, but not always, represents upper GI pathology.

PATHOPHYSIOLOGY

- ▶ ASA and NSAIDs (including both COX-1 and COX-2 inhibitors) inhibit mucus membrane protective PG synthesis, increasing risk for gastric and duodenal ulcers, and, less frequently, ulcers in small bowel and colon.
- ▶ Plavix, heparin, and Coumadin can cause asymptomatic lesions to become symptomatic.
- ▶ *Helicobacter pylori* bacteria compromise the gastric mucosal defense against acid.
- ▶ Structural abnormalities of the GI tract increase probability of bleeding.
- ▶ Chronic liver disease and cirrhosis frequently predispose to upper GIB due to portal HTN and formation of esophageal varices.

CLINICAL PRESENTATION

- ▶ Classic signs of upper GIB include hematemesis, coffee-ground emesis, and/or melena.
- ▶ Classic sign of lower GIB is hematochezia (up to 10% of hematochezia is caused by upper GIB).
- ▶ Weakness, light-headedness, syncope, and altered mental status are also common presentations.

TABLE 37-1.
DIFFERENTIAL DIAGNOSIS OF GIB

Melena/hematemesis	Hematochezia
Peptic or duodenal ulcer disease	Diverticulosis (~30%)
Gastritis	Colonic AVMs (~20%)
Esophageal varices	Colitis (~15%)
Mallory-Weiss tear	Colon cancer or post-polypectomy (~10%)
Erosive esophagitis secondary to GERD	Upper GIB (~10%)
	Hemorrhoids or rectal varices (~5%)
AVM	Small intestine disease, including Crohn's disease, AVMs, Meckel's diverticula, and tumors (uncommon)
	Aortoenteric fistula (rare)

DIFFERENTIAL DIAGNOSIS

▶ See Table 37-1.

EMERGENCY DEPARTMENT MANAGEMENT

Diagnosis

▶ Decreased HCT and/or positive rectal exam may be only signs in subtle cases.

▶ Frequently, > 20:1 ratio of BUN to creatinine, especially in upper GIB.

▶ T&S/cross-match with initial labs (should generally include PT, PTT, electrolyte, and LFTs as well as HCT).

▶ Anoscopy may reveal source of bleeding in hematochezia, especially in cases with stable HCT.

▶ Orthostatic vital signs may aid detection of under-resuscitated patients.

▶ NG lavage may help detect upper GIBs when presenting sign is not hematemesis. A negative lavage does not entirely rule out an upper source; however, upper GIB is unlikely if there is return of bile but no blood or coffee grounds.

Treatment

General

▶ Volume resuscitation.

▶ Central access or two large-bore peripheral IVs required for resuscitation.

▶ Transfusion is required for hypotension, ongoing bleeding, HCT < 30, especially in patients with coronary disease.

▶ Transfusion with FFP as required for elevated INR.

Upper Gastrointestinal Bleed

▶ Intubation for airway protection may be required for severe upper GIB.

▶ For ongoing upper GIB thought to be secondary to peptic or NSAID-associated ulcer disease, IV Protonix, 80 mg IV bolus over 15 minutes followed by 8 mg/hour infusion reduces re-bleeding rates.

▶ For ongoing upper GIB secondary to varices, endoscopic sclero-therapy is treatment of choice, successful in 60–90%.

▶ Medication adjuncts to endoscopy for variceal bleeds temporize or improve endoscopy's efficacy.

  • Vasopressin via central line (which decreases splanchnic blood flow).

    ○ 0.3 units/minute for 30 minutes, may be increased by 0.3 units/minute twice, until side effects or bleeding controlled.

    ○ May need NTG drip to keep SBP > 100.

  • Octreotide, longer acting than somatostatin, less studied but likely equivalent, may be preferred agent.

    ○ 50 mcg bolus followed by 50 mcg/hour

Lower Gastrointestinal Bleed

▶ With ongoing hematochezia, a well-resuscitated patient may undergo colonoscopy as early as 2 hours following GoLYTELY prep via NGT.

▶ Tagged RBC scan may localize and demonstrate ongoing bleeding amenable to angiography in a patient with ongoing lower GIB not stable enough to await colonoscopy.

  • These patients may also be considered for surgical resection.

▶ Actively bleeding sites on hemorrhoidal varices frequently found in liver failure patients can be clamped and then tied with slowly absorbing suture.

  • Medical adjuncts, as in esophageal varices, may be helpful.

Disposition

▶ Patients with any significant ongoing bleeding should be admitted to ICU.

▶ Patients at highest risk for adverse outcome are those with comorbidities.

▶ Patients without significant comorbidities may be admitted to a step-down bed if vital signs are normal.

▶ Healthy patients not admitted should have repeat HCT prior to discharge.

▶ Observation center protocols for stable patients with probable lower GIB may be utilized.

CHAPTER 38

HEPATITIS

Cemal B. Sozener

▶ Hepatitis is defined as inflammation of the liver with hepatocellular necrosis.

▶ Most patients presenting to the ED present with hepatitis as a result of either viral etiology or alcohol ingestion.

VIRAL HEPATITIS

▶ Viral hepatitis is an infection of the liver as a result of infection with one of several viral agents (A, B, C, D, E, and G) that have been identified to cause hepatitis.

▶ Poses a significant public health problem, and currently there are only vaccines available for hepatitis A and B.

Clinical Presentation

▶ Presentation may range in severity from inconsequential asymptomatic infection to fulminant liver failure.

▶ Typically starts with viral prodromal phase, which includes fever (typically low-grade), myalgias, malaise, arthralgia, fatigue, and anorexia. GI symptoms are also common with nausea, vomiting, and occasionally diarrhea or constipation. Abdominal pain is typically limited to the RUQ and is mild and constant.

▶ Liver tenderness is usually present, and just over 50% of livers affected by hepatitis are enlarged. Splenomegaly is present in approximately 15% of reported cases.

▶ If jaundice develops, it typically occurs 5–10 days following the initial symptoms. Most cases usually do not develop jaundice.

▶ The acute phase of the illness usually lasts approximately 2–3 weeks with complete clinical recovery in 9–10 weeks with hepatitis A and in 16 weeks with hepatitis B.

▶ 5–10% of cases may be more prolonged with approximately 1% of these cases leading to fulminant liver failure.

▶ With hepatitis B, C, D, and G, there is a chance of developing chronic hepatitis, which is defined as having elevated serum transaminase levels for over 6 months.

Emergency Department Management

▶ Expect striking elevations in AST and ALT levels early in the disease with subsequent elevations in bilirubin and alkaline phosphatase. WBC is usually normal to low. Prolonged PT typically indicates more severe disease and correlates with increased mortality.

▶ A standard hepatitis panel that we most often use in the ED typically includes IgM anti-hepatitis A virus, hepatitis B surface antigen (HBsAg), IgM anti-hepatitis B core antigen (anti-HBc), and anti-hepatitis C virus.

▶ In general, treatment of acute hepatitis is supportive. Avoid alcohol consumption and other hepatotoxins. Hospitalization is recommended for marked or severe symptoms.

▶ Encephalopathy or severe coagulopathy heralds acute hepatic failure, and hospitalization is required for those with PT prolongation, bilirubin > 20 mg/dl, intractable vomiting, hypoglycemia, immunosuppression, or age > 45.

HEPATITIS A

▶ Acquired from oral contact, mainly fecal-oral transmission.

▶ Symptom onset appears to be more abrupt with an incubation period of approximately 2–6 weeks.

▶ Mostly a self-limited infection, however, cases of fulminant liver failure and death have been documented.

Diagnosis

▶ Acute infection is confirmed by presence of IgM anti-hepatitis A virus.

▶ Presence of IgG anti-hepatitis A virus indicates either previous infection or previous hepatitis A vaccination.

Treatment

▶ Immune globulin is recommended for all close contacts of patients acutely infected with hepatitis A.

▶ Hepatitis A vaccine is recommended for persons planning to travel to endemic regions or with risk factors for developing hepatitis A.

HEPATITIS B

▶ Virus present in blood, saliva, semen, and vaginal secretions and generally considered to be transmitted via contaminated blood products, sexual contact, or mother to fetus during delivery.
▶ Symptom onset between 4 weeks and 6 months.
▶ Risk of fulminant hepatitis is low (< 1%); however, chronic hepatitis occurs in up to 10% of patients and can lead to cirrhosis and hepatocellular carcinoma.
▶ Hepatitis B vaccine has made a significant impact on the prevalence of the disease in the United States.

Diagnosis

▶ Acute infection is confirmed by the presence of HBsAg, which is the first serologic marker to appear.
▶ Antibody to HBsAg (anti-HBs) appears next and persists indefinitely.
▶ Hepatitis B e antigen indicates maximal viral replication and infectivity.
▶ Presence of the antibody to hepatitis e antigen along with HBsAg indicates the end of viral replication and the soon-to-occur resolution of the disease.
▶ Antibody to HBc (anti-HBc) begins 1–2 weeks following the detection of HBsAg and can serve as a marker for current or recent infection even in the absence of any other markers.
▶ The IgM anti-HBc is present in the first 4–6 months of the infection, whereas the IgG antibody is present in patients with either complete recovery or chronic infection.
▶ Presence of only anti-HBs in the absence of the other markers indicates previous successful vaccination.

Treatment

▶ Hepatitis B immunoglobulin (HBIG), when given in large doses followed by hepatitis B vaccine within 7 days of exposure, may be protective or attenuate the severity of the disease.

▶ Progression to chronic hepatitis is less of a risk for immuno-competent individuals; however, much higher risk exists if disease acquired as an infant.

HEPATITIS C

▶ Transmission of virus primarily through contact with blood and blood products. IV drug use remains the greatest source of transmission.
▶ Symptom onset usually 6–8 weeks after virus transmission.
▶ Chronic infection as a result of hepatitis C infection is relatively common, occurring in 50–80% of those with acute infection. Cirrhosis may develop in as many as 20% of these individuals.

Diagnosis

▶ Diagnosis made by detecting antibodies to hepatitis C virus and confirmed in some cases by using an assay to detect hepatitis C RNA.

Treatment

▶ Treatment with interferon alpha has been shown to decrease the risk of chronic hepatitis.
▶ Chronic hepatitis develops in > 80% of these patients over time.

HEPATITIS D

▶ Also known as the delta agent and can cause hepatitis only with current or previous infection with hepatitis B. Felt to be transferred via percutaneous exposure.
▶ Relatively rare in the United States.

Diagnosis

▶ Diagnosis is made by detecting the antibody to hepatitis D antigen, or in some cases, detection of hepatitis D RNA in the serum.

Treatment

▶ Supportive

HEPATITIS E

▶ Rare virus in the United States; occasionally reported in travelers to India, Mexico, the Middle East, and Southeast Asia.

▶ Pathogenesis is felt to be similar to hepatitis A, except more severe clinically.

Diagnosis

▶ Diagnosis made using enzyme immunoassays that detect IgM and IgG antibodies. These assays are not readily available and would need to be referred to the CDC.

Treatment

▶ Supportive

ALCOHOLIC HEPATITIS

▶ Alcoholic hepatitis is defined as acute or chronic inflammation and necrosis of the liver caused by alcohol consumption.

▶ Reversible cause of liver disease, but the leading cause of cirrhosis in United States.

▶ Greater alcohol consumption combined with longer duration of drinking increases a patient's risk of developing alcoholic cirrhosis.

Clinical Presentation

▶ Presentation ranges from asymptomatic to critical illness. Patients typically have an enlarged liver with nausea, vomiting, fever, abdominal pain, jaundice, and possible encephalopathy.

▶ Typically follows period of heavy or binge drinking.

Management

▶ Liver enzymes are typically elevated with AST:ALT ratio 2:1. AST is rarely elevated > 300 U/L.

▶ Alkaline phosphatase and bilirubin are typically elevated.

▶ Markedly elevated bilirubin level and PT indicate more severe disease.

▶ Ultrasound exam and CT of the abdomen can be helpful in detecting ascites and excluding biliary obstruction.

▶ Treat with abstinence from alcohol, vitamin replenishment (especially folate and thiamine), IVF rehydration with dextrose-containing fluids, as well as provide good nutrition.

▶ Methylprednisolone administration appears to reduce mortality in patients with advanced alcoholic hepatitis.

▶ Hospitalization is required for all but the mildest of cases.

CHAPTER 39

ESOPHAGEAL EMERGENCIES

Nathaniel S. Bowler

ESOPHAGEAL FOREIGN BODIES AND ESOPHAGEAL IMPACTION

▶ FBs can be categorized into food boluses, blunt objects, sharp objects, and other miscellaneous objects such as narcotic packs and button batteries.

▶ Peak incidence of FB ingestions in children is age 6 months to 3 years.

▶ FBs in the esophagus can frequently lead to obstruction.

▶ The most common cause of esophageal obstruction in adults is food bolus; coins are the most common cause in children.

Pathophysiology

▶ < 1% of all FBs result in perforation, but with sharp objects, the incidence increases to as much as 35%.

▶ Impaction of an FB in the esophagus usually occurs at one of four sites: at the upper esophageal sphincter, the aortic arch, the left mainstem bronchus, or the lower esophageal sphincter.

▶ Obstruction in the mid- to lower esophagus is the most common, affecting ≤ 50% of ingestions.

Clinical Presentation

▶ Symptoms of esophageal FB include dysphagia, odynophagia, and chest pain.

▶ History is often the key to diagnosis; those unable to provide a good history (young children, the mentally or psychologically impaired) may present with choking, refusal to eat, vomiting, drooling, wheezing, bloodstained saliva, or respiratory distress.

▶ Those with an esophageal FB or food impaction may only experience mild discomfort with a partial obstruction, or may manifest severe distress in the case of a complete obstruction.

- Sialorrhea (drooling or excessive salivation) and regurgitation are classic symptoms of complete esophageal obstruction and can lead to aspiration.

- The most serious result of esophageal FB or impaction is esophageal perforation, and these patients can present with crepitance in the mediastinal or cervical regions, peritonitis, tachycardia, fever, or bloody saliva.

▶ FBs lodging beyond the stomach present with signs and symptoms consistent with bowel obstruction.

Management

▶ ABCs: a large esophageal FB impinging on the trachea or the inability to handle secretions due to complete obstruction can rapidly cause airway compromise and requires emergent intervention.

▶ Esophageal impaction initial therapy includes 1 mg glucagon IV to help relax the lower esophageal sphincter.

- Clinical studies show varying efficacy of glucagon.

▶ Indications for emergent endoscopy include complete obstruction, sharp or > 6 mm FB, and button batteries.

▶ AP and lateral X-ray views of the affected area should be obtained to localize the object; most FBs can be identified on plain films.

- Coins seen above the diaphragm on a chest or neck X-ray can be localized to either the esophagus or the trachea by their orientation:
  ○ Esophageal FBs will be seen flat/horizontal facing the film in a PA view.
  ○ Tracheal FBs will be seen on edge in the PA view.

- Other methods of diagnosing and localizing swallowed FBs include direct or indirect laryngoscopy, swallow studies, endoscopy, and CAT scan.

▶ 80–90% of ingested materials that enter the stomach pass the GI tract spontaneously.

▶ Swallowed objects < 2 cm usually pass without difficulty in adults, whereas objects > 6 cm in length often obstruct the second part of the duodenum and usually require endoscopic removal.

▶ Sharp FBs that are in the esophagus or are able to be retrieved from the stomach or proximal duodenum should be removed immediately by endoscopy due to risk of perforation.

▶ Button batteries lodged in the esophagus are a medical emergency due to the high risk of perforation with pressure necrosis and should be immediately removed endoscopically; if the battery has passed into the stomach, it may be allowed to pass spontaneously with monitoring.

▶ All other esophageal FBs or impactions that do not exhibit signs of complete obstruction (vomiting, inability to handle saliva, severe distress) can initially be observed to allow for spontaneous passage but should never remain in the esophagus for longer than 24 hours due to increased risk of perforation.

▶ Ingested sharp objects that are not able to be retrieved can be followed with daily radiographs; surgery is considered when an object fails to progress for 3 days.

▶ All other objects can be followed expectantly with instructions to return for vomiting, abdominal pain, fever, hematemesis, melena, or rectal bleeding.

ESOPHAGEAL PERFORATION

▶ The most common causes of esophageal perforation include FBs, trauma, caustic ingestions, Boerhaave's syndrome, and iatrogenic rupture due to esophageal instrumentation.

▶ Boerhaave's syndrome is caused by a sudden increase in the intraluminal pressure due to rapid stretching of the esophagus, usually from forceful vomiting or retching.

Clinical Presentation

▶ Acute esophageal perforation is a medical emergency and may present with frank shock in up to 25% of cases.

▶ May have history of heavy drinking, alcoholism, PUD, or any recent esophageal instrumentation.

▶ The classic triad in esophageal perforation is pain, fever, and subcutaneous or mediastinal air.

▶ Hamman's sign (mediastinal crunching sound heard on auscultation) often can be heard due to mediastinal emphysema.

Management

▶ A CXR may demonstrate pneumomediastinum, mediastinal widening, pleural effusion.

▶ Lab testing is initially normal but eventually may demonstrate leukocytosis and acidosis due to developing sepsis.

▶ Esophageal contrast studies are the diagnostic modality of choice.

▶ CT scan is extremely sensitive and specific. Water-based contrast should be used.

▶ All patients with known or suspected esophageal perforation should be started on broad-spectrum antibiotics.

▶ In iatrogenic cases that are caught early, a non-surgical approach is sometimes entertained, although a surgical consult should always be initiated.

▶ Perforations from Boerhaave's syndrome, non-contained perforations, or perforations with an associated PTX or retained FB require surgical intervention.

CHAPTER 40

ANORECTAL EMERGENCIES

Michael Mikhail

HEMORRHOIDS

▶ Most common cause of hematochezia
▶ Associated with constipation, straining, pregnancy, and obesity

Clinical Presentation

▶ Internal: usually cause painless, bright red bleeding with defecation.
▶ External: present with palpable mass, pruritus, pain if becomes thrombosed.
▶ Evidence of hemorrhoidal bleeding does not exclude other causes of rectal bleeding, and further investigation may be warranted in patients whose symptoms suggest proximal colon pathology.

Management

▶ Conservative medical management of hemorrhoids can be accomplished in the majority of patients.
▶ Bleeding internal hemorrhoids: sitz baths, bulk laxatives, or stool softeners.
▶ External hemorrhoids: sitz baths, bulk laxatives, high-fiber diet, topical steroids, and systemic analgesics.
▶ Acutely thrombosed (< 48 hours) and severely painful external hemorrhoids should be treated with an elliptical excision of the clot, under local anesthesia or conscious sedation. Wound is left open and patient discharged with stool softeners, sitz baths, and analgesia.
▶ Surgical intervention is indicated for continued bleeding, intractable pain, incarceration, or strangulation.

ANORECTAL ABSCESSES

▶ Infection of deep tissues around the dentate line. Includes perianal (most common), ischiorectal, intersphincteric, and supralevator abscesses.

▶ Most common in males aged 20–45.

▶ Usually mixed aerobic-anaerobic infections.

▶ Abscesses originate in the anal crypts with gland obstruction and spread to involve the surrounding or deep spaces.

Clinical Presentation

▶ A hot, red, tender area adjacent to the anal verge is usually easily palpated with or without fluctuance. Fever and leukocytosis are uncommon.

▶ Pain and tenderness without a palpable or visible mass suggest a deeper space infection or anorectal fistula.

▶ Fistulas may complicate an abscess (most commonly ischiorectal).

Management

▶ Most simple perianal abscesses may be incised and drained in the ED with an elliptical incision. Adequate local anesthesia is often difficult to achieve, and conscious sedation is usually necessary. Loculations should be broken up with a finger. Antibiotics need only be considered for immunocompromised patients or associated significant cellulitis. Should have surgical follow-up as outpatient.

▶ Deep space abscesses should be drained in the OR.

▶ Fissures require surgical excision, which may be done as an outpatient.

ANORECTAL FISSURE

▶ Longitudinal tear of the anal canal (90% posterior midline)

▶ Most common cause of painful rectal bleeding

Clinical Presentation

▶ Severe pain with defecation associated with hematochezia. Usually painless between bowel movements, so patient often avoids defecating.

▶ Most are visible to inspection by spreading the buttocks and applying gentle traction on the skin around anus.
▶ Skin tag at anal verge suggests a chronic fissure.

Management

▶ Sitz baths, high-fiber diet, local analgesic, and hydrocortisone lotions provide symptomatic relief and alleviate sphincter spasm.
▶ Topical NTG has also been successfully used to relax the internal sphincter.
▶ Fissures that do not respond to conservative treatment may require surgical repair.

PILONIDAL ABSCESS

▶ A painful mass arising in the intergluteal region overlying the lower sacrum and coccyx, which is a result of an ingrown hair provoking an FB reaction and infection of the pilonidal cleft
▶ Predominantly in men (80%), rare after age 45

Clinical Presentation

▶ A painful abscess, midline about 5 cm cephalad from the anus, is the most common finding.
▶ Abscess may spontaneously drain or form a second tract.

Management

▶ Acute abscesses should be incised (elliptical), drained, and packed in the ED.
▶ Patients should be discharged with follow-up in 2 days for repacking of wound.
▶ Surgical referral recommended for definitive care.

CHAPTER 41

APPROACH TO HEMATURIA

Rahul K. Khare and Christopher R. H. Newton

▶ Gross hematuria: blood visible to the naked eye.
▶ Microscopic hematuria: > 3–5 RBCs/hpf.
▶ Many substances in urine may mimic appearance of hematuria [myoglobin, foods (e.g., blackberries and blueberries), drugs (e.g., rifampin [RIF] and Pyridium), food dyes].
▶ Painless gross hematuria is malignancy until proven otherwise.

DIFFERENTIAL DIAGNOSIS
▶ See Table 41-1.

CLINICAL PRESENTATION
▶ Dysuria, frequency → UTI.
▶ Fever, chills, flank pain or tenderness → pyelonephritis.
▶ Sexually active and vaginal or penile discharge → STD urethritis.
▶ History of analgesic abuse → papillary necrosis.
▶ Hypotension, tachycardia, fatigue, fever → urosepsis.
▶ Recent travel to Africa or Middle East → schistosomiasis.
▶ Recent strep infection → post-streptococcal glomerulonephritis.
▶ FH of deafness → Alport's syndrome.
▶ Rash, abdominal pain, and arthritis → Henoch-Schönlein purpura.
▶ Abdominal mass with gross hematuria → Wilm's tumor.
▶ AF with flank tenderness → embolic renal infarction.
▶ Consider risk factors for cancer: age > 40, alcohol and tobacco use, occupational exposures (e.g., benzenes, dyes), pelvic radiation, and cyclophosphamide.

TABLE 41-1.
DIFFERENTIAL DIAGNOSIS OF HEMATURIA

Infection (20%)
Nephrolithiasis (25%)
Neoplasm (up to 20% > 40 years old)
Glomerulonephritis (more common in children)
Renal trauma
BPH
Anticoagulation (warfarin) or primary coagulopathy (hemophilia)
Sickle cell disease
Exercise induced

▶ Anticoagulation alone should not cause hematuria unless there is underlying pathology.

DIAGNOSIS

Urine

▶ Clean catch specimen appropriate for most (consider a catheter specimen for menstruating females).

▶ Dipstick is a commonly used screening test but has high false-positive and false-negative results.

▶ UA: RBC with leukocytes → likely infectious etiology.

▶ UA: red cell casts, dysmorphic red cells, proteinuria → glomerular etiology. Will need further work-up, which usually can be done as an outpatient.

Lab Tests

▶ BUN/creatinine (for renal failure, pre- and post-renal determination)

▶ CBC (leukocytosis, anemia, thrombocytopenia)

▶ PT/PTT (for those on warfarin therapy or liver failure)

Renal Imaging

▶ Is unnecessary for asymptomatic hematuria in the ED

▶ Non-contrast CT used for evaluation of stones

▶ Retrograde urethrogram, cystogram, or IV contrast CT for traumatic hematuria

TREATMENT AND DISPOSITION
Gross Hematuria

▶ Stabilize vitals, may require transfusion, bladder irrigation with a large-bore Foley catheter (18G) or 3-way irrigating Foley

Disposition
▶ Consider admission for significant anemia and/or hemodynamic compromise.
▶ If discharged, should be referred to urologist for further evaluation and work-up. Foley catheter is often left in to prevent urinary retention caused by clots.

Microscopic Hematuria

▶ Unless complicated by renal failure or other pathology, the work-up is usually done as an outpatient in the primary care setting.
▶ If a specific diagnosis is made, it should be treated appropriately.
▶ With or without a specific diagnosis, referral to primary care is necessary for re-testing and further evaluation to rule out underlying malignancy.

CHAPTER 42

URINARY TRACT INFECTIONS AND PYELONEPHRITIS

David Renken

PATHOPHYSIOLOGY

► Usually an ascending infection.
► Shorter urethra in women makes them more prone to UTI.
► Increased with sexual activity, pregnancy, and instrumentation.
► Urinary obstruction increases risk (e.g., prostatic hypertrophy, kidney stone, vesicoureteral reflux).
► Bacteria
   • > 80% *Escherichia coli*
   • 10% *Staphylococcus saprophyticus*
   • *Proteus, Klebsiella, Enterobacter* also common

CLINICAL PRESENTATION

► Urgency, frequency, dysuria, fever, and pain are most common presenting complaints.
► Upper tract infections and pyelonephritis more commonly have fever in association with flank pain and vomiting.
► Upper tract infections more likely:
   • With fever, obstructive risk, or structural abnormality
   • With concurrent chronic illness (diabetes, immunosuppression, sickle cell disease)
   • Recurrent infection (3 UTIs or pyelonephritis in past year)
   • Duration of symptoms > 7 days
► Women who need pelvic exam
   • History of pelvic complaints (discharge, multiple sexual partners)
   • Normal UA with urinary symptoms
► Abnormal vital signs (fever, tachycardia, hypotension) should raise suspicion for systemic infection, including infection with obstructing ureteral stone.

TABLE 42-1.
DIFFERENTIAL DIAGNOSIS OF UTIs AND PYELONEPHRITIS

Kidney stone	PID
STD	Other pelvic pathology (cyst, torsion)
Appendicitis	Prostatitis
Epididymitis	Testicular torsion

DIFFERENTIAL DIAGNOSIS

▶ See Table 42-1.

EMERGENCY DEPARTMENT MANAGEMENT

Diagnosis

▶ Symptomatic patients with frequency, dysuria, urgency, and suprapubic pain may be treated on the basis of presentation, but if there is question of diagnosis, obtain UA.

▶ Clean catch midstream UA
  • Epithelial cells indicate contamination and require repeat specimen (consider catheterized specimen).
  • Leukocyte esterase has sensitivity of 75–96% and specificity of 94–98%.
  • Nitrite test is specific (92–100%), but not sensitive (40–85%).
  • In combination, these tests detect about 80% of specimens with $\geq 10^5$ colony-forming units.
  • Pyuria common with UTI, > 10 WBC/hpf.
  • Hematuria may be seen with UTI, microscopic or gross in association with pyuria.
  • Bacteruria alone requires treatment in pregnancy.

▶ Pyelonephritis has associated flank pain, fever, nausea, and vomiting with associated cystitis symptoms.

▶ Send urine culture in men, obstruction, pregnancy, upper tract infection, treatment failure, immunocompromised, and recent instrumentation.

▶ Imaging tests in patients with suspected ureteral stone or sepsis include non-contrast CT scan or ultrasound to evaluate for fluid collection or hydronephrosis.

Treatment

▶ Asymptomatic bacteruria in pregnancy
  • Ampicillin or cephalexin, 500 mg qid × 7–10 days
▶ Simple cystitis
  • SMX-TMP DS bid × 3 days
  • Nitrofurantoin macrocrystals, 100 mg qid × 3 days
  • Ciprofloxacin, 250 mg bid × 3 days
        plus
  • Pyridium, 100–200 mg tid × 3 days, for symptom control
▶ Pyelonephritis
  • Ciprofloxacin, 500 mg bid × 10 days
  • SMX-TMP DS bid × 10 days
▶ Inpatient treatment
  • Ciprofloxacin, 400 mg IVPB q12h
        or
  • Gentamicin, 4–5 mg/kg
        plus
  • Ampicillin, 1–2 g IVPB q4–6h

Disposition

▶ Asymptomatic bacteruria in pregnancy may be treated as an outpatient with culture and follow-up.
▶ Simple cystitis treated as an outpatient with routine follow-up and no urine culture unless in high-risk group.
▶ Complicated or recurrent cystitis (> 3 episodes/year) may be treated as outpatient with close follow-up, urine culture, and possible urologic referral.
▶ Pyelonephritis without hemodynamic compromise and tolerating oral medications may be treated with oral antibiotics, urine culture, and primary care follow-up.
▶ Pyelonephritis with hemodynamic compromise, inability to take oral medications, immunocompromise, pregnancy, or urinary obstruction should be treated with IV antibiotics and admission.
▶ Urinary infection with obstructing kidney stone and systemic illness requires urologic consultation.

CHAPTER 43

ACUTE RENAL FAILURE

Colin F. Greineder

▶ Acute decline in renal function with resultant hemodynamic and metabolic derangements due to loss of homeostasis and accumulation of normally excreted waste products.

▶ Regularly cited figures are 50% reduction in GFR/creatinine clearance, or alternatively, 50% increase in serum creatinine over baseline.

PATHOPHYSIOLOGY

▶ ARF is exceedingly broad and is best broken up anatomically into pre-renal, intrinsic renal, and post-renal etiologies.

▶ Pre-renal failure (40–80%)
  • Hypovolemia (most common cause)
  • Cardiorenal syndrome (decreased cardiac output with poor renal perfusion)
  • Intravascular depletion (third spacing, decreased oncotic pressure)
  • Renovascular disease (atherosclerosis, fibromuscular dysplasia, embolic disease)

▶ Intrinsic (10–50%)
  • Glomerular disease [post-infectious, vasculitis, collagen vascular disease, primary glomerulonephritis (GN)]
  • Tubular disease (ischemic or nephrotoxic acute tubular necrosis, rhabdomyolysis, hemoglobinuria)
  • Interstitial disease (allergic interstitial nephritis, infiltrative, infectious)
  • Small-vessel vascular disease (TTP, HUS, malignant HTN)

▶ Post-renal (2–5%)
  • Ureteral disease (retroperitoneal tumor or fibrosis, stricture, trauma)
  • Bladder outlet and urethral disease (BPH, neurogenic bladder, trauma, cancer)

CLINICAL PRESENTATION

▶ History and physical should be directed toward distinguishing between pre-renal, intrinsic renal, and post-renal causes.

Pre-Renal Failure

▶ Poor PO intake, fluid losses (vomiting, diarrhea), or increased insensible losses (fever, tachypnea)
▶ Orthostasis or orthostatic hypotension
▶ History or symptoms of cardiac failure, cirrhosis, burns, pancreatitis, or other concomitant diseases leading to decreased renal blood flow

Intrinsic Renal Failure

▶ Recent pharyngeal or skin infection
▶ Recent period of hypotension
▶ Nephrotoxic (e.g., aminoglycoside) or acute interstitial nephritis (AIN)-inducing (e.g., methicillin) drug exposure
▶ Use of ACE inhibitor
▶ Recent radiocontrast study (2–3 days prior)
▶ Features of nephrotic (edema, hypoalbuminemia, hypercholesterolemia) or nephritic (HTN, hematuria, edema) syndromes
▶ Rhabdomyolysis or massive hemolysis (with hemoglobinuria)
▶ Rash, joint pain, history or FH of collagen vascular disease or vasculitis

Post-Renal Failure

▶ High-risk patients:
  • Elderly males, children with recurrent UTIs, females with history of gynecologic surgery, patients with metastatic cancer or history of pelvic irradiation, and patients with recent trauma

EMERGENCY DEPARTMENT MANAGEMENT
Diagnosis

▶ Mainly based on lab studies reflecting reduction in GFR.
▶ Most commonly utilized indicator is increase in P^{Cr}, although this is a surrogate marker of creatinine clearance.
▶ It is important to ask patients for their baseline creatinine or get old records to determine their baseline.

Ancillary Testing

▶ Microscopic UA
  - Normal urine sediment (i.e., no cells or casts) suggestive of pre- or post-renal etiologies.
  - Other findings may include red cell casts (suggestive of GN), eosinophils (suggestive of AIN), positive urine dip for blood but no red cells (consistent with myoglobinuria or hemoglobinuria), or granular casts (non-specific but suggestive of ATN).
    ○ FeNa

$$(U^{Na} / P^{Na}) / (U^{Cr} / P^{Cr}) \times 100$$

    ○ FeNa directly reflects tubular sodium handling and is useful in differentiating pre-renal (FeNa < 1%) from intrinsic (FeNa > 1%) failure.
  - Renal ultrasound
    ○ Has become preferred test for evaluation for post-renal obstruction and hydronephrosis, with sensitivity > 95%
  - CT scan
    ○ Non-contrast CT scan is widely used and has almost entirely replaced IVP in diagnosis of nephrolithiasis, given ~100% sensitivity for intra-renal or ureteral stones.
  - Renal biopsy
    ○ Generally indicated only once an intrinsic etiology of renal failure has been confirmed

Treatment

▶ Primary prevention
  - Recognizing patients at high risk for developing renal failure and avoiding iatrogenic insults (IV contrast) that may precipitate full ARF are the most important interventions that EM physicians can make.
  - Prevention of concomitant insult
    ○ Preventing additional insults in the patient with established ARF or CRF should be a priority.
    ○ Avoiding interventions that may worsen the patient's homeostatic imbalance (volume overload, possibly resulting in the need for emergent dialysis).

► Specific treatments
  • Treatment of ARF is generally supportive, with exception of those cases in which there is a readily identifiable reversible cause (generally pre- and post-renal etiologies).
► Supportive care and emergent dialysis
  • Main goal for the ED physician is to identify and correct potentially life-threatening derangements associated with renal failure.
    ○ Volume overload
    ○ Hyperkalemia
    ○ Metabolic acidosis
    ○ Uremia
  • When these derangements do not respond to standard treatment modalities or compromise patient stability, emergent dialysis is required.

Disposition

► Patients with ARF are admitted to the hospital.
► Early nephrology notification or consultation for possible emergent dialysis.
► Appropriate site of admission may vary between telemetry or ICU depending on concomitant disease processes and severity of secondary derangements (e.g., hyperkalemia or severe acidosis).

CHAPTER 44

COMMON COMPLICATIONS OF CHRONIC RENAL FAILURE

Neal Chawla

HEMODIALYSIS
Arteriovenous Fistula/Graft Complications

► Fistula should be treated with great care to avoid infection, bleeding, thrombosis.
► BP cuffs and tourniquets should not be applied to arm with fistula.
► Avoid using fistula or graft for blood draws unless absolutely necessary.

Stenosis and Thrombosis
► Most common problem.
► Grafts have higher rate of stenosis than fistulas.
► Loss of bruit and thrill.
► Consult a vascular surgeon, as these often need surgical revision.
► Can often be treated within 24 hours by angiographic clot removal (80% effective), angioplasty (80% effective but 55–70% re-stenose in a year), or thrombolysis (90% effective).

Infection
► Grafts have higher incidence of infection than fistulas.
► Can present with sepsis: fever, hypotension, elevated white count.
► Most common: *Staphylococcus aureus.*
► Usually require admission.
► Vancomycin, 1 g IV, is drug of choice for coverage and long half-life (5–7 days) in dialysis patients.
  • Cefazolin may be needed for VRE.
► Gentamicin or aztreonam usually added to cover against gram-negatives.

Hemorrhage

▶ Can be from aneurysm, anastomosis rupture, or over-anticoagulation.

▶ Start with digital pressure for 5–10 minutes and observe 1–2 hours.

▶ Continued bleeding may require a tourniquet.

▶ Consult vascular surgeon if bleeding cannot be controlled.

▶ If concern for over-anticoagulation with heparin, can give protamine.

• Protamine, 0.01 mg/IU heparin, given during dialysis

• Protamine, 10–20 mg, if unknown amount of heparin given

Vascular Insufficiency

▶ Steal syndrome where blood shunted from nutrient arteries instead to venous side of access

▶ Presents with exercise pain, non-healing ulcers, and cool, pulseless digits

▶ Diagnosis by Doppler or angiography

▶ Requires surgical repair

Complications during Hemodialysis

Hypotension

▶ Most frequent complication, 10–30%.

▶ Most common cause is excessive ultrafiltration and resulting decreased circulating volume and impaired compensation.

▶ Consider pericardial or cardiac disease, volume status, infection, GI bleed.

▶ Treat with stopping hemodialysis (HD) and placing patient in Trendelenburg position.

▶ Treatment includes small fluid boluses if unresponsive; may require further work-up for possible cause.

Dialysis Disequilibrium

▶ Signs and symptoms: nausea, vomiting, HTN at the end of dialysis

▶ Can progress to seizure, coma, death

▶ Believed to be due to large fluid shifts leading to cerebral edema

▶ Usually resolves over a few hours as fluids redistribute

▶ Can be managed with mannitol or hypertonic saline

▶ Diagnosis of exclusion; first consider more emergent causes

Air Embolism
▶ Can cause pulmonary, cerebral, or arterial symptoms.
▶ Traditionally, place in left side down and Trendelenburg to trap air in right ventricle or hyperbaric chamber.

Peritonitis
▶ Most common complication of peritoneal dialysis (PD).
▶ Patients on average experience one episode every 15 months.
▶ Mortality 2.5–12.5%.
▶ Signs include fever, abdominal pain, and rebound tenderness.
▶ Cloudy peritoneal fluid and abdominal pain strongly suggest peritonitis.
▶ Dialysate fluid should be sent for cell count and differential, Gram's stain, and culture.
  • 100 WBC with > 50% neutrophils suggests peritonitis.
▶ Mostly *Staphylococcus* or *Streptococcus* species but can be gram-negatives, anaerobic, or fungi.
▶ Treatment:
  • Begin with a few rapid exchanges.
  • Add heparin to decrease fibrin clot formation.
  • Antibiotics can be given into dialysate.
    ○ Vancomycin and either a cephalosporin, aminoglycoside, or aztreonam for gram-negative coverage.
  • Treatment usually for total of 10–14 days.
  • Decision to admit is usually clinical; many treated as outpatient.
  • If patient takes insulin by intra-peritoneal route, dose may have to be transiently increased for a few days.
▶ If antibiotic therapy is failing or patient experiences many episodes of peritonitis, Tenckhoff catheter may need to be removed.

Catheter Site Infections
▶ Usually around a PD catheter entrance/exit site.
▶ Commonly *Staphylococcus* or *Pseudomonas*.
▶ Can use first-generation cephalosporin or fluoroquinolone.
▶ Instruct patients to keep site clean with iodine or peroxide.

Hernias
▶ Abdominal wall hernias estimated in 10–15% of patients.

► Dialysis patients at increased risk due to chronically increased intra-abdominal pressures.

► Treatment is immediate repair due to high risk of incarceration.

LAB ABNORMALITIES IN RENAL FAILURE

► Cardiac markers may be falsely elevated (myoglobin and troponin).

• Serial cardiac enzymes are recommended with increasing markers consistent with MI.

► Pancreatic enzymes can be elevated up to 3 times the normal.

► Metabolic acidosis:

• Can be due to decreased acid excretion, namely, ammonium.

• Bicarbonate buffers this, and as a result, can be decreased to 12–20 mEq/L.

• Many advocate giving bicarbonate, or alternatively, adding bicarbonate in dialysate.

► Hyperkalemia:

• CHF patients often tolerate slightly higher levels of potassium and do not get ECG changes until later.

• However, potassium can rise rapidly in patients with renal failure.

• Dialysis is the treatment of choice for hyperkalemia in CHF but may temporize with insulin/glucose, Kayexalate, and calcium (see Chap. 171 for dosing).

CHAPTER 45

NEPHROLITHIASIS

Neal Chawla

▶ 12% of general population, males > females.
▶ Most commonly occurs in those aged 30s–50s.
▶ One-third have recurrence within a year, one-half within 5 years.

PATHOPHYSIOLOGY

▶ 75% are either calcium oxalate or calcium phosphate.
- Increased calcium intake and hyperparathyroidism can predispose.
▶ 15% are magnesium-ammonium-struvite (phosphate).
- Usually result of recurrent UTI (proteus)
▶ 10% are uric acid stones.
- Increased risk in patients with gout
▶ 1% are cysteine, caused by an inborn metabolic error.
▶ Most common sites for obstruction are
- Renal calyx
- Ureteropelvic junction
- Ureterovesical junction, which has the smallest diameter
▶ < 5 mm stones have 90% chance of passing within 4 weeks.
▶ 5–8 mm stones have 15% chance of passing.
▶ > 8 mm stones have 5% chance of passing.

CLINICAL PRESENTATION

▶ Patients usually describe acute onset of severe unilateral flank pain that radiates anteroinferiorly around abdomen.
▶ May be associated with nausea, vomiting, diaphoresis.
▶ Patient is often unable to find a comfortable position and has a hard time lying still.
▶ Gross hematuria present in up to one-third of patients.
▶ History of fever and chills is concerning for infected stone.

▶ If peritoneal signs exist or there is significant abdominal tenderness, another etiology of abdominal pain must be pursued.

▶ CVA tenderness is common, but consider pyelonephritis if patient has a fever.

▶ Look for rash to exclude herpes zoster and consider pelvic exam in females when diagnosis is uncertain.

EMERGENCY DEPARTMENT MANAGEMENT
Diagnosis
Urinalysis

▶ 85% have hematuria; therefore, a negative UA does not exclude diagnosis of urinary calculi.

▶ A few WBCs are common, but if > 5 WBCs, consider possibility that urine is infected and send culture.

Lab Studies

▶ CBC not usually required unless concerned for infection or anemia.

▶ BUN/creatinine if patient at risk for nephrotoxicity or if planning a contrast study.

▶ Uric acid, calcium, and phosphorus levels may suggest type of stone, but do not need to be done emergently.

▶ Pregnancy test should be sent on all women of childbearing age.

Imaging

▶ Indications: no prior history of stone, diagnosis is unclear, concern for infection, patients > 50 years old when there is concern for AAA, persistent pain.

▶ May be deferred in young, healthy patients with a classic presentation and prior history of nephrolithiasis.

▶ IVP has been traditionally the gold standard; however, in many institutions, it is being replaced by non-contrast helical CT.

▶ Ultrasound is preferred in pregnant patients.

▶ Non-contrast helical CT
  • 95–97% sensitive and 96–98% specific.
  • Secondary signs can also be picked up: ureteral dilatation, perinephric fat stranding, and renal enlargement.
  • Advantages: no contrast needed, rapid, may pick up other disease processes, and can detect AAAs, but not 100%.

- Disadvantages: does not evaluate renal function or provide details about degree of obstruction, and higher cost than most other studies.

▶ IVP
- 64–90% sensitive, 94–100% specific.
- Can provide information about renal function and anatomic morphology.
- After IV contrast given, obtain scout film and then repeat at 5, 10, and 20 minutes.
- Location of stone can often be determined.
- Disadvantages
  - ◦ IV contrast risks nephrotoxicity and allergic reaction.
    - ■ Patients with renal insufficiency or diabetes have 9% chance of nephrotoxicity.
  - ◦ Time, especially if serial delayed images are required; this can take hours.

▶ Ultrasound
- 63–85% sensitive and 79–100% specific for detection of stones.
- 98% sensitive and 100% specific for hydronephrosis, which may be due to stones.
- Advantages are non-invasive, no IV dye or radiation, and no side effects.
- Helpful in patients who are pregnant or have a contrast dye allergy and are not candidates for CT or IVP.
- Stones < 5 mm are not easily detected.

▶ KUB X-ray
- 29–58% sensitive and 69–74% specific.
- 85% of stones are radiopaque, but they are usually very small and can be shadowed by bone and soft tissues.
- Greatest utility in assessing location of previously identified calculi.

Treatment

▶ Major goal is pain control.
- Do not delay pain control while waiting for test results.

▶ Use a combination of narcotics and NSAIDs.
- Ketorolac, 30 mg IV
- Morphine, 2–10 mg IV or
- Dilaudid, 1–2 mg IV

▶ Anti-emetics, if indicated.
▶ IVF hydration, but bolus fluids to flush out stone are **not** beneficial.
▶ If there is evidence of an infected stone, IV antibiotics and urology consult should be obtained.
▶ Preliminary studies show beneficial effects of CCBs, which are used to prevent ureterospasm.
  • Nifedipine (Procardia XL), 30 mg PO q day for 5–10 days

Disposition

▶ Indications for admission
  • Intractable pain or vomiting
  • Infection with obstruction or sepsis
  • Solitary kidney or transplanted kidney with obstruction
▶ Patients with irregular, proximal stones over 5–6 mm should be discussed with urology and, if discharged, have close follow-up.
▶ Safe to discharge patients with small stones, no evidence of infection, and adequate pain control.
▶ Discharge first-time calculi patients with urology follow-up, urinary strainer/container.
▶ Discharge with instructions for analgesia and maintaining hydration.

CHAPTER 46

TESTICULAR EMERGENCIES

Marquita N. Hicks

► A thorough history and physical can help distinguish most causes of scrotal swelling.
► The history should include the following:
  • Characteristics of pain and/or swelling
  • Associated signs and symptoms (nausea, vomiting, abdominal pain)
  • Recent trauma
  • Sexual activity
► Genital exam
  • Palpate testis, spermatic cord, and epididymis for tenderness, fluid, or subcutaneous emphysema.
  • Transillumination can distinguish between a fluid-filled cavity and a mass.

DIFFERENTIAL DIAGNOSIS FOR THE ACUTE SCROTUM

► See Table 46-1.

Testicular Torsion

► Testicular torsion is a urologic emergency.
  • Delay in diagnosis can result in loss of testicle.
► Occurs in two peak periods: first year of life and puberty, when testicles are rapidly changing in size

Pathophysiology

► Torsion results from the spermatic cord twisting, leading to ischemia.
► During torsion of the testis, obstruction of venous return occurs initially.
► As twisting persists, venous thrombosis is followed by arterial thrombosis.

TABLE 46-1.
DIFFERENTIAL DIAGNOSIS FOR THE ACUTE SCROTUM

Testicular torsion	Testicular neoplasm
Epididymitis	Hydrocele
Orchitis	Varicocele
Trauma	Scrotal abscess
Incarcerated hernia	Torsion of a testicular/epididymal appendage

▶ May be precipitated by trauma, sex, or exercise.

Clinical Presentation

▶ Classically presents with sudden onset of severe unilateral testicular pain.
  • May have referred pain to the abdomen, thigh, flank, or hip.
▶ Other symptoms include nausea and vomiting (20–30%), abdominal pain (20–30%), fever (16%), and urinary frequency (4%).
▶ The affected testicle appears high in the scrotum, has a transverse axis, and is tender to palpation.
▶ Swelling and edema of the affected skin.
▶ Absent cremasteric reflex (if reflex present, does not rule out torsion).

Management

▶ Emergent urologic consultation for surgical exploration, if strong clinical suspicion.
▶ UA and CBC are usually unremarkable.
▶ Diagnostic studies
  • Color Doppler ultrasound is the test of choice when diagnosis is in question.
    ○ Along with demonstration of arterial blood flow to the testicle, it can provide information about scrotal anatomy and other testicular disorders (epididymitis).
    ○ Sensitivity 86% and specificity 100% for torsion.
▶ If immediate surgical intervention is not available, manual detorsion (opening the book) of the testis should be attempted.
  • Manual detorsion successful in 30–70%.
▶ Testicular salvage is close to 100% if detorsion occurs within 6 hours of pain. However, it decreases to < 20% if delayed > 12 hours.

▶ Viability of the affected testicle after detorsion is assessed while contralateral orchiopexy is performed. If the testis is deemed viable, it is anchored to the scrotal wall.

Epididymitis

▶ Most common misdiagnosis for testicular torsion

Pathophysiology
▶ Usually results from the spread of infection from the urethra or bladder via retrograde ascent
  • Among sexually active men < 35 years old, most common cause is *Chlamydia trachomatis* or *Neisseria gonorrhoeae.*
  • Gram-negative organisms associated with UTIs occur more frequently in men age > 35 years old.
  • In the prepubertal male, commonly secondary to a viral infection or chemical irritation.
▶ Complications of untreated acute epididymitis include abscess, testicular infection, chronic pain, and infertility.

Clinical Presentation
▶ Typically presents with a gradual onset of pain during a period of hours to days.
▶ A history of UTI symptoms, such as dysuria, may precede the pain.
▶ Localized, tender epididymis at the superior aspect of the testicle.
  • The testicle is non-tender unless the infection is complicated by an epididymo-orchitis.
▶ A reactive hydrocele may be appreciated on transillumination.
▶ External urethral orifice should be inspected and the urethra milked for possible discharge.
▶ A cremasteric reflex is usually present.
▶ A prostate exam should be performed carefully, keeping in mind that the primary infection may be spread by a vigorous massage.

Management
▶ Lab evaluation
  • Clean catch UA and culture
    ○ UA may reveal evidence of infection.
  • Urethral swab or urine PCR for gonorrhea and chlamydia
▶ Scrotal imaging
  • Doppler ultrasound reveals increased blood flow to the scrotum.

▶ Treatment is symptomatic relief of pain and treatment of suspected infection.
  • < 35 years old:
    ○ Ceftriaxone, 250 mg IM × 1 and
    ○ Azithromycin, 1 g PO × 1, or doxycycline, 100 mg PO × 7 days
  • Sexual partners should be referred for evaluation and treatment.
  • Avoid sexual intercourse until patient and his partners have completed their course of antibiotics and symptoms have resolved.
  • > 35 years old:
    ○ SMX-TMP (Bactrim DS), 1 tab PO bid × 14 days or
    ○ Ciprofloxacin, 500 mg PO bid × 14 days
  • However, if STD is likely, patients should be treated as if they have an STD.
  • Pre-pubertal patients should be given antibiotics against gram-negative bacilli and *Pseudomonas*.
  • Other symptomatic treatments include bed rest, scrotal support, analgesics, and ice packs.
▶ Follow-up with a urologist should also be arranged, especially in the pre-pubertal male.
  • Return to the ED or follow up with the urologist if symptoms do not improve within 3 days.
▶ Swelling or tenderness may persist for up to 8 weeks after completion of antibiotic therapy.

Orchitis

▶ Orchitis is an acute infection of the testis.

Pathophysiology
▶ Etiology may be viral, bacterial, or mycobacterial pathogens.
  • The most common bacterial pathogens are *Escherichia coli*, *Klebsiella*, and *Pseudomonas*.
  • Viral etiology is most commonly associated with mumps or enteroviral infection.
  • Granulomatous orchitis occurs most often in immunocompromised host associated with syphilis, mycobacterial, and fungal disease.
▶ Rare without a preceding epididymitis.

Clinical Presentation

▶ Viral orchitis typically presents with testicular pain and swelling approximately 5 days after parotitis and onset of testicular symptoms.

▶ If the orchitis is pyogenic, the patient may present with a toxic appearance.

▶ Exam may reveal a reactive hydrocele and/or a swollen, tender testis associated with an epididymitis.

Management

▶ Lab studies:
  • UA and culture
  • Blood cultures if toxic appearing
▶ Scrotal imaging:
  • Color ultrasonography
▶ Treatment of orchitis is typically supportive.
  • Ice packs, analgesics, bed rest, and scrotal elevation.
  • Antibiotic therapy: If bacterial orchitis is suspected, cover with same antibiotics as epididymitis.
▶ Treatment of pyogenic orchitis should be considered in any high-risk or immunocompromised patient and started on antibiotics with emergent urologic consultation.

CHAPTER 47

PRIAPISM

Marquita N. Hicks

▶ Prolonged engorgement or erection of the penis that persists beyond or is unrelated to sexual stimulation.

▶ Priapism is a true urologic emergency, with the goal of therapy being detumescence in under 12 hours from time of onset of symptoms.

▶ Biphasic peaks of incidence between 5 and 10 years and between 20 and 50 years but can occur at any age.

▶ Risk factors:

• History of psychogenic or neurogenic erectile dysfunction.

• Hematologic disorders such as sickle cell anemia (10–63% of cases with increased prevalence in pediatric population) and leukemia.

• Perineal trauma (12%).

• Many medications (approximately 20% of cases); most commonly those producing alpha-adrenergic blockade or serotonergic receptor stimulation.

  ○ Many antidepressants, antipsychotics, hydroxyzine, prazosin, anticoagulants, oral and injectable medications for pre-existing erectile dysfunction, cocaine, and alcohol

• More than one-third of cases are idiopathic.

PATHOPHYSIOLOGY

▶ Classified into two types: low-flow (ischemic or veno-occlusive) and high-flow (arterial or non-ischemic) priapism.

▶ High-flow priapism results when blood inflow is increased beyond capacity of venous outflow system.

• Result of perineal trauma, such as a straddle injury. Cavernous artery is injured by compression against the pubic bone, resulting in uncontrolled blood inflow to the penis.

• May present on a delayed basis from the original injury.

▶ Low-flow priapism results from venous outflow obstruction (most common).
  • Impaired venous drainage from medication side effects, sludging due to sickled red cells, hyperviscosity syndromes, or mass effect.
  • This is a compartment syndrome that results in progressive tissue ischemia and ultimately irreversible damage beginning after 12 hours.

CLINICAL PRESENTATION

▶ High-flow priapism
  • Semi-rigid penis that may be described as a persistent morning erection
  • Little or no associated pain
  • History of perineal or penile trauma
  • May have history of recent sexual activity without detumescence
▶ Low-flow priapism
  • Rigidly erect penis with tense corpora cavernosa but with soft glans.
  • Intense pain.
  • History frequently reveals risk factors, although up to one-third of cases are idiopathic.

DIFFERENTIAL DIAGNOSIS

▶ Normal penile erection from sexual arousal
▶ Urethral FB
▶ Peyronie's disease
▶ Erection due to spinal cord injury
▶ Penile implants

EMERGENCY DEPARTMENT MANAGEMENT
Diagnosis

▶ Clinical diagnosis based on history and physical exam.
▶ Penile blood gases may help to discriminate type if clinically uncertain.
  • Low-flow: low pH, low O_2, high CO_2

- High-flow: normal pH, high O_2, low CO_2
  - In high-flow priapism, penile Doppler ultrasound should be performed to demonstrate arterial injury and/or arterial fistula.

Treatment

▶ High-flow priapism
  - Observation and pain management
  - Urologic consultation
▶ Low-flow priapism: urologic emergency that necessitates immediate therapy and early consultation
  - Hydration, pain control (consider parenteral routes and dorsal penile block), relief of urinary obstruction
  - Treatment
    - Cavernosal aspiration and irrigation.
    - Parenteral vasodilators such as terbutaline, 0.25–0.50 mg IV every 4 hours.
    - Intracavernosal injection of alpha agonists such as phenylephrine in repeated doses of 0.1 ml/minute of a 500 mcg/ml phenylephrine solution for a total infused dose of 1 mg.
    - Priapism persisting for longer than 24 hours in an individual with sickle cell anemia despite treatment with O_2, hydration, and analgesics is an indication for an exchange transfusion.
    - Surgical shunt if pharmacologic measures fail.

CHAPTER 48

APPROACH TO ALTERED MENTAL STATUS

Sara Chakel

► **Altered mental status** includes a variety of symptoms, including impairment of level of consciousness (coma, stupor, obtundation, lethargy) or impaired cognition (confusion, agitation, psychosis, memory loss).

► Life-threatening processes, including hemodynamic instability, often present as an altered mental status. Assess vital signs early and often.

► Diminished level of consciousness indicates global pathology affecting the entire ascending reticular activating system or both cerebral hemispheres.

► Impaired cognition may be caused by either focal or global pathology.

DIFFERENTIAL DIAGNOSIS

► **Traumatic** (usually sudden in onset)
  • Focal injuries such as cerebral contusion/SAH, subdural or epidural hematoma
  • Global injuries such as diffuse axonal injury or generalized brain edema with raised ICP

► **Vascular** (usually sudden in onset)
  • Focal events such as ischemic stroke; hypertensive, vasculopathic, or coagulopathic intracranial hematoma; or SAH
  • Global events such as global cerebral ischemia, from hypoperfusion or hypoxemia

► **Infectious** (usually rapid to gradual in onset)
  • Focal processes such as brain abscess, septic emboli, subdural empyema, or focal encephalitis
  • Global processes such as meningitis, diffuse encephalitis, or sepsis

▶ **Toxic** (usually rapid to gradual in onset)
- Rarely focal presentations such as extrapyramidal effects or dystonia from neuroleptics
- Usually global symptoms such as diminished level of consciousness from sedative/hypnotics; agitation from sympathomimetics; confusion from alcohols, salicylates, or anticholinergics; or other adverse effects of psychiatric medications. Also from withdrawal states (alcohol, opioids, benzodiazepines)

▶ **Environmental** (usually rapid to gradual in onset)
- Hyperthermia or hypothermia can result from exposure to extreme conditions alone or in combination with extreme exertion (as in athletes), poor innate compensatory mechanisms (such as occur in the very young and the elderly), or use of medications that impair temperature regulation (such as anticholinergics).

▶ **Metabolic** (variable onset from rapid to prolonged)
- A broad category usually with global symptoms from endocrine disorders (diabetic ketoacidosis, hyperosmolar hyperglycemic non-ketotic coma, hypoglycemia, hyper- or hypothyroidism, adrenal insufficiency), organ failure (uremia, liver failure/hyperammonemia), electrolyte abnormalities (especially hyponatremia), hereditary disorders (such as porphyria), or nutritional deficiencies (Wernicke's encephalopathy)

▶ **Neoplastic** (usually gradual to insidious in onset)
- Focal presentation from local mass effect and cerebral compression
- Global presentation from diffuse edema, hydrocephalus, or paraneoplastic syndrome

▶ **Neuropsychiatric** (variable onset from sudden to prolonged)
- Focal presentations from partial seizures or Todd's phenomenon, or atypical migraines
- Global presentations such as generalized seizures, post-ictal states, neurodegenerative disorders, or primary mental illnesses such as depression, mania, or other psychosis

EMERGENCY DEPARTMENT MANAGEMENT

▶ Primary survey
- Assess vital signs. Ensure ABCs. Provide C-spine stabilization if traumatic cause of altered mental status is suspected.

► Consider the "coma cocktail"
  • Treatments that can safely be given empirically for suspected conditions prior to diagnostic confirmation
    ○ O_2, given in all, but not helpful unless patient is hypoxic.
    ○ **Thiamine, 100 mg IV,** prior to glucose in suspected thiamine deficiency (malnourished elderly or alcoholic patients) to treat or prevent Wernicke's encephalopathy.
    ○ **Dextrose (50%), 50 cc IV,** for hypoglycemia.
    ○ **Naloxone, 0.4–2.0 mg IV,** for suspected opiate intoxication with hypoventilation. Continued observation required after reversal because half-life of naloxone is generally shorter than the intoxicant.
    ○ Flumazenil should *not* be considered part of the coma cocktail, as it is contraindicated in habitual benzodiazepine users or patients with possible polysubstance overdose, and can precipitate status epilepticus.
► Key elements of the history
  • History is usually important to the diagnosis, but patients with altered mental status are, by definition, limited historians.
    ○ If patients are brought by EMS, do not let crew depart until a careful report has been obtained.
    ○ Obtain from patient, family members, caregivers, and past medical records. Use all resources available to obtain this history.
    ○ Onset of symptoms gradual or abrupt? Constant, progressive, or fluctuating?
    ○ Known recent trauma, environmental, or drug exposure or other ingestion?
    ○ Associated symptoms such as headache, seizure, dizziness, diplopia, or vomiting?
    ○ Past medical history including baseline mental status, previous similar symptoms, and possible precipitating illnesses such as diabetes, HTN, thyroid disease, psychiatric problems, or immunosuppression.
    ○ Prescription, over-the-counter, and herbal medications (especially those that are psychoactive) including compliance and recent changes in dosage or use.
    ○ Social history, including drug or alcohol abuse, and HIV risk factors.

▶ Physical exam
- A careful head-to-toe exam is important. Be complete, but check the following in particular.
- Vital signs are crucial. Hemodynamic instability can indicate cerebral hypoperfusion. Tachycardia or hypoventilation can suggest specific toxidromes. Abnormal temperatures (high or low) can suggest infection, environmental exposures, or metabolic pathology.
- Level of consciousness: several nomenclatures and scores available.
  - AVPU: *a*lert, responds to *v*oice, responds to *p*ain, *u*nresponsive.
  - GCS: a scale from 3 (worst) to 15 (best); the sum of three scores given for best eye opening, verbal response, and motor response (see Chap. 78).
  - Colloquial terms are imprecise and are applied variably, but one interpretation is: coma (unresponsive to any stimulus), stupor (some response to vigorous stimulus), obtundation (decreased alertness with some response to voice or touch), lethargy (arousal diminished but maintained spontaneously).
- Orientation and cognition: easy to misjudge if systematic approach is not used. Best evaluated by the formal Mini-Mental Status examination or some abbreviated version (Table 48-1). In general, confusion with disorientation suggests delirium rather than psychosis.
- Trauma: Look for signs of traumatic injury, including scalp hematoma, and signs of basilar skull fracture (hemotympanum, periorbital ecchymosis, and postauricular ecchymosis, i.e., Battle's sign).
- Eye exam: Check pupillary size and reactivity (dilated or pinpoint pupils can suggest toxins or pontine hemorrhage, asymmetric blown pupil can be a sign of impending uncal herniation, and bilateral fixed pupils can suggest diffuse brain injury). In alert patients, check extraocular movements for gaze palsy or deviation. In comatose patients, look for doll's eyes (brainstem reflex moving eyes away from direction of sideways rotation of the head) or perform caloric testing of vestibulo-ocular reflex (nystagmus resulting from unilateral irrigation with warm or cold water, cold causes

TABLE 48-1.
A QUICK MENTAL STATUS EXAM

Orientation	"What is today's date? Where are you?" Ask the patient to be as specific as possible.
Attention	"Spell the word WORLD, and then spell it backwards" or "What is 100 minus 7? What is 7 from that? What is 7 from that?"
Short-term memory	"Remember three words (tree, orange, honesty)." Ask patient to recall at end of exam.
Abstraction	"What does 'don't count your chickens before they are hatched' mean to you?"
Visuospatial	Draw a circle. Have the patient draw numbers on the circle like the face of a clock.

beating to opposite side, warm to same side). Absence of brainstem reflexes in comatose patients suggests brain death.

- Oropharynx and skin: Dry mucus membranes can indicate anticholinergics or dehydration. Look for rashes indicative of infections (like meningococcemia) or drug reactions (like serotonin syndrome).

- Musculoskeletal and vascular exam: Check neck for meningismus, arms and legs for stiffness and clonus. Asymmetrical pulses can suggest dissection.

- Complete neurologic exam: Obviously, in addition to the findings mentioned, the most complete exam with which the patient will cooperate must be performed of the cranial nerves, vision, speech, language, motor strength, sensation, cerebellar function, and gait. Examine for extinction: Focal deficits can be subtle but revealing. Multifocal deficits suggest embolic disease.

▶ **Lab tests** are rarely diagnostic in altered mental status, but as in the physical exam, a broad net is often warranted.

- Basic metabolic panel can show hyponatremia, uremia, or suggest anion-gap acidosis (alcohols, salicylates, and ketoacidosis can cause altered mental status).

- CBC with platelets can show critical anemia. Leukocytosis is neither sensitive nor specific for infection.

- Hepatic causes of mental status changes may be associated with changes in liver enzymes or ammonia levels.

- UA and urine culture may help identify otherwise occult infections, especially in the elderly or disabled.

- LP is usually diagnostic for CNS infections and SAH. If the patient has mental status changes, a head CT is warranted prior to LP.
- Other potentially useful tests include TSH, carboxyhemoglobin level, and tests for other specific toxins such as ethanol or salicylates. The value of screening urine or serum for drugs of abuse is less clear and should be driven by clinical suspicion.

▶ **Medical imaging tests**
- Brain CT performed without contrast is the preferred initial imaging test for patients with traumatic injury, focal neurologic findings, or signs of increased ICP. Contrast CT is more sensitive for early or subtle neoplastic disease.
- Advanced brain imaging such as MRI is rarely needed in the ED evaluation of altered mental status but can be useful in selected patients suspected to have encephalitis, intracranial venous thrombosis, or certain ischemic stroke syndromes.
- CXR may identify otherwise occult infection causing altered mental status in the elderly or disabled.

▶ **Electrophysiologic studies**
- ECG can suggest arrhythmia as the source of embolic disease, cardiogenic causes of hypoperfusion, or certain toxic ingestions.
- EEG is the only way to identify non-convulsive status epilepticus when suspected in otherwise unexplained coma, especially in patients with known seizures.

TREATMENT AND DISPOSITION

▶ Further disease-specific treatment and consultation based upon findings in the initial diagnostic evaluation
▶ Disposition
- Admission: Patients with persistent mental status changes require admission for further diagnosis and treatment and frequent neurologic re-evaluation.
  ○ Initiate appropriate treatment and consultation in the ED.
  ○ Hemodynamic monitoring for high-risk patients or those with unstable vital signs.
  ○ Intensive care for patients with unstable neurologic exam.
- Discharge: Patients with reversible known etiology who have returned to baseline mental status (e.g., those with ethanol intoxication) can be safely discharged.

CHAPTER 49

APPROACH TO HEADACHE

Christopher R. Schmelzer and Christopher R. H. Newton

▶ Common presentation with very broad differential diagnosis.
▶ Goal of ED care is to exclude potentially life-threatening causes while alleviating symptoms.

DIFFERENTIAL DIAGNOSIS
▶ **Subarachnoid hemorrhage (SAH)**
  • Classic presentation is sudden onset of severe headache (i.e., thunderclap headache). Presentation can be global, although often described as occipitonuchal and may include an element of nuchal rigidity (70%).
  • Neurologic exam may include focal findings, however, is usually normal.
▶ **Meningitis**
  • Classic presentation of fever, headache, and stiff neck. Bacterial etiology is often rapidly progressive, with deteriorating mental status and evolving neurologic findings. Viral meningitis typically presents with more indolent course and less impressive findings.
▶ **Temporal arteritis**
  • Should be considered in all patients over the age of 50 (F > M). Classically a dull, aching temporal pain that may include jaw claudication, temporal tenderness and unilateral blindness
▶ **Migraine**
  • Recurrent headache of vascular origin. Common presentation is of unilateral headache that may also be associated with nausea, vomiting, photo- and phonophobia. Patient may also present with visual phenomena including flashing lights and zigzag lines. Complex or basilar migraines may present with transient focal neurologic deficits.

▶ **Cluster**
  • Rare, classically presenting as ice pick or "hot poker in eye." Most patients describe unilateral severe headache, with rapid onset lasting a mean of 45 minutes. Attacks occur several times daily for days to weeks followed by remission. Often with associated autonomic findings on the ipsilateral side including rhinorrhea, ptosis, and lacrimation.

▶ **Trigeminal neuralgia**
  • Paroxysms of pain in the distribution of the trigeminal nerve, most commonly the maxillary and mandibular divisions. Most commonly seen in the age range of 50–70. Pain episodes are commonly triggered by touch, chewing, or temperature change. A diagnosis of exclusion, and exam must rule out other causes of facial pain including otitis, glaucoma, and herpes zoster.

▶ Other causes to consider include
  • Acute angle glaucoma, brain tumor, abscess, subdural hematoma, vertebral dissection, pseudotumor cerebri, cerebral venous thrombosis, post LP, and headache secondary to HTN.

EMERGENCY DEPARTMENT MANAGEMENT
Diagnosis

▶ Detailed history and exam are often all that is needed for diagnosis in the ED.

▶ Concerning features that warrant testing and further work-up include
  • Sudden onset or worst headache of life
  • Fever and/or immunocompromised patient
  • Focal neurologic findings (although these may be part of complex migraine, must be assumed to be abnormal especially if first presentation)
  • Patients > 65 years old or history of cancer
  • Any history of trauma—particularly if using anticoagulants
  • Visual loss
  • Altered level of consciousness

▶ **Lab:**
  • ESR in patients > 60 years old (usually > 50 mm/hour, often > 100 mm/hour)

- • PT, PTT if patient is on Coumadin
- • CBC, blood cultures if considering meningitis
- ▶ **Head CT:** for trauma, mental status changes, focal neurologic deficits, worst headache of life, history of cancer, or immunocompromised. MRA may also be needed in equivocal LP for the evaluation of SAH.
- ▶ **LP:** diagnostic for meningitis and also SAH. Remember to measure opening pressure to exclude pseudotumor cerebri (normally < 20 cm).

Treatment

- ▶ Prochlorperazine, 10 mg IV, or other antiemetic.
- ▶ Hydration with NS.
- ▶ Consider opiates if unresponsive to initial therapy.
  - • Morphine sulphate, 2–10 mg IV
  - • Dilaudid, 1–2 mg IV
- ▶ Cluster headaches: 100% O_2, antiemetics, hydration.
- ▶ Temporal arteritis: admit for IV steroids.
- ▶ Meningitis: IV antibiotics and admission if suspect bacterial etiology.
- ▶ SAH: Surgical vs. endovascular approach depends on site and also neurosurgical expertise.

Disposition

- ▶ Vast majority of headache patients can be discharged to home after symptomatic treatment and exclusion of life-threatening pathology.

◑ PEARLS
- • A normal neurologic exam does not exclude life-threatening pathology.
- • Always measure visual acuity and IOP in patients with visual changes and a headache. Always consider glaucoma even in patients without visual changes.
- • A normal head CT does not exclude SAH—it should always be followed by an LP.
- • Only 12% of thunderclap headaches turn out to be SAH.

CHAPTER 50

APPROACH TO SEIZURES

Manya Faith Newton

▶ Seizures are the clinical manifestations of abnormal, synchronous, and sustained firing of a population of cortical neurons.

▶ Although convulsions are most common, the physical manifestation of a seizure depends on the area of brain cortex involved.

▶ 10% of the population will have at least one seizure in their lifetime.

▶ 1% of people have epilepsy (recurrent seizures).

PATHOPHYSIOLOGY

▶ Primary epilepsy is genetic or idiopathic in origin. All other causes are considered reactive or secondary.

▶ Electrolyte derangement (including hypoglycemia, hyponatremia, hypernatremia).

▶ Infectious (usually meningitis or encephalitis).

▶ Toxicologic (commonly alcohol or benzodiazepine withdrawal, but many other drugs can cause seizures).

▶ Trauma. (Most post-traumatic seizures occur within 24 hours and are benign in minor brain injury. Onset of seizure after 1 week is associated with recurrent seizures.)

▶ Neurodegenerative.

▶ Stroke.

▶ Brain tumors.

▶ Endocrine and metabolic.

▶ Pregnancy.

CLINICAL PRESENTATION

▶ Seizures are classified based upon their physical or EEG manifestations.

• Generalized seizures have initial activation of neurons throughout both cerebral hemispheres. These include tonic-clonic, absence, atonic, or myoclonic seizures.

- Partial (also called focal) seizures have initial activation of a limited population of neurons in part of one hemisphere. Partial seizures can be simple or complex. Simple indicates preservation of consciousness, and complex indicates altered consciousness.

▶ Generalized convulsive (tonic-clonic or grand mal) seizures.
  - Seizure is characterized by LOC and convulsions (stiffening, a muscular hypertonic state, then usually rhythmic, violent contractions of multiple, bilateral, symmetric muscle groups).
  - Post-ictal state is characterized by coma gradually replaced by confusion and drowsiness. Todd's paralysis is a transient, self-limited focal paralysis or hemiparesis mimicking stroke. Post-ictal symptoms usually improve within minutes or hours but may occasionally be prolonged.

▶ Absence (petit mal) seizures.
  - Cessation of normal activity followed by a non-convulsive dissociative state.
  - Classified as typical or atypical. Typical are sudden in onset, terminate abruptly, and rarely exceed 10 seconds in duration. Atypical generally exceed 10 seconds, are more gradual in onset and recovery, and have less marked alterations in consciousness.
  - Usually without any aura or post-ictal symptoms.

▶ Atonic seizures (drop attacks).
  - Sudden loss of muscle tone in multiple postural muscle groups.
  - Consciousness is usually impaired, although recovery is rapid.
  - May be preceded by myoclonic jerks or accompanied by tonic episodes, but other post-ictal symptoms are absent.

▶ Myoclonic seizures.
  - Single or repetitive, symmetrical, rapid, and forceful muscle contractions. Often involve only the face and shoulder but may also involve the trunk and distal extremities. No LOC.

▶ Simple partial (focal) seizures.
  - Seizures most typically are ipsilateral focal clonic movements but may also manifest as sensory auras (visual, auditory, olfactory, somatosensory, or gustatory), autonomic phenomena (sweating and flushing, pupillary dilatation), or cognitive symptoms (déjà vu, hallucinations).
  - Consciousness is retained.

- May progress to generalized seizure as neurons are recruited to aberrant activity.
- Not followed by post-ictal symptoms.
► Complex partial.
  - Seizures typically begin with a motionless stare or arrest of activity followed by automatisms, gestures, eye movements, or speech disturbances. Consciousness is always altered.
  - Higher cortical functions are often preserved, including the ability to continue rote tasks, drive an automobile, or play a musical instrument.
  - Post-ictal symptoms may occur.
► Secondary manifestations and complications.
  - Seizures may cause shoulder dislocation or fractures resulting from forceful convulsions, tongue biting, or other traumatic injuries resulting from falling.
  - Skeletal muscle pain or injury (including lactic acidosis and rhabdomyolysis) may result from prolonged convulsions.
  - Aspiration during a seizure may cause pneumonitis.
  - Convulsions may cause hyperthermia, which may mimic fever.

EMERGENCY DEPARTMENT MANAGEMENT OF STATUS EPILEPTICUS

► Status epilepticus is generalized tonic-clonic seizure activity that is continuous, or involves serial seizures with no return to baseline between seizures.
► ABC. Obtain reliable venous access. Intubate if necessary. Realize that paralytics will stop convulsions but will not break the seizure. Avoid long-lasting paralytics that will mask further seizure by preventing convulsions. Patients who inadvertently get long-lasting paralytics, or require them to assist ventilation, require emergent EEG monitoring.
► Stop the seizure.
► First-line agents: benzodiazepines.
  - **Lorazepam (Ativan), 2–4 mg IV** (0.05 mg/kg in children), repeat after 10 minutes if not effective, or **diazepam (Valium), 5–10 mg IV** (0.2–0.5 mg/kg in children), repeat after 10 minutes if not effective.
  - Other routes, including rectal, ET, or intraosseous, can be used if venous access cannot be obtained.

- • If rapid titration is ineffective, add second-line agent.
- ▶ Second-line agents: anti-arrhythmics and barbiturates.
  - • Route: IV is the only route appropriate in status epilepticus.
  - • Agent: no clear evidence of superiority for any specific agent:
    - ○ **Phenytoin (Dilantin), 2 g IV** (10–20 mg/kg in children), infused at 50 mg/minute, or
    - ○ Fosphenytoin (Cerebyx), 2 g phenytoin equivalent IV (10–20 mg/kg in children), infused at 150 mg/minute (may also be given intramuscularly, but this is suboptimal in status), or
    - ○ **Phenobarbital, 1–2 g IV** (10–20 mg/kg in children), repeat in 15 minutes if needed.
  - • Other class IB anti-arrhythmics (like lidocaine) are as effective as phenytoin.
- ▶ Etiology-specific therapy: Provide concurrently with anticonvulsants.
  - • Dextrose, 1 amp D50W slow IVP for hypoglycemia
  - • Pyridoxine (vitamin B_6), 1–5 g IV (70 mg/kg maximum for children), for isoniazid (INH) overdose
  - • Magnesium, 4–6 g IV bolus, for eclampsia
- ▶ Other agents: Newer agents recently promoted for the treatment of seizures include valproate sodium (Depacon) and propofol (Diprivan). After ET intubation, refractory seizures may also be terminated with barbiturate coma or general inhalational anesthetics.
- ▶ Neurology consultation and admission are advisable.
- ▶ EEG monitoring is required for refractory seizures.

EMERGENCY DEPARTMENT MANAGEMENT OF NEW-ONSET SEIZURE

- ▶ The goal of the ED evaluation of a new-onset seizure is to search for a treatable precipitating event requiring specific therapy.
- ▶ An accurate and thorough history is critical. Obtain and document a description of the seizure if it was witnessed. Recent cessation of alcohol use? Other toxic ingestions or new medications? FH of epilepsy? Concurrent symptoms or illness? History of malignancy, comorbid conditions, or trauma?
- ▶ Examine the patient from head to toe. Check vital signs. Hemodynamic instability can suggest cerebral hypoperfusion or cer-

tain toxidromes. Document level of consciousness and mental status. Evaluate for traumatic injuries that may have precipitated or resulted from the seizure. Pupillary response can indicate toxins or intracranial abnormalities. Dry mucus membranes can suggest anticholinergics. Look for a meningococcal rash. Check the neck for meningismus. A complete neurologic exam of the cranial nerves, vision, speech, language, motor strength, sensation, cerebellar function, and gait is important to exclude any focal deficits.

▶ Brain CT scan is indicated in any patient with new-onset seizure and persistent or prolonged symptoms, recurrent episodes, traumatic injury, or focal neurologic deficits. LP is indicated in any patient whose presentation is consistent with meningitis, encephalitis, or SAH.

▶ Serum electrolytes, including a basic metabolic panel, calcium, and magnesium, are indicated in the evaluation of new-onset seizure. In suspect cases, tests for specific toxins such as ethanol or salicylates can be useful. The value of screening urine or serum for drugs of abuse is less clear and should be driven by clinical suspicion. CBC, osmolarity, liver enzymes, and other tests can also be used selectively.

▶ Admission is indicated in patients with status epilepticus, persistent or recurring neurologic abnormalities, or in whom an underlying condition requiring inpatient treatment is identified.

▶ Although practice styles vary, neurologic consultation in the ED and admission are generally not indicated in patients with a single isolated new-onset seizure without any persistent symptoms or deficits.

▶ Patients who can be safely discharged do not need to be started on antiepileptic medications but must be advised not to drive for 6 months, or until evaluated and cleared by a neurologist. Referral to a neurologist and consideration of an outpatient EEG are appropriate.

EMERGENCY DEPARTMENT MANAGEMENT OF BREAKTHROUGH SEIZURE

▶ Breakthrough seizures are common in many patients with primary epilepsy. The goal of the ED evaluation is to determine if the present episode was typical and to identify a possible precipitant for the breakthrough.

▶ If the patient's history does not suggest an event typical of the patient's breakthrough seizures, a broader evaluation is warranted. Typical events can have a focused evaluation.

▶ Sub-therapeutic levels of antiepileptic medications are a common cause of breakthrough seizures. Serum levels of phenytoin, phenobarbital, valproic acid, and carbamazepine can generally be obtained in the ED and can be used to confirm sub-therapeutic levels.

▶ Test blood glucose and basic electrolytes.

▶ Brain CT is not needed in the evaluation of breakthrough seizure unless complicated by prolonged symptoms or significant head trauma.

▶ Check for new medications with potential interactions with anticonvulsants.

▶ Check for changes in anticonvulsant dosing regimens.

▶ If anticonvulsant is being given as a suspension, make sure it is being shaken well before being given (unshaken bottles lead to inadequate doses when the bottle is new and toxic doses when the bottle is close to empty).

▶ Provide counseling if the breakthrough seizure is the result of non-compliant behaviors, such as missed medication or any form of substance abuse.

▶ Patients with isolated breakthrough seizures, without persistent symptoms or deficits, can be safely discharged. Follow-up with their neurologist is indicated, but neurology consultation is only needed in the ED for questions regarding necessary changes in dosing of anticonvulsants.

CHAPTER 51

ISCHEMIC STROKE

Phillip A. Scott

▶ Stroke is the third leading cause of death and the leading cause of disability in the U.S.
▶ There are 700,000 new cases of stroke annually, with estimated costs exceeding $40 billion.

PATHOPHYSIOLOGY

▶ A sudden onset of a neurologic deficit that is either embolic, thrombotic, or lacunar in nature.
▶ Risk factors include HTN, coronary or peripheral atherosclerotic disease, AF, diabetes, age, elevated cholesterol, smoking, oral contraceptives, and history of prior stroke or TIA. Males have higher risk than females, and black patients have greater risk than white patients.

CLINICAL PRESENTATION

▶ **Anterior cerebral artery syndrome**
  • Hemiparesis with greater involvement of the leg than face or arm
  • Urinary incontinence, primitive reflexes (grasp and suck) often present
▶ **Middle cerebral artery syndrome**
  • Most common stroke syndrome.
  • Weakness of the face and arm greater than the leg, often with cortical sensory loss.
  • Aphasia localizes the lesion to dominant hemisphere.
  • Inattention, extinction on double simultaneous sensory or visual testing, or neglect may be the only indication of non-dominant hemisphere stroke.

- Homonymous hemianopia and conjugate eye deviation may also be found.
▶ **Posterior cerebral artery syndrome**
  - Homonymous hemianopia secondary to visual cortex involvement.
  - Patient often unaware of the deficit until formally tested.
  - Minimal motor involvement; light touch and pinprick loss may be severe.
▶ **Vertebrobasilar artery syndrome**
  - Hallmark is crossed symptoms: ipsilateral cranial nerve palsy and contralateral hemiplegia.
▶ **Cerebellar infarction**
  - Sudden inability to walk or stand.
  - Complaints of headache, nausea, vomiting, and central vertigo.
  - Cranial nerve findings may also be present.
  - One-third of patients develop significant edema, causing a decreased level of consciousness, typically after a stable period of 6–12 hours. Surgical decompression and/or medical treatment of elevated ICP may be life-saving.
▶ **Lacunar syndromes**
  - Pure motor strokes, with variable presentations but often causing equal deficits of the face, arm, and leg. Cortical sensory deficits are absent. May cause subtle findings such as the clumsy hand–dysarthria syndrome.

DIFFERENTIAL DIAGNOSIS
▶ See Table 51-1 for non-ischemic strokes and stroke mimics.

TABLE 51-1.
DIFFERENTIAL DIAGNOSIS OF ISCHEMIC STROKE

TIA	Epidural hematoma
Intracerebral hemorrhage	Subdural hematoma
SAH	Tumor
Conversion disorder	Meningitis/encephalitis
Hypoglycemia	Hypertensive encephalopathy
Seizure with Todd's paralysis	Wernicke's encephalopathy
Complex (hemiplegic) migraine	Multiple sclerosis
Bell's palsy	Drug toxicity (phenytoin, lithium)
Abscess or septic emboli	

EMERGENCY DEPARTMENT MANAGEMENT
Diagnosis

▶ **Diagnostic neurologic exam:** Acute ischemic stroke is diagnosed by physical exam. A very rapid but thorough exam is essential to determine the severity of deficit and to help identify stroke mimics.

- Mental status and function, including level of consciousness, language, memory, and ability to follow commands. Aphasia can be subtle and fluid; ask patients to name common objects and repeat phrases.
- Cranial nerves, including gaze deviation, and facial strength and sensation. Sparing of the forehead in unilateral facial weakness indicates central pathology. Check visual fields by confrontation.
- Motor strength, in both proximal and distal muscle groups, in upper and lower extremities, and in both flexors and extensors. Pronator drift is a sensitive indicator of upper-extremity weakness.
- Sensory exam should be interpreted in view of the patient's ability to cooperate.
- Cerebellar function can be assessed by finger-to-nose or heel-to-shin tests and by observing rapidly alternating movements. Deficits should only be attributed to ataxia if they are out of proportion to weakness.
- Subtle weakness, ataxia, rigidity, and sensory defects can be identified by observing gait, toe-walking, heel-walking, tandem walking, and Romberg tests.

▶ **ED stroke imaging:**

- Brain CT scan without contrast is the initial standard imaging modality in patients with symptoms of acute ischemic stroke. The purpose of the CT is to identify alternative diagnoses, including hemorrhage. Ischemic lesions do not become hypodense for 6–72 hours and are often not visible on initial CT evaluation.
- Advanced brain imaging with CT angiography, CT perfusion imaging, MRI with diffusion and perfusion weighted sequences, MRA, and transcranial Doppler imaging are diagnostic in acute stroke and are being studied for use in acute stroke evaluations, but do not usually change emergent management of the patient.

TABLE 51-2.
CRITERIA FOR IV THROMBOLYSIS IN ACUTE STROKE

Diagnosis of stroke with measurable neurologic deficit, which is not resolving spontaneously or minor in nature.
Onset of symptoms < 3 hours before beginning treatment.
No head trauma or prior stroke (any type) in previous 3 months.
Symptoms not suggestive of SAH.
No history of any prior intracranial hemorrhage.
No MI in the past 3 months.
No seizure with post-ictal residual neurologic impairments.
No major surgery in the previous 14 days.
No GI or GU hemorrhage in previous 21 days.
No arterial puncture at a non-compressible site in previous 7 days.
No evidence of active bleeding or acute trauma (fracture) on exam.
SBP < 185 mmHg **and** diastolic BP < 110 mmHg.
Not taking oral anticoagulants or, if taking, INR ≤ 1.5.
If receiving heparin in previous 48 hours, a PTT must be normal.
Blood glucose ≥ 50 mg/dl (2.7 mmol/L).
Platelet count ≥ 100,000/mm.

Treatment

▶ In stroke patients who present within 3 hours of symptom onset, the goal of treatment is to re-establish cerebral blood flow with IV thrombolytic agents. Effective reperfusion at later time points in selected patients using IA endovascular approaches is possible and is an unproven treatment option at some centers.

▶ Most stroke patients are not eligible for IV or IA therapy. The goal of treatment in these patients is to optimize chances of recovery by preventing recurrent stroke and minimizing secondary brain injury from cerebral hypoperfusion, hyperthermia, or hyperglycemia.

▶ **Thrombolytic therapy in stroke:**

- Determine eligibility strictly. Table 51-2 outlines inclusion and exclusion criteria for the use of IV tPA. Protocol violations are associated with worse outcomes. Consent for treatment should include discussion about the potential risks and benefits of the treatment.

- Use the time "last known to be normal" as the onset time to determine eligibility, not the time the symptoms were first noticed.

- Treat HTN if > 185/110 mmHg—see Table 51-3 for guidelines.

TABLE 51-3.
POST r-tPA BP MANAGEMENT IN ACUTE STROKE

A. Monitor BP every 15 minutes.
B. If SBP is > 180 mmHg or if diastolic BP is 105–140: Give labetalol, 10 mg IV over 1–2 minutes. The dose may be repeated or doubled every 10–20 minutes, up to 300 mg. Alternatives include an initial labetalol dose followed by an infusion at a rate of 2–8 mg/minute. If BP not controlled, consider sodium nitroprusside infusion.
C. If diastolic BP is ≥ 140 mmHg: Infuse sodium nitroprusside at a rate of 0.5 mcg/kg/minute and titrate to desired pressure.

- If eligible, treat with tPA as early as possible.
  - **Alteplase (Activase), 0.9 mg/kg (maximum dose 90 mg)** with 10% given as a bolus over 1 minute, and the remainder given over 60 minutes via infusion pump. (Note that this is lower than the dose used in acute MI and that other thrombolytics used in patients with MI are not approved for use in patients with stroke.)
- Control of HTN after treatment with tPA is important too. Table 51-3 presents post-treatment BP control guidelines.
- In the NINDS trials, patients treated with r-tPA were at least 30% more likely to have minimal or no disability 3 months after the event, compared with those who received placebo.
- Patients treated with tPA had a symptomatic hemorrhage rate of 6.4% vs. 0.6% for placebo. Risk of bad outcome without treatment and of hemorrhage with treatment increases with age and stroke severity.
- There was no change in mortality in tPA-treated patients compared to placebo.
- Post-hoc analyses do not support withholding therapy from any patient on the basis of suspected stroke subtype, age, clinical deficit, or CT findings of early ischemic changes.
- Watch for signs of hemorrhage. Should hemorrhage be suspected, discontinue tPA infusion, obtain an immediate brain CT, send blood for PT/PTT/INR, CBC with platelets, T&S, and fibrinogen. If CT shows hemorrhage, transfuse 6 units each of platelets and cryoprecipitate and obtain emergent hematology and neurology/neurosurgery consults as needed.

- Compliance with protocols derived from the NINDS trials is critical. Studies of protocols using other thrombolytic agents, longer treatment windows, or in which protocol violations were frequent demonstrate less benefit and more complications.

▶ **BP management in stroke:**
  - Optimal BP management in patients with acute stroke is not clear and is the subject of ongoing investigations. Initially high or low BP, and large increases or decreases in BP, are associated with worsened outcomes.
  - Antihypertensive agents are not recommended in acute stroke unless the SBP is > 220 mmHg or unless the diastolic BP is > 120 mmHg, or unless specifically indicated because of thrombolytic therapy, AMI, hypertensive encephalopathy, arterial dissection, or hemorrhagic transformation.
  - In stroke patients not treated with tPA but requiring antihypertensive therapy, the goal is a gradual reduction of BP by 15%. Avoid precipitous BP lowering.
  - For SBP > 220 or DBP 121–140 mmHg, give **labetalol, 10–20 mg IV** over 1 minute, repeated or doubled every 10 minutes (maximum dose 300 mg), or **nicardipine (Cardene), 5 mg/hour IV** infusion as initial dose; increase 2.5 mg/hour every 5 minutes to maximum of 15 mg/hour.
  - For DBP > 140 mmHg, treat with **nitroprusside, 0.5 mcg/kg/minute IV;** carefully titrated continuous invasive BP monitoring is recommended.
  - Low BP can be treated with gentle volume expansion using NS. Agents to raise BP, including phenylephrine, are under investigation but are not yet indicated in standard care.

▶ **Temperature control in stroke:**
  - Hyperthermia is a complication of certain types of stroke and is associated with worse neurologic outcomes.
  - Treat temperature elevations with
    ○ Acetaminophen (APAP), 1 g PO/PR every 4 hours, and/or with
    ○ Surface or endovascular cooling devices
  - Mild hypothermia to 33° C is under investigation but is not yet indicated in ischemic stroke.

▶ **Control of serum glucose in stroke:**
  - Treat excessive glucose levels with insulin to maintain serum glucose of < 300 mg/dl. Avoid hypoglycemia.

▶ **Anticoagulation:**
  • Emergent anticoagulation to improve neurologic outcome or prevent early recurrent stroke is not recommended.
▶ **Antiplatelet therapy:**
  • ASA therapy should begin within 48 hours with 325 mg in patients who are not treated with thrombolytic therapy.
  • Clopidogrel (Plavix) and ASA combined with dipyridamole (Aggrenox) were variably more effective than ASA alone in preventing recurrent stroke or death. Studies have not evaluated their use in the acute setting, however.

Disposition

▶ Patients with acute stroke are generally admitted to the hospital.
▶ Patients with minor, completed strokes are candidates for an ED clinical decision unit.
▶ ICU admission is indicated for patients treated with tPA or patients with cerebellar or large hemispheric strokes at risk for cerebral edema.
▶ Neurologic consultation is indicated in the ED when the diagnosis is unclear or further evaluation is required (e.g., arterial dissection, migrainous infarct, unusual hematologic conditions).

CHAPTER 52

TRANSIENT ISCHEMIC ATTACK

Phillip A. Scott

▶ Definition: brief episode of neurologic dysfunction with symptoms lasting < 1 hour without evidence of acute infarction.
▶ 25% of TIA patients have a recurrent TIA or stroke, cardiovascular event, or death within 90 days of the initial event—5% experience a stroke within 48 hours of the initial event.

PATHOPHYSIOLOGY

▶ TIAs occur from plaque ulceration or embolism of platelet aggregates.
▶ Small-vessel disease, cardiac dysrhythmias, and hypotension are other causes.

RISK FACTORS AND DIFFERENTIAL DIAGNOSIS

▶ See Chap. 51.

CLINICAL PRESENTATION

▶ Carotid artery syndrome (Contralateral monoparesis or hemiparesis, numbness, tingling, aphasia, or hemianopia; temporary monocular blindness is known as amaurosis fugax.)
▶ Vertebrobasilar artery syndrome (Vertigo, dizziness, ataxia, nausea and/or vomiting, dysarthria, dysphagia, and perioral numbness may occur. Diplopia may result from loss of conjugate gaze.)
▶ Drop attacks (Basilar artery TIAs cause brief paretic spells with the patient dropping to his or her knees. There is no LOC, distinguishing it from true syncope.)
▶ Transient global amnesia (Rapid development of retrograde memory loss with preservation of self-identity.)

EMERGENCY DEPARTMENT MANAGEMENT
Diagnosis

▶ Focus on identifying whether the deficit involves the anterior or posterior circulation and the source of the TIA, and ruling out other causes.

▶ Recognize patients at the highest risk of a subsequent stroke, including those whose symptoms are more severe or of longer duration, as well as those with "crescendo" TIAs (repetitive events with progressive frequency, usually occurring within a 72-hour period).

▶ Diagnosis of TIA is usually based entirely on history. The neurologic exam in patients with TIAs is most often completely normal.

▶ Brain CT scan is indicated to evaluate for evidence of subacute or previous ischemic or hemorrhagic stroke, and to exclude other causes of focal deficits.

▶ Cardiac evaluation in the ED need only include a 12-lead ECG. Transthoracic or TEE need not be performed in the ED, but should be obtained urgently to identify cardioembolic disease.

▶ Carotid arteries should be evaluated urgently by duplex ultrasonography or other imaging modality in patients with anterior circulation TIAs without contraindications for vascular surgery, although this does not need to be performed in the ED.

Treatment

▶ Medical therapy is indicated for patients with posterior circulation TIAs, those with anterior circulation TIAs who have < 50% stenosis on carotid duplex scanning, and patients not eligible for endarterectomy.

▶ ASA (50–325 mg/day) reduces the incidence of stroke, MI, and death from all vascular causes in patients with TIAs.

▶ Dipyridamole (200 mg bid) has a small additional protective effect when used with low-dose (50 mg/day) ASA (Aggrenox®), as does clopidogrel (Plavix®).

▶ Anticoagulation with heparin lacks a rigorous scientific basis. If used at all, it should be reserved for "high-risk" patients such as those with crescendo, vertebrobasilar or recurrent TIAs failing maximal antiplatelet therapy, or known high-grade carotid stenosis. Neurologic consultation is recommended prior to initiation.

▶ Adjusted-dose oral anticoagulation with warfarin is indicated in patients with TIA due to AF. A target INR of 2.0–3.0 is recommended.

▶ Carotid endarterectomy improves outcomes in symptomatic patients with high-grade (70–99%) stenosis. In randomized trials, patients with endarterectomy had a 17% reduction in the risk of ipsilateral stroke after 2 years, compared with medical treatment.

▶ Carotid and intracranial angioplasty and stenting for symptomatic stenoses are currently under evaluation in prospective trials as an alternative approach to surgery.

Disposition

▶ Patients with new anterior circulation TIAs, who are potential surgical candidates, should not be discharged without arranging expeditious evaluation of the carotid arteries.

▶ Because of the increased short-term risk of stroke, it may be optimal to admit TIA patients to an inpatient or observation bed, particularly in the setting of high-risk presentations.

▶ Patients discharged home should have rapid follow-up and clear instructions on stroke signs and symptoms to ensure rapid return.

CHAPTER 53

SUBARACHNOID HEMORRHAGE

Thomas G. Greidanus

- ► SAH occurs in 30,000 patients per year in the U.S.
- ► Patients with SAH make up about 1% of all patients with headache in the ED.
- ► Sudden-onset, severe "thunderclap" headaches that may spontaneously improve.
- ► Most often caused by rupture of a cerebral aneurysm or AVM.

PATHOPHYSIOLOGY

- ► SAH is common in traumatic brain injury. Traumatic SAH is pathophysiologically distinct from non-traumatic hemorrhage and is discussed in Chap. 78.
- ► Non-traumatic SAH is caused by rupture of saccular or berry aneurysms (80%) or AVMs, mycotic aneurysms, or bleeding related to other vascular pathology, including angioma, neoplasm, coagulopathies, or cortical thrombus.
- ► Familial cerebrovascular aneurysmal disease is common and may be associated with other syndromes including Ehlers-Danlos syndrome, coarctation of the aorta, polycystic kidney disease, Marfan's syndrome, or fibromuscular dysplasia.
- ► Aneurysms may be present in 0.5–5.0% of the population, usually at the circle of Willis.
- ► Most cases of SAH occur in patients between 40 and 60 years of age. Young patients are more likely to have AVMs than aneurysms.
- ► Incidence is higher in women than in men.
- ► Mortality in SAH is 25%; severe morbidity is present in 50% of survivors.

CLINICAL PRESENTATION

▶ The presentation of SAH is highly variable, ranging from "sentinel" headaches, which are difficult to distinguish from benign headaches, to neurologically devastated patients presenting in coma.

▶ Sentinel (i.e., warning) headaches occur in 50% of patients with SAH, although the SAH is often not diagnosed at the time of the sentinel headache.

▶ Sentinel headaches are often described as the sudden onset of a "thunderclap" headache, which is often described as the worst in the patient's life.

▶ Sentinel headaches are generally not associated with any focal neurologic deficits, and prognosis is markedly improved if aneurysms are diagnosed and treated at this stage.

▶ More severe presentations of SAH can be associated with meningeal irritation and nuchal rigidity, syncope, photophobia, vomiting, and focal or global neurologic abnormalities.

▶ The aneurysm itself can cause specific focal neurologic deficits from cranial nerve compression with abnormal extraocular movements, gaze deviation or palsy, or monocular vision loss.

▶ In larger SAH, seizures and coma are common.

▶ Grade according to Hunt and Hess scale:
  • Grade 0: unruptured aneurysm
  • Grade 1: asymptomatic or minimal headache
  • Grade 2: moderate to severe headache, no neurologic deficits except cranial nerve palsy
  • Grade 3: mild altered mental status (confused, drowsy), mild focal deficit
  • Grade 4: moderate to severe hemiparesis and depressed level of consciousness
  • Grade 5: comatose or posturing

DIFFERENTIAL DIAGNOSIS

▶ See Chap. 49.

EMERGENCY DEPARTMENT MANAGEMENT
Diagnosis

▶ Patients with Hunt and Hess grade 3 to 5 SAH are readily diagnosed in the ED. The challenge in the ED is distinguishing patients with Hunt and Hess grade 1 and 2 SAH from the many similar patients with benign headache.

▶ In patients with focal neurologic deficits or diminished level of consciousness, brain CT without contrast has a high diagnostic yield and should be the initial diagnostic test.

▶ In patients with headache, but no focal deficits and a normal level of consciousness, brain CT can still be used as the initial diagnostic test but is inadequate to exclude SAH. LP should always follow a negative CT if SAH is considered.

▶ An acceptable alternative is to perform an LP as the initial diagnostic test in patients with possible SAH without neurologic abnormalities.

▶ Brain CT misses 2–7% of all patients with SAH and gets less sensitive for SAH more than 24 hours after onset of symptoms.

▶ LP findings of SAH include grossly bloody CSF or xanthochromia, or RBCs on CSF cell counts (there is no definite lower limit of positivity with regard to number of RBCs present; in a nontraumatic tap, 50–75 RBCs may be positive for SAH). Traumatic taps cannot be definitively interpreted, but RBC counts usually decrease between tubes 1 and 4 after traumatic tap. RBC counts that do not decrease are suggestive of SAH rather than (or despite) a traumatic tap.

▶ CT angiography and MRA are now being used selectively to aid with diagnosis at some centers.

Treatment—Supportive

▶ Patients with coma or diminished consciousness require ET intubation.

▶ Seizure prophylaxis is commonly used for patients with SAH: **phenytoin (Dilantin), 1 g IV** infused at 50 mg/minute, or **fosphenytoin (Cerebyx) 1 g phenytoin equivalents IV** infused at 150 mg PE/minute.

▶ Delayed vasospasm is a common cause of secondary injury; to reduce risk of vasospasm, calcium channel blockade should be started urgently with nimodipine, 60 mg PO q4h. Treatment does not need to begin in the ED.

▶ Optimal management of BP in patients with acute SAH is unknown, but treatment of extremes of HTN and hypotension is common.

▶ Provide IVF hydration to maintain an adequate fluid status.

► As in other forms of brain injury, avoid hyperthermia and hyperglycemia.

Treatment—Definitive

► Emergent neurosurgical consultation is required for all patients with SAH.
► Cerebral angiography is done emergently after diagnosis of SAH to assess vascular anatomy, current bleeding site, and for the presence of other aneurysms.
► Repair of aneurysms by craniotomy and clipping, or increasingly by endovascular coiling or balloons, may be performed emergently or may be delayed for several days at the discretion of the treating neurosurgeon.

Disposition

► All patients with acute SAH should be admitted to the hospital.
► Patients with Hunt and Hess grades 1 and 2 may be admitted to a stroke unit or any other unit where close neurologic checks can be performed.
► Patients with Hunt and Hess grades 3 to 5 should be admitted to an ICU.

CHAPTER 54

MENINGITIS

Colin F. Greineder

▶ Inflammation of leptomeninges, in particular the CSF in subarachnoid space and ventricles, most commonly due to infection.

▶ All meningeal infections are considered urgent conditions, but in particular, acute bacterial meningitis is a true emergency, with collection of diagnostic specimens and prompt initiation of antibiotic therapy being standard of care in the ED.

BACTERIAL MENINGITIS

▶ Mortality and morbidity of bacterial meningitis are significant, with a case-fatality rate of close to 25% and with permanent neurologic sequelae in 25% of survivors.

▶ Incidence of disease and frequency of organism vary by age of the patient (Table 54-1).

▶ Influence of vaccination. In the mid-1980s, the median age of patients with bacterial meningitis was 15 months, and *Haemophilus influenzae* caused > 40% of cases in all age groups. HIB vaccine was introduced in 1991, and by mid-1990s, overall incidence was reduced by 55%, median age was 25 years, and *Streptococcus pneumoniae* was the most common pathogen. With the recent introduction of childhood pneumococcal vaccination, the epidemiology may be changing again.

▶ The vast majority of cases result from hematogenous spread of bacteria, although direct spread from contiguous sites of infection (OM, sinusitis, brain abscess) or portals of entry (open skull fracture, neurosurgical devices) is also possible.

Clinical Presentation

▶ Meningitis has a variable but often rapidly progressive presentation. Early diagnosis and treatment are thought to improve prognosis.

TABLE 54-1.
INCIDENCE AND FREQUENCY OF ORGANISM BY AGE

Age	Incidence per 100,000	Major pathogens
Neonates (< 1 month)	180	Group B streptococcus (70%) Listeria Escherichia coli S. pneumoniae
1 month to 2 years	14.6	S. pneumoniae (45%) Neisseria meningitidis (30%) Group B streptococcus (20%)
2–29 years	1.8	N. meningitidis (60%) S. pneumoniae (30%)
30+ years	~2	S. pneumoniae (60–70%) Listeria (5–15%)

▶ Classic symptoms are headache and the classic triad of fever, neck stiffness, and altered mental status. Other symptoms include nausea, vomiting, focal neurologic deficits, seizures, rash, and photophobia. While fulminant cases (perhaps 25% of adult cases) may be easy to identify clinically, the absence of a classic presentation does not exclude meningitis.

▶ 95% of patients with meningitis have at least two of four elements of headache, fever, neck stiffness, or altered mental status.

▶ Classical bedside physical exam findings of meningismus have very low sensitivity: nuchal rigidity (30%), Kernig's sign (painful knee extension with hip flexed, 5%) and Brudzinski's sign (hip flexion with neck flexion, 5%)—even in a subset of patients with moderate meningeal inflammation (> 100 WBCs/ml of CSF).

Emergency Department Management

Diagnosis

▶ Diagnosis depends on evaluation of the patient's CSF. LP is the diagnostic test for meningitis and should be performed as soon as possible upon arrival in the ED.

▶ Routine blood and serum tests, such as a CBC, basic metabolic panel, and blood cultures, are commonly performed but are non-diagnostic in meningitis.

▶ Evaluation of CSF. Meningitis is diagnosed by cell counts, Gram's stain, and antigen panels or cultures of the CSF. Typical

TABLE 54-2.
TYPICAL LP FINDINGS IN DIFFERENT FORMS OF MENINGITIS

Parameter	Bacterial	Viral	Cryptococcal (HIV associated)	Tuberculous
Opening pressure	↑↑	↑	↑↑	↑
CSF WBC	> 500/μL	< 500/μL	< 50/μL	< 500/μL
Predominant cell type	PMNs	Lymphocytes	Variable	Mononuclear cells
CSF glucose	Decreased	Normal	Normal	Decreased
CSF protein	Increased	Normal	Normal	Increased (can be extremely high)

- LP results for bacterial, viral, and other meningitides are shown in Table 54-2.
- ▶ Brain CT imaging is generally not indicated in the evaluation of patients with suspected meningitis. CT imaging should be performed in patients with altered mental status, focal neurologic deficits, immunosuppression, seizures, age > 60 years, or previous CNS diseases.

Treatment
- ▶ Antibiotics should be empirically administered immediately after performance of LP. A bactericidal antibiotic that penetrates CSF should be given. ED arrival to time of antibiotic delivery (door to needle time) should be as short as possible. Consider steroid use with the first dose of antibiotics.
- ▶ If LP is delayed (to obtain a CT scan, for example), obtain blood cultures (which may provide causative organism in 50–75% of cases), and then immediately administer empiric antibiotics prior to the CT scan and LP.
- ▶ Empiric antibiotic therapy includes meningeal doses of a broad-spectrum, third-generation cephalosporin like **ceftriaxone (Rocephin),** 2 g IV (50 mg/kg IV in children).
- ▶ In patients suspected of having antibiotic-resistant *S. pneumoniae,* **vancomycin,** 1 g IV (10–20 mg/kg IV in children).
- ▶ In young infants (< 3 months), immunocompromised individuals receiving chemotherapy or high-dose steroids, and possibly

older patients (> 60 years old), add coverage for *Listeria*: **ampicillin,** 1–2 g IV (50 mg/kg IV in children).

▶ In patients with nosocomial infection or immunosuppression, give cephalosporins with increased gram-negative and pseudomonal coverage such as **ceftazidime (Fortaz),** 1 g IV (30–50 mg/kg IV in children), or **cefepime (Maxipime),** 1–2 g IV (50 mg/kg IV in children).

▶ Steroids are now recommended in both adults and children with acute bacterial meningitis. **Dexamethasone,** 10 mg IV (0.2 mg/kg in children).

VIRAL MENINGITIS

▶ While viral meningitis generally presents with a more indolent onset and less severe symptoms than bacterial infection, CSF is essential in differentiating between the two (see Table 54-2).

▶ Even after LP, diagnosis can be unclear due to overlap of CSF findings—e.g., neutrophils may predominate in first 24 hours of viral infection and mononuclear cells occasionally predominate in bacterial meningitis.

▶ Majority of cases in the United States caused by enteroviruses (coxsackievirus A and B, echovirus, etc.), although HSV-2 is increasingly recognized as a causative agent.

▶ Because clinical experience suggests some benefit from antiviral therapy in HSV-2 meningitis but not with any of the other viruses, efforts to identify HSV-2 infection should be made, and if suspected, may be treated with **acyclovir,** 10 mg/kg IV q8h or 800 mg PO five times/day.

▶ HSV-2 meningitis may be associated with primary or recurrent HSV infection—85% of the primary cases are associated with genital lesions that precede meningeal symptoms by several days.

▶ DNA PCR has emerged as superior test for detecting HSV in CSF, with positive results as early as 1 day after onset and published sensitivity and specificity > 95%.

▶ Patient with viral meningitis need not be admitted to the hospital, but disposition and treatment of patients with suspected viral meningitis depend on confirming that the infection is not bacterial and making certain that symptoms are sufficiently controlled.

▶ When diagnosis is unclear, admission with empiric antibiotics is appropriate, with subsequent discharge if CSF cultures return negative.

CRYPTOCOCCAL MENINGITIS IN AIDS PATIENTS

▶ Cryptococcal meningoencephalitis is an important opportunistic infection in immunosuppressed patients, in particular those with AIDS, in whom it often leads to the identification of underlying HIV infection.

▶ Infection almost always occurs in patients with CD4 counts < 100/μl.

▶ Due to reduced inflammatory response, the clinical presentation is usually mild (headache, fever, malaise) and indolent (developing over the course of 1–2 weeks).

▶ Likewise, CSF findings (see Table 54-2) are often unimpressive.

▶ Thankfully, high burden of organisms means adjunctive tests are usually positive: India ink preparation in ~60% and cryptococcal antigen assay in > 90% of cases.

▶ Untreated cryptococcal meningoencephalitis is fatal, and antifungals should be initiated in the ED, generally a combination of IV amphotericin and PO fluconazole.

TUBERCULOUS MENINGITIS

▶ TB meningitis, while rare in the U.S. (< 500 cases/year), is fatal if untreated, and clinical outcome depends on the stage at which treatment is initiated.

▶ Most important for the emergency physician is to understand what populations are at risk and what laboratory means exist for diagnosis, so that appropriate samples can be collected and treatment initiated when TB meningitis is in the differential.

▶ Current lab diagnostic methods are neither simple nor entirely satisfactory, meaning none is employed in routine screening of CSF samples. Rather, most laboratories restrict testing to those cases in which there is physician suspicion for TB and a lymphocytic or monocytic predominance on cell count.

▶ Acid-fast staining of CSF is highly specific but requires large volumes of CSF (~10 cc) and has poor sensitivity (10–35%), unless serial samples are tested.

▶ CSF culture, which has acceptable sensitivity and specificity, has a detection time of approximately 3 weeks.

▶ Treatment should be initiated immediately if strong clinical suspicion of infection and generally consists of standard combination of isoniazid (INH), rifampin (RIF), and pyrazinamide (PZA), with consideration of additional drugs if there is concern for resistance.

CHAPTER 55

BELL'S PALSY

Robert F. McCurdy

▶ Rapid-onset idiopathic unilateral facial weakness
▶ Accounts for 60–75% of cases of acute facial palsies

CLINICAL PRESENTATION

▶ Unilateral paralysis or paresis of upper and lower facial muscles.
▶ Onset of symptoms is typically abrupt and evolves in < 48 hours.
▶ May follow a recent URI.
▶ Associated symptoms include
  • Facial, ear, or mastoid pain
  • Hyperacusis secondary to involvement of stapedius muscle
  • Decreased tearing
  • Alteration of taste
  • Numbness or tingling of the cheek/mouth

DIFFERENTIAL DIAGNOSIS

▶ See Table 55-1.

EMERGENCY DEPARTMENT MANAGEMENT
Diagnosis

▶ Bell's palsy is a clinical diagnosis utilizing history and physical exam.
▶ Physical exam
  • The primary purpose of the physical exam is to determine if the patient's facial weakness is central or peripheral.
  • Facial weakness causes flattening of the furrows of the forehead and the nasolabial fold and is usually obvious upon observation. Weakness is further demonstrated by testing the patient's response to questions.

TABLE 55-1.
DIFFERENTIAL DIAGNOSIS OF BELL'S PALSY

Stroke or TIA
Ramsay Hunt syndrome
Tumor
Botulism
Traumatic neurapraxia
Multiple sclerosis
Lyme disease

- Demonstration of facial weakness is elicited by directing a patient to "close your eyes" to test upper facial muscles, or to "show me your teeth" to test lower facial muscles.
- Complete paralysis of the forehead and upper facial muscles is only possible in facial nerve palsy and thus distinguishes central from peripheral etiologies.
- Partial sparing of the forehead occurs in facial weakness secondary to stroke or other central causes because of crossed cortical fibers.
- In Bell's palsy, the patient is unable to completely close the eye on affected side. On attempted eye closure, the eye rolls upward and inward (Bell phenomenon).
- Otalgia and vesicular rash of the ear associated with facial nerve palsy indicate herpes zoster eruption (Ramsay Hunt syndrome).

▶ Imaging
- Imaging studies are not indicated in the acute setting for patients with symptoms of Bell's palsy.
- MRI is the test of choice for evaluation of patients with progressive worsening of symptoms or failure to improve over 8–10 weeks.
- Emergent consultation is not indicated in the ED for patients with Bell's palsy.

Treatment

▶ Corticosteroids
- Use of steroids is widespread but controversial, as most patients fully recover without intervention.
- Prednisone was superior to acyclovir in a randomized trial comparing the two treatments, and other observational data

suggest that corticosteroid treatment may shorten the course and lessen the severity of symptoms.

- Relatively safe in absence of co-morbid conditions such as diabetes, HTN, and PUD.
- **Prednisone,** 60–80 mg PO once per day for 7 days.

▶ Antivirals
- Use of antiviral agents is also common, but of unproven benefit.
- Acyclovir plus prednisone showed some incremental benefit compared with prednisone alone in one randomized trial.
- Relatively good safety profile.
- **Acyclovir,** 400 mg PO five times per day for 7–10 days, or valacyclovir, 1 g PO twice per day for 7–10 days, or famciclovir, 750 mg tid for 7–10 days.

▶ Eye care
- Essential to prevent irritation, discomfort, and keratitis from dry eyes and inability to close eye
- Hourly saline drops or eye patch while awake
- Ophthalmic ointment and/or eye patch at night

PROGNOSIS

▶ Over 70% of patients will have full recovery within 6–8 weeks.
▶ In up to 15% of patients, recovery does not begin until 3–6 months after onset of symptoms.
▶ Severity of symptoms directly correlates with likelihood of full recovery.
▶ Factors associated with poorer prognosis include diabetes, HTN, and age > 60 years.
▶ Long-term sequelae include residual facial weakness, dysesthesia, loss of smell, facial spasms, and tics.

DISPOSITION

▶ Patients with acute Bell's palsy should be referred to their primary care physicians for follow-up within 7–10 days.
▶ Patients with persistent symptoms may be referred to an ENT specialist.
▶ Patients with eye complications should be referred urgently to an ophthalmologist.

CHAPTER 56

APPROACH TO VAGINAL BLEEDING— NONPREGNANT

Lisa M. Schweigler

▶ Mean age for menarche 12.5 years and menopause 51 years in United States
▶ Menorrhagia—menstrual blood loss > 80 ml or > 6 consecutive days of flow
▶ Metrorrhagia—abnormal bleeding at irregular intervals/between cycles

NORMAL MENSTRUAL CYCLE

▶ Estrogen secreted by ovarian follicle during first 14 days of menstrual cycle (follicular phase) → endometrial proliferation.
▶ Ovulation induced by FSH/luteinizing hormone (LH) surge from pituitary around day 14.
▶ Estrogen and progesterone secreted by corpus luteum in second 14 days (luteal phase) maintain endometrium for possible implantation.
▶ In absence of embryonic HCG, corpus luteum involutes → hormonal withdrawal causes loss of endometrial blood supply and bleeding.

DIFFERENTIAL DIAGNOSIS

▶ Dysfunctional uterine bleeding, polycystic ovarian syndrome (PCOS), hypothyroidism, atrophic endometrium, infection, FB, trauma, excessive exercise, oral contraceptives (breakthrough or withdrawal bleeding), IUDs, neoplastic, coagulation disorders, uterine prolapse

CLINICAL PRESENTATION

▶ Key history points: amount of bleeding, presence of clots (indicates brisk bleeding), menstrual history, parity, contraception, sexual activity, past medical/surgical history, trauma, medications, hygiene practices

▶ Hemodynamic instability → genital tract lacerations, coagulation disorders, PID with sepsis

▶ Irregular menstrual cycles → anovulatory cycles/dysfunctional uterine bleeding

▶ Obesity, acne, hirsutism → PCOS, adrenal hyperplasia

▶ Galactorrhea → hyperprolactinemia

▶ Fatigue, cold intolerance, hair loss → hypothyroidism

▶ Abdominal/uterine pain/tenderness, fever → endometritis, PID

▶ Discharge, cervical motion tenderness → PID

▶ Adnexal mass → PID, estrogen-secreting ovarian cyst/tumor

▶ Friable cervix → cervicitis, cervical cancer

▶ Enlarged uterus → fibroids, adenomyosis

▶ Easy bruising, purpura → coagulation disorders

▶ Fatigue, weight loss → malignancy

DIAGNOSIS

▶ **Must** rule out pregnancy, trauma, coagulopathy, infection, FB.

▶ Dysfunctional uterine bleeding most common, but diagnosis of exclusion.

▶ Physical exam:
  • Evaluate for hemodynamic instability → vital signs, orthostatics.
  • Complete pelvic exam to determine source of bleeding (also consider GI, urinary), evaluate for pelvic tenderness and masses.
    ○ Posterior vaginal fornix common site of coital injury

▶ Lab studies:
  • Urine/serum pregnancy test.
  • Consider CBC, PT, PTT, and T&S if heavy or prolonged bleeding.
  • Wet prep and cultures especially if mucopurulent discharge.

▶ Imaging usually **not** needed in nonpregnant vaginal bleeding.
  • Consider ultrasound in ED if bleeding associated with abdominal pain → ovarian cysts, tubo-ovarian abscess, and fluid in cul-de-sac.

TREATMENT AND DISPOSITION

▶ Gynecology referral if diagnosis unclear, if further work-up or long-term management required, and for all postmenopausal bleeding as high incidence of malignancy

Hemodynamically Unstable

▶ Resuscitation.

▶ Immediate gynecology consult (e.g., repair of complex lacerations, immediate D&C).

▶ Uterine packing increases risk of infection.

▶ Consider giving conjugated estrogen if life-threatening hemorrhage not due to tumor/not amenable to surgical intervention.

▶ Admit if there is ongoing instability or significant hemorrhage requiring blood transfusion.

Lacerations

▶ Repair simple genital tract lacerations if > 2 cm in length and/or actively bleeding.

▶ Vaginal mucosa and perineal muscle laceration: 3-0 Vicryl.

▶ Skin laceration: 4-0 Vicryl.

▶ External anal sphincter laceration: Recommend gynecologist to repair.

Atrophic Vaginitis

▶ Must follow up to rule out malignancy (Pap smear).

▶ Topical vaginal estrogen: estradiol vaginal tablets, 10–25 mcg at night.

Dysfunctional Uterine Bleeding

▶ Hormonal stabilization of endometrium if hemodynamically stable (dysfunctional uterine bleeding):

   • Estrogen therapy: oral conjugated estrogen (Premarin), 2.5 mg qid or 25 mg IV q2–4h × 24 hours (similar efficacy) → when bleeding stops add medroxyprogesterone, 10 mg/day. Continue both estrogen and progesterone for 7–10 days → stop for withdrawal bleed.

     ◦ Oral contraceptive therapy: ethinyl estradiol, 35 mcg, and norethindrone, 1 mg, 4 tabs for 7 days or slow taper:

                 4 tabs for 2 days → 3 tabs for 2 days → 2 tabs for 2 days → 1 tab for 3 days.

- ○ Progesterone therapy: medroxyprogesterone, 10 mg/day for 10 days.
- ○ Antifibrinolytic therapy: tranexamic acid, 0.3–1.0 g every 8 hours for 3 days (reduces vaginal bleeding).
- ▶ Long-term medical therapy rarely started in ED. Includes OCPs, NSAIDs (via change in PG levels, start first day of period, continue until bleeding stops/pain resolves).

CHAPTER 57

APPROACH TO VAGINAL BLEEDING—PREGNANT

Lisa M. Schweigler

GESTATIONAL AGE < 20 WEEKS

▶ Spontaneous abortion: 50–60% embryonic chromosomal abnormalities, maternal factors [e.g., advanced age, history of previous abortions, other medical disorders, infections (e.g., UTI)]

Differential Diagnosis

▶ Spontaneous abortion
  • Threatened: vaginal bleeding without cervical dilatation
  • Inevitable: vaginal bleeding with cervical dilatation
  • Incomplete: not all products of conception (POC) are passed
  • Complete: all POC are passed
  • Missed: fetal death without passage of fetal tissue for 3–4 weeks
  • Septic: infection during any stage of abortion
▶ Ectopic pregnancy (see Chap. 58)
▶ Complications from elective abortion
▶ Gestational trophoblastic disease (GTD)
▶ Implantation bleeding

Clinical Presentation

▶ Spontaneous abortion: abdominal pain, passing of tissue, vaginal bleeding
▶ Elective abortion complications: abdominal pain, fever, inconsistent history if illegal
▶ GTD: more common in Asian women, often associated with hyperemesis, early pregnancy-induced HTN, uterus large for GA

Management

▶ Hemodynamic stabilization. 2–3 L IVF if tachycardic, orthostatic, or hypotensive.

▶ Careful pelvic exam to determine source of bleeding, whether cervical os is open, adnexal mass → ectopic or heterotopic (1 in 30,000).

▶ All retrieved tissue needs to be sent for pathology (to evaluate for GTD, chromosomal abnormalities, ensure tissue not just heavy clots seen with ectopic, etc.).

▶ Lab evaluation: CBC, coagulation studies, serum beta-HGC, T&S, UA.

▶ Correlate beta-HGC with GA by dates/ultrasound.

▶ Give Rho D immune globulin (RhoGAM) if Rh negative:
  • 50 mg IM for spontaneous abortion < 12 weeks gestation
  • 300 mg IM/IV for vaginal bleeding > 12 weeks gestation

▶ Imaging: transabdominal or transvaginal ultrasound (see below).

▶ Obstetric/gynecologic consult: hemodynamically unstable, persistent heavy bleeding, significant drop in HCT, infection, retained POC → emergent surgical evacuation of uterus.

▶ Non-viable IUP in hemodynamically stable patient: admission for D&C vs. methotrexate vs. 1-week outpatient follow-up depending on patient/physician comfort.

▶ Threatened abortion: outpatient follow-up with serial beta-HGC if hemodynamically stable.

▶ Completed abortion: outpatient follow-up.

▶ Vaginal bleeding instructions if discharged: return for soaking > 1 pad/hour for 6 hours, pain, fever.

Ultrasound

▶ Looking for
  • Free intra-abdominal fluid, adnexal mass → ectopic
  • Gestational sac, fetal pole, fetal heartbeat → IUP

▶ Beta-HGC > 1500 IU/ml → IUP should be visible on transvaginal ultrasound

▶ Beta-HGC > 6500 IU/ml → IUP should be visible on transabdominal ultrasound

▶ Days from last menstrual period:
  • 36 → yolk sac
  • 41–47 → heartbeat

▶ Transvaginal ultrasound interpretation (Table 57-1)

TABLE 57-1.
TRANSVAGINAL ULTRASOUND INTERPRETATION

Viable IUP	Yolk sac without fetus at estimated GA < 5 weeks
	Fetal pole < 5 mm at estimated GA < 7 weeks
	Fetal pole > 5 mm with fetal heartbeat
Non-viable IUP	Fetal pole > 5 mm without fetal heartbeat
	Sac abnormalities: large (mean diameter > 25 mm without embryo, > 20 mm without yolk sac), irregular, low-lying, containing debris
	Open cervical os
	Echogenic material in endometrium without gestational sac

GESTATIONAL AGE > 20 WEEKS

▶ Usually presents directly to labor and delivery triage
▶ Automatic obstetrics consult
▶ Fetal heart tone monitoring: fetal distress → tachycardia, lack of variability, variable/late decelerations, bradycardia
▶ Tocometry

Differential Diagnosis

▶ Bloody show
▶ Placenta previa: placenta implanted over cervical os
▶ Vasa previa: umbilical cord inserts in placental membrane, tributary vessel below presenting fetal part near cervical os
▶ Abruptio placentae: premature separation of normally implanted placenta
▶ Postpartum hemorrhage
  • Uterine atony: failure of uterus to contract appropriately
  • Retained POC: failure of complete placental separation/expulsion
  • Vaginal/cervical trauma
  • Uterine inversion
  • Coagulation defects
  • Amniotic fluid embolism
▶ Uterine rupture

Clinical Presentation

▶ Bloody show: painless, GA appropriate for spontaneous onset of labor, no continued bleeding, no fetal distress.

▶ Placenta previa: painless bleeding, usually stops in 1–2 hours. Risk factors include increased age, multiparity, and prior C-section.

▶ Abruptio placentae: painful bleeding, continuous, significant fetal distress. Risk factors include maternal HTN, trauma, and cocaine use.

▶ Vasa previa: painless bleeding, significant fetal distress.

▶ Coagulation defects: easy bruising/bleeding.

▶ Amniotic fluid embolus: dyspnea, evidence of disseminated intravascular coagulation.

▶ Uterine rupture: painful bleeding, significant abdominal pain.

▶ Uterine atony: boggy uterine fundus.

Management

▶ Call obstetrics consult as soon as possible.

▶ Hemodynamic stabilization: Mother takes priority. Two large-bore IVs.

▶ Blood products as appropriate for blood loss and coagulation disorders.

▶ No cervical/bimanual exam until placenta previa/vasa previa has been excluded.

▶ Careful speculum exam to evaluate for bulging membranes, vasa previa, postpartum vaginal/cervical lacerations; cervical lacerations > 2 cm/actively bleeding require repair (see Chap. 56).

▶ If suspect spontaneous onset of labor and bloody show only, consider sterile cervical exam to evaluate effacement, dilation, station.

▶ Transabdominal ultrasound to evaluate location of placenta.

▶ Labs: CBC, coagulation studies, T&S/type & cross (6 units), renal function, disseminated intravascular coagulation panel if suspecting abruptio placentae or amniotic fluid embolus, Kleihauer-Betke with history of trauma to evaluate for feto-maternal hemorrhage.

▶ Uterine atony:
  • Uterine massage
  • Oxytocin, 20–30 units/L at 200 cc/hour IV

▶ Ultrasound may be helpful to evaluate for postpartum retained POC (absence of normal uterine stripe).

CHAPTER 58

ECTOPIC PREGNANCY

Nathaniel S. Bowler

▶ Leading cause of pregnancy-related death in first trimester, accounting for up to 13% of all pregnancy-related deaths.

▶ Rate of heterotopic pregnancy (IUP and ectopic pregnancy at the same time) varies from 1 in 3000 to 1 in 8000 at baseline to 1–3% in women taking fertility agents.

▶ Risk factors for ectopic pregnancy include previous ectopic pregnancy, documented tubal pathology, in utero diethylstilbestrol (DES) exposure, history of STDs, infertility, multiple sexual partners, smoking, previous pelvic or abdominal surgery, vaginal douching, and an early age of first intercourse.

PATHOPHYSIOLOGY

▶ Ectopic pregnancy occurs when a fertilized ovum implants anywhere outside the endometrium of the uterus.

▶ 97% of ectopic pregnancies occur in the fallopian tube (55% ampulla, 25% isthmus, 17% fimbria). The remaining 3% are located in ovarian, cervical, or other extrauterine sites.

CLINICAL PRESENTATION

▶ Classic triad of symptoms for the patient with ectopic pregnancy is amenorrhea, abdominal pain, and vaginal bleeding.

▶ Most patients have abdominal pain of varying intensity, usually located in the lower quadrants.

▶ Pain may be located in the left shoulder in patients with ruptured ectopics due to irritation of the diaphragm by intra-peritoneal blood, Kehr's sign.

▶ Vaginal bleeding is a common symptom and may range from spotting to profuse.

▶ Hypotension or tachycardia may indicate a ruptured ectopic and a need for aggressive resuscitation.

TABLE 58-1.
DIFFERENTIAL DIAGNOSIS OF ECTOPIC PREGNANCY

Salpingitis	Dysfunctional uterine bleeding
Threatened or incomplete abortion	Adnexal torsion
Ruptured corpus luteum	Degenerative uterine leiomyoma
Appendicitis	Endometriosis

▶ Physical exam may demonstrate peritoneal signs, an adnexal mass, cervical motion tenderness, and unilateral or bilateral abdominal or pelvic tenderness.

- Adnexal masses are noted in < 10% of affected patients, and pelvic exam may be completely normal in up to 10%.

DIFFERENTIAL DIAGNOSIS
▶ See Table 58-1.

EMERGENCY DEPARTMENT MANAGEMENT
Diagnosis
▶ Every reproductive-age female presenting with abdominal pain, syncope, hypotension, or altered mental status should be screened for pregnancy.

▶ Lab studies include CBC, blood type and cross-matching, Rh status, and a quantitative beta-HCG. The mainstay of inclusion or exclusion of the diagnosis of ectopic pregnancy involves ultrasound and beta-HCG values.

▶ The level of beta-HCG at which an IUP is expected to be seen on ultrasound is approximately 6500 mIU/ml for trans-abdominal ultrasound or 1000–1500 mIU/ml for the trans-vaginal approach.

▶ The discriminatory zone refers to the beta-HCG level at which an IUP should be visible if present. See Table 58-2.

▶ A trans-vaginal ultrasound can be helpful even if the beta-HCG is below the discriminatory zone because IUPs and ectopic pregnancies can sometimes be identified at levels below 1500 mIU/ml.

▶ Ultrasound findings highly suspicious for ectopic pregnancy include a beta-HCG above the discriminatory zone with an empty uterus, an adnexal mass that is not a simple cyst and is

TABLE 58-2.
BETA-HGC LEVEL CORRELATION WITH STRUCTURES SEEN ON VAGINAL ULTRASOUND

Beta-HCG level (mIU/ml)	Days gestation	Structure visualized (trans-vaginal ultrasound)
1000–1500	35–37	Gestational sac
2500	37	Yolk sac (seen in gestational sac > 9 mm)
5000	40	Fetal pole (seen in gestational sac > 16 mm)
17,000	45	Fetal heart beat

separate from the ovary, a moderate to large amount of fluid in the cul-de-sac, or any echogenic fluid that could indicate blood.

Treatment

▶ Place two large-bore IVs.

▶ Immediate gynecologic consultation and urgent laparotomy are warranted for all hemodynamically unstable patients in whom a ruptured ectopic pregnancy is a likely cause.

▶ In stable patients, treatment should be dictated by the gynecologic consultant and can be either surgical or medical.

▶ In certain cases, ectopic pregnancy can be medically treated with methotrexate.

  • Indications include an adnexal mass < 3–4 cm in diameter, hemodynamic stability, desire for future fertility, and a stable or rising beta-HCG level that is < 15,000 mIU/ml.

  • Methotrexate therapy should always be initiated and managed by a gynecologist. Dosage: methotrexate, 50 mg/m^2 IM or IV × 1.

▶ Ectopic pregnancies that do not meet the criteria for medical therapy are treated surgically, most commonly using a laparoscopic approach.

Disposition

▶ Patients meeting criteria for medical therapy may be discharged home with close follow-up with gynecology.

▶ In patients with a beta-HCG level below the discriminatory zone, one must maintain a high clinical suspicion for ectopic pregnancy with close follow-up either in gynecology clinic or a return to the ED to have a repeat beta-HCG level drawn in 48 hours.

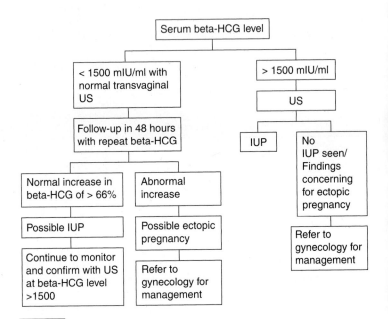

FIGURE 58-1.

Use of beta-HCG for patients with suspected ectopic pregnancy.

► Beta-HCG levels in normal early pregnancy double every 1.4 days to 2.1 days, slowing down after reaching 10,000 mIU/ml (Figure 58-1).

CHAPTER 59

PELVIC INFLAMMATORY DISEASE

Geetika Gupta

▶ Spectrum of inflammatory infections of the upper female genital tract:
  • Endometritis, salpingitis, tubo-ovarian abscess, pelvic peritonitis
▶ PID affects 11% of women of reproductive age.
▶ PID leads to a 7- to 10-fold increased risk for ectopic pregnancy.
▶ Risk factors:
  • Early onset of intercourse, multiple sexual partners, IUD insertion, and tobacco smoking

PATHOPHYSIOLOGY

▶ Microorganisms spread directly by ascending from the vagina and cervix. The cervix produces mucus that usually protects against upward spread, but bacteria may penetrate the cervical mucus and cause widespread infection.
▶ Most common organisms are *Chlamydia trachomatis* and *Neisseria gonorrhoeae.*

CLINICAL PRESENTATION

▶ Symptoms:
  • Lower abdominal pain, vaginal discharge (75%), or bleeding
  • May also complain of dysuria or dyspareunia
▶ Pain:
  • Present in more than 90% of documented cases
  • Dull, aching, and constant; starts usually a few days postmenses, worsened with movement, exercise, or coitus
  • Usually lasts < 7 days; if lasting > 3 weeks, then PID is less likely the correct diagnosis

TABLE 59-1.
DIFFERENTIAL DIAGNOSIS OF PID

Appendicitis
Ovarian torsion
UTI/pyelonephritis
Ectopic pregnancy
Endometriosis
Ruptured ovarian cyst
Abortion, threatened
Gastroenteritis

► Temperature > 38° C (30%), nausea, and vomiting manifest late in the clinical course of the disease.
► Exam:
  • Cervical motion tenderness, uterine or adnexal tenderness
  • May have obvious discharge on speculum exam (sensitivity of pelvic exam only 60%)

DIFFERENTIAL DIAGNOSIS
► See Table 59-1.

EMERGENCY DEPARTMENT MANAGEMENT
Diagnosis
► Treat presumptively in high-risk patients with
  • Uterine, adnexal, or cervical motion tenderness
  • Abdominal tenderness
► Other criteria in support of PID diagnosis:
  • Temperature > 100.4° F or 38° C.
  • Leukocytosis > 10,000 WBC/mm^3.
  • Purulent material in the peritoneal cavity obtained by culdocentesis or laparoscopy.
  • Pelvic abscess or inflammatory complex detected by bimanual exam or by ultrasonography.
  • Patient is a sexual contact of a person known to have an STD.
  • Positive culture or DNA probe of chlamydial or gonorrheal infection in patients with pelvic or lower abdominal pain.
► Delay in diagnosis or treatment can result in infertility and chronic pelvic pain.

Treatment

▶ IV regimen A
  • Cefotetan, 2 g IVPB q12h or cefoxitin, 2 g IVPB q6h, **plus**
  • Doxycycline, 100 mg PO or IVPB q12h × 14 days
▶ IV regimen B
  • Clindamycin, 900 mg IVPB q8h, **plus**
  • Gentamicin, 2 mg/kg loading dose, then 1.5 mg/kg q8h
▶ Oral regimen A
  • Ofloxacin, 400 mg PO bid × 14 days or levofloxacin, 500 mg PO qd × 14 days, **plus/minus** for better anaerobic coverage
  • Metronidazole, 500 mg PO bid × 14 days
▶ Oral regimen B
  • Ceftriaxone, 250 mg IM single dose, **plus**
  • Doxycycline, 100 mg PO q12h × 14 days, **plus/minus** for better anaerobic coverage
  • Metronidazole, 500 mg PO bid × 14 days

Disposition

▶ Indications for hospitalization:
  • Severe illness or nausea and vomiting precluding outpatient treatment
  • Failure of outpatient management
  • Pelvic abscess on ultrasound
  • Non-compliance
  • Immunodeficiency
  • Pregnancy
▶ Mild cases in patients with good follow-up can be treated as outpatient.
▶ Remind patient to inform all sexual partners.

CHAPTER 60

COMPLICATIONS IN LATE PREGNANCY

Geetika Gupta

PREECLAMPSIA

▶ BP > 140/90 with proteinuria (> 300 mg/24 hours) and generalized or pedal edema or weight gain of at least 5 lb over 1 week.
▶ Cause of preeclampsia is unknown, however, possibly related to placental dysfunction that may lead to systemic vasospasm, ischemia, and thrombosis.
▶ Risk features:
  • Pre-pregnancy HTN, obesity, NIDDM, previous history, multiple fetuses, primigravida, advanced maternal age, FH, crack/cocaine use

Clinical Presentation

▶ Usually presents after 20 weeks' gestation, with a variety of complaints.
  • Headache, visual changes, confusion, upper abdominal pain, and jaundice.
  • Decreased UO.
  • If untreated, may proceed to HELLP syndrome or eclampsia.
▶ HELLP occurs in 5–10% of patients with preeclampsia.
  • Hemolytic anemia, elevated liver enzymes, and low platelets.
  • Variant of preeclampsia.
  • Consider in all patients > 20 weeks with RUQ/epigastric pain.

Management

▶ Goals of treatment are to limit maternal and fetal morbidity and mortality.
▶ Lab evaluation:
  • CBC may reveal hemolytic anemia or thrombocytopenia due to HELLP syndrome.

- Creatinine may be elevated due to dehydration or renal dysfunction.
- LFTs may be elevated secondary to HELLP syndrome.
- PT/PTT help rule out disseminated intravascular coagulation.
- UA should be done to look for protein.

▶ If there is concern for preeclampsia, patients should be admitted to the hospital with an immediate obstetric evaluation.

▶ HTN and proteinuria may be caused by chronic primary HTN, but this is a diagnosis of exclusion and may only be considered after preeclampsia has been excluded.

▶ Severe preeclampsia should be admitted to Labor and Delivery for magnesium sulfate and delivery if > 34 weeks, or for administration of betamethasone along with concomitant magnesium sulfate if < 34 weeks.

▶ Treatment:
- Reduce BP to DBP of 90.
  - Hydralazine, 2.5 mg IV push slow, then 5–10 mg IV push slow q10min
  - Labetalol, 20 mg IV push slow, then 40–80 mg IV push slow q20min, maximum dose 300 mg

▶ Consider CT of the head with neurologic complaints.

▶ Ultrasound and fetal monitoring.

▶ The definitive treatment for preeclampsia is delivery of fetus.

ECLAMPSIA

▶ Preeclampsia complicated by seizures or coma, usually after 20 weeks' gestation.

▶ Maternal mortality rate is 8–36%; fetal mortality rate is 13–30%.

Clinical Presentation

▶ Symptoms
- Seizure (100%), headache (80%), generalized edema (50%), and vision disturbance (20%)

▶ Signs
- HTN (SBP > 160 or DBP > 110) and tachycardia
- Mental status changes
- Papilledema

Management

► Definitive treatment is delivery of the fetus, and all other therapy should be regarded as temporizing prior to patient going to OR.
► Same initial work-up as preeclampsia.
► Head CT to look for intracranial hemorrhage or CVAs.
► Magnesium sulfate is initial drug of choice to terminate seizures.
  • Loading dose, 4–6 g in 100 ml of fluid over 20 minutes.
  • Then 2 g/hour drip initially up to a maximum of 4 g/hour.
  • Follow deep tendon reflexes (DTRs) and watch for respiratory depression.
► Benzodiazepines can be used for seizures that are not responsive to magnesium sulfate.
  • Lorazepam, 1–2 mg IV
► After initial loading dose of magnesium sulfate, up to 15% of patients are still hypertensive.
  • Hydralazine, 2.5 mg IV push slow, then 5–10 mg IV push slow q10min
► These patients should be placed in an ICU for close monitoring of BP.

PRETERM LABOR

► Contractions of sufficient strength and frequency to effect progressive effacement and dilation of the cervix between 20 and 37 weeks' GA.
► Accounts for 70% of neonatal morbidity.
► Risk factors include PPROM, abruption, multiple gestation, polyhydramnios, incompetent cervix, infection, uteroplacental insufficiency, uterine structural abnormality, assisted reproductive technology, and previous preterm delivery.

Management

► In patients with significant contractions, the cervix should be examined by the emergency physician.
  • Obstetrics consult
  • Admission for monitoring

- Tocolysis
  - Magnesium sulfate
    - See above for dosing.
  - Indomethacin if < 32 weeks
    - 50 mg PO loading dose followed by 25 mg q6h for a total of 48 hours
- Fetal lung maturation
  - Glucocorticoids (< 34 weeks): betamethasone, 12.5 mg IV q24h for 2 doses
- GBS prophylaxis (all patients with unknown GBS status or culture positive)
  - Penicillin G, 5 million U IV, then 2.5 million U IV q4h, or clindamycin, 600 mg IV q6h for patients who are allergic to penicillin

PREMATURE RUPTURE OF MEMBRANES

▶ GA < 37 weeks with SROM and no onset of labor
▶ Occurs in approximately 10% of pregnancies, 90% of which progress to spontaneous labor within 24 hours

Clinical Presentation

▶ Leakage of clear fluid.
▶ Pooling of fluid in the vagina.
▶ Ferning of vaginal fluid.
▶ Nitrazine paper turns blue in contact with the vaginal fluid.
  - Blood contamination or recent intercourse can falsely turn Nitrazine blue.

Management

▶ Speculum exam only.
▶ Obstetrics consult.
▶ Admit and initiate bed rest with steroid administration if < 32 weeks.
▶ Continuous fetal HR monitoring if > 34 weeks.
▶ Antibiotics:
  - Reduces infant and maternal morbidity
    - Ampicillin, 2 g IV q6h, and erythromycin, 250 mg IV, **or**
    - Ampicillin/sulbactam, 3 g IVPB q6h

▶ Tocolysis:
  • Magnesium sulfate (see above for dosing) if < 32 weeks for benefit of steroid administration
▶ Fetal lung maturation:
  • Betamethasone (see above for dosing)
▶ Treat for group B streptococcus (GBS) prophylaxis in all patients with unknown GBS status or culture positive (see above for dosing).

CHAPTER 61

MASTITIS

Ellen C. Walkling

▶ Mastitis is commonly observed during lactation (10% of breast-feeding mothers).
▶ Most common in first 6 weeks post-partum, but up to 33% occur > 6 months post-partum.
▶ Progresses to abscess in 5–10%.

PATHOPHYSIOLOGY

▶ Lactational mastitis is a cellulitis of the mammary glands and interlobular connective tissue caused by stasis of milk due to incomplete drainage (duct obstruction, missed feedings) and cracked or abraded nipples allowing bacterial entry.
▶ Microorganisms are generally *Staphylococcus aureus* and strepto-cocci from infant's nose and *Escherichia coli.*
▶ Non-lactational mastitis organisms are *S. aureus*, gram-negatives, and anaerobes.
 • Assume ducts are blocked by cancer until proven otherwise.

CLINICAL PRESENTATION

▶ Obstructed milk duct
 • Gradual onset of mild local tenderness, redness, and occasionally mass
▶ Mastitis
 • Local findings of erythema (often in wedge-shaped distribution), edema, exquisite tenderness, warmth, firmness; often with sudden-onset systemic symptoms of fever, chills, rigors, myalgias, malaise, and flu-like symptoms
▶ Abscess
 • May be deep or difficult to palpate due to compartmentalized structure of breast; patients may appear toxic.

EMERGENCY DEPARTMENT MANAGEMENT

Diagnosis

▶ Systematic breast exam, upright with arms over head for inspection and axillary palpation, then supine with arm above head and pillow under shoulder for palpation.

▶ Ultrasound may be useful to identify abscess.

▶ Milk culture may be helpful if recurrent.

Treatment

▶ Warm compresses, increased fluid intake, bed rest.

▶ NSAIDs for analgesia:
  • Ibuprofen, 600 mg q6h PRN pain

▶ For obstructed duct, localized massage.

▶ For lactational mastitis and abscesses, empty breast completely and regularly by nursing, expressing, or pumping.
  • Mother should continue breast feedings, and she should be given reassurance that this is not harmful to the baby.

▶ Oral antibiotics for 10–14 days:
  • Dicloxacillin, 500 mg PO qid
  • Cephalexin, 500 mg PO qid
  • For penicillin allergic, erythromycin, 333 mg PO bid

▶ I&D of abscesses are usually necessary.

▶ If superficial, can be done in ED under local anesthetic with incision radiating from nipple.
  • Small lactational and subareolar abscess may respond to antibiotics without drainage.

▶ For nipple irritation or cracks in lactating women, refer to lactation consultant and avoid irritants. Air-dry nipples after feeds and apply breast milk or lanolin. Can use 1% cortisone on cracks after feeds.

Disposition

▶ Generally outpatient treatment unless patient has abscess, appears toxic, has diabetes, or is immunocompromised.

▶ Follow-up required in 1–3 days to ensure resolution.

▶ For failed outpatient treatment, admit for IV antibiotics.

▶ For chronic infections and for any non-lactational mastitis, always consult a breast surgeon.

CHAPTER 62

SEXUAL ASSAULT

Marquita N. Hicks

▶ Sexual assault includes all forced or inappropriate sexual contact with or without penetration of the mouth, vagina, or anus.
▶ Three key elements: threat or use of force, evidence of sexual contact, and lack of consent.
▶ Up to 25% of women and 7.5% of men report rape or sexual assault over their lifetime.
▶ In the U.S., almost 700,000 sexual assaults occur per year, but it is estimated that only about 15% are reported.
▶ Goals of ED treatment:
  • Identification, documentation, and treatment of any injuries
  • Detection and prophylaxis of STD and pregnancy
  • Forensic evidence collection
  • Provision of emotional support and referrals for psychological follow-up
  • Guidance in the initiation of the legal process should the patient desire

EMERGENCY DEPARTMENT MANAGEMENT

▶ Ensure the patient's privacy by rapidly providing a quiet, private area. Allow the patient to contact a support person if desired.
▶ Evaluate for injuries that require immediate attention.
▶ Obtain consent for medical treatment and for forensic evidence collection to complete the rape kit.
▶ Obtain a focused history including pertinent history of the assault. The patient should be warned that questions may be very personal.
  • Gynecologic history including last menstrual period, use of contraception, and last consensual intercourse
  • Pertinent details of the assault
    ○ Number of perpetrators

- ○ Time and location of the assault
- ○ Type of sexual contact including use of condoms, ejaculation
- ○ Occurrence of any physical violence or use of weapons
- ○ Use of any alcohol or drugs by the patient or alleged perpetrator(s)
- Activities since the assault that may influence physical evidence found, such as showering, urinating, brushing teeth, changing clothes

▶ Physical exam should be carefully performed in order to identify and document presence of any injuries. Consider photographing injuries for the medical record.
- Document patient's emotional state.
- Careful skin examination for abrasions, lacerations, contusions.
- Identify foreign material and consider use of an ultraviolet light (Wood's lamp) as semen will fluoresce.
- Petechiae and ruptured retinal vessels may suggest strangulation.
- Oral exam for tears of the frenulum, broken teeth, and contusions of the palate.
- Bite marks, particularly on the breasts and genitals.
- Speculum exam should use water as a lubricant only.
  - ○ Close inspection of the perineum
  - ○ Evidence of trauma such as tears and abrasions
  - ○ Pooled secretions in the posterior fornix of the vagina
- Anal/rectal exam as directed by the history.
  - ○ Rectal tone.
  - ○ Consider anal wash in situations of anal penetration (5–10 cc of sterile saline instilled into rectum then aspirated after 2 minutes).

▶ Evidence collection proceeds through the use of a standardized rape kit.
- Collection of victim's clothes
- Careful documentation of all injuries/physical exam findings
- Collection of hair samples
- Collection of swabs for DNA evidence at sites of penetration

▶ Lab testing:
- As indicated by victim's injuries.
- Consider HIV, RPR, and hepatitis serologies.
- Pregnancy testing.

▶ Prophylactic treatment:
  • Only 30% of sexual assault victims follow up after their initial assessment, so, rather than waiting for culture results, prophylactic treatment should be considered.
  • STDs: gonorrhea, chlamydia, bacterial vaginosis, *Trichomonas* are the most common infections transmitted after a sexual assault.
    ◦ Ceftriaxone, 125 mg IM, **plus**
    ◦ Metronidazole, 2 g PO × 1 dose, **plus**
    ◦ Azithromycin, 1 g PO × 1 dose, or doxycycline, 100 mg PO bid × 7 days
  • HIV:
    ◦ Risk from a single sexual encounter is 1%, but there are documented cases of HIV being acquired from sexual assaults.
    ◦ Current recommendation is baseline testing and follow-up at 3, 6, and 12 months post-exposure.
    ◦ If prophylaxis is desired in a high-risk setting such as an assault by a known HIV-positive assailant, current therapy is zidovudine, 300 mg bid, and lamivudine, 150 mg bid, for 28 days. Addition of a protease inhibitor may also be considered.
  • Pregnancy:
    ◦ Occurs in 1% of sexual assault victims.
    ◦ Evaluate for pre-existing pregnancy.
    ◦ If within 72 hours of assault, use standard post-coital contraception regimes, such as levonorgestrel (Plan B).
  • Hepatitis B:
    ◦ Hepatitis B vaccination should be considered.

DISPOSITION

▶ Ascertain that the patient has a safe destination and friends or family for support.
▶ Arrangements for medical follow-up 1–2 weeks later if uninjured, and otherwise as dictated by physical injuries. Follow-up considerations include repeat STD and HIV testing.
▶ Referrals for counseling and crisis hotlines.

CHAPTER 63

APPROACH TO PEDIATRIC FEVER

Hadar Tucker

▶ Fever is defined as rectal temperature > 100.4° F (38° C). Rectal or oral temperatures should be measured in young children.
▶ Infants who were febrile at home but not in the ED warrant the same evaluation they would have received if they had been febrile in the ED.
▶ Fever is a marker of underlying illness. Response to antipyretics does not distinguish children with serious bacterial illness from those with viral infections.
▶ Neonates and immunocompromised patients may present with hypothermia rather then fever in the presence of a serious bacterial infection.

GENERAL APPROACH

▶ The initial approach to fever is guided by the patient's age, immunization status, and how sick the child looks (toxicity). Clinical assessment of toxicity is less reliable in infants < 4–12 weeks and immunocompromised children.
▶ Toxic-appearing children need a full sepsis evaluation and usually empiric treatment for possible bacterial illness (sepsis evaluation: blood, urine, CSF analysis and cultures ± stool cultures, and CXR).
▶ *Toxicity* is a clinical judgment. Toxic infants frequently have lethargy, poor perfusion, cyanosis, tachycardia or bradycardia, and hypo- or hyperventilation. Poor perfusion can be assessed by capillary refill > 2–3 seconds. Factors to consider in assessing infant mental status include irritability, poor eye contact, and failure to interact with their environment.
▶ LP is needed when bacterial meningitis cannot be excluded clinically. Children > 3 months with bacterial meningitis almost always appear toxic; the exceptions are those children exam-

ined during the first day of illness and severely immunocompromised children.

AGE-SPECIFIC APPROACH TO FEVER

Neonates (< 4 Weeks of Age)

▶ Neonates with fever should receive a complete sepsis evaluation regardless of whether they have a viral source for their fever (blood, urine, and CSF cultures, along with a CXR, UA, CBC, and CSF analysis). These children always require hospital admission.

▶ Remember to obtain a maternal history of group B streptococcus (GBS), TORCH, or other perinatal infections: "Was mom being treated for anything?"

▶ Febrile neonates are usually treated with
  • Ampicillin, 200 mg/kg/day IV divided into doses q4–6h (to treat *Listeria*) along with **either**
  • Gentamicin, 5–7.5 mg/kg/day IV divided into doses q8–12h, **or**
  • Cefotaxime, 100–200 mg/kg/day IV divided into doses q6–12h (ceftriaxone is relatively contraindicated in this group due to biliary stasis).
  • Add acyclovir, 30 mg/kg/day IV divided into doses q8h if there is reason to suspect herpes virus infection.
  • Consider adding vancomycin, 40–60 mg/kg/day IV divided into doses q6h if there is a high local prevalence of penicillin-resistant streptococci.

4–12 Weeks of Age with No Obvious Source of Infection on Physical Exam

▶ The Philadelphia and Rochester criteria (Table 63-1) identify a low-risk group among febrile 8- to 12-week-old children who can be treated as outpatients without antibiotics. Low-risk children by these criteria have < 1% chance of serious bacterial illness. If all criteria are met, the Rochester criteria do not mandate CSF analysis; in practice, many physicians routinely include an LP for CSF analysis in the evaluation of all febrile children in whom they cannot clinically exclude meningitis.

▶ Another option for non-toxic children aged 8–12 weeks who are low risk based on history and ED evaluation is to discharge home after 50 mg/kg of ceftriaxone (IV/IM), pending culture

TABLE 63-1.
ROCHESTER CRITERIA

A. Well-appearing infant
B. No skeletal, soft tissue, skin, or ear infections
C. Full-term birth (> 37 weeks)
D. No prior illness
   1. No prior hospitalizations
   2. Not hospitalized longer than mother after delivery
   3. No prior antibiotics
   4. No history of hyperbilirubinemia
   5. No chronic or underlying illness
E. CBC normal
   1. WBC normal (5000–15,000/mm^3)
   2. Bands < 1500/mm^3
F. Other lab findings
   1. If diarrhea is present, fecal leukocytes < 5/hpf
   2. Urine WBCs < 10/hpf

results. All febrile children aged 4–12 weeks who are discharged from the ED should be re-evaluated within 24 hours.

▶ Controversies:

- Evaluation and management of well-appearing children aged 4–8 weeks. Safest approach in this group is to proceed with septic work-up and admission.
- Whether an LP is mandatory in children aged 4–12 weeks with an apparent bacterial source of infection (pyelonephritis, cellulitis, omphalitis, pneumonia). Safest approach is to do an LP on any child < 12 weeks who will be treated with antibiotics.
- The approach to febrile children between 4 and 12 weeks with an obvious viral source (e.g., bronchiolitis).
  - 4- to 8-week-old children in this group usually need at least a catheterized UA and culture.

▶ Febrile children with any exam findings suggesting pneumonia should have a CXR obtained. Children < 12 weeks with pneumonia usually require admission.

12 Weeks to 24 Months

▶ Well-appearing children > 12 weeks with an obvious viral source of fever rarely need lab evaluation.

▶ Examples of obvious viral sources are viral exanthems (e.g., chicken pox), bronchiolitis, non-streptococcal exudative pharyngitis, or pharyngitis associated with viral lesions. Note: Obvious pharyngitis is sometimes missed by not getting a good look at the posterior pharynx in an uncooperative child.

▶ Caution with fever in children who appear sick or have not had their first three sets of immunizations: Viral URI and OM are so common that they may occur at the same time as other sources of fever. Many serious illnesses mimic gastroenteritis.

▶ Fully immunized (DPT × 3, HIB × 3, Prevnar × 3), non–toxic-appearing children have a very low incidence of serious bacterial infection (< 1%). Urine culture is the most useful lab test in these children.

▶ Catheterized urine should be obtained from girls and non-circumcised boys < 24 months, and circumcised boys < 12 months who present with fever in the absence of an obvious source by history and physical exam.

▶ In clinical practice, there is a gray area between *toxic* and *non-toxic*. Some practitioners use an elevated peripheral WBC count as a marker for bacterial disease in this subset of sick children; currently, there are little data to either support or refute this approach. In general, the more toxic the child, the more extensive the evaluation and follow-up.

▶ Occult bacteremia: positive blood cultures obtained from non–toxic-appearing children without obvious source for their fever.

▶ Before the widespread use of the pneumococcal vaccine, the incidence of bacteremia in immunized children was ~3%. Most (80–90%) of the positive cultures grew strains of streptococcal pneumonia included in the current vaccine. Most streptococcal pneumonia bacteremia cleared even without treatment.

▶ The current incidence of bacteremia is thought to be < 1% in fully immunized children. Children who seem toxic or are not immunized are at higher risk for bacteremia. Children with very high fevers may also be at increased risk for bacteremia.

▶ Radiologic evaluation for pneumonia is controversial. In children > 3 months, no single physical finding reliably predicts pneumonia. It is difficult to distinguish bacterial from viral pneumonias by CXR. Most clinicians either test or empirically treat children > 3 months clinically suspected of having pneumonia. Consider a CXR in a febrile child without obvious source for fever and a peripheral WBC count > 20,000 even without clinical evidence of pneumonia.

CHAPTER 64

APPROACH TO PEDIATRIC DEHYDRATION

Amy Shirk

▶ Dehydration is a loss of body water and salt.
▶ Infectious gastroenteritis is the most common cause of pediatric dehydration.

PATHOPHYSIOLOGY

▶ Infants have an increased BSA leading to increased insensible losses.
▶ Infant kidneys have immature collecting tubules that do not maximally concentrate urine.
▶ Infants have higher caloric and water requirements.

CLASSIFICATION OF DEHYDRATION

▶ Dehydration is commonly classified as
  • Isotonic: Water and salt are lost in equal concentrations.
  • Hypotonic: Salt is lost in greater concentration than water. Often occurs when only free water is used to replace salt and water loss. Na < 130.
  • Hypertonic: Free water is lost in a greater proportion than salt. Due to the increased level of intracellular dehydration in these children, their fluid deficits must be replaced more slowly to avoid a rapid fluid shift that may precipitate cerebral edema.

CLINICAL PRESENTATION

▶ Mild: 5% or 50 ml/kg fluid loss, dry mucus membranes, normal vital signs, oliguria
▶ Moderate: 10% or 100 ml/kg loss, tachycardia, stable BP, marked oliguria, sunken eyes and fontanelle, decreased skin turgor, irritable or lethargic

▶ Severe: 15% or 150 ml/kg loss, tachycardia, hypotension, poor perfusion, extreme lethargy

MANAGEMENT
Oral Rehydration Therapy

▶ Oral rehydration therapy (ORT) relies on the coupled transport of sodium and glucose in the intestine.

▶ It is successful in treating dehydration secondary to gastroenteritis in 90% of children.

▶ Oral rehydration solutions (ORS) have glucose concentrations that do not exceed the sodium concentration in millimoles by more than 2:1.

▶ Small volumes of fluid (5 cc) are administered every 5 minutes.

▶ Children in the mildly dehydrated category with 5% fluid loss are given 50 ml/kg of ORS plus ongoing losses over 4 hours.

▶ Moderate dehydration with a 10% fluid loss is replaced as 100 ml/kg of ORS plus ongoing losses over 4 hours.

▶ Ongoing losses are estimated at 10 ml/kg/stool.

▶ Age-appropriate feedings are slowly reintroduced once the child is rehydrated.

▶ ORT is labor intensive and time consuming and requires willing parents.

Intravenous Fluid Therapy

▶ Any child with signs of circulatory instability warrants immediate IV volume resuscitation.

▶ The initial phase of management of moderate to severe dehydration consists of a 20 ml/kg bolus of an isotonic fluid such as 0.9% NS.

Rehydration in Isotonic Dehydration

▶ The initial fluid bolus of 20 ml/kg accounts for 2% of body mass or 2% of the fluid deficit. The remainder of the deficit should be replaced over the next 8 hours.

Rehydration Plan in Hypertonic Dehydration

▶ Infants who are suffering from hypertonic dehydration must have their fluid deficits replaced more slowly to prevent fluid shifts that may result in cerebral edema.

▶ Fluid bolus is subtracted from the overall deficit, and the remaining deficit is added to the maintenance fluid requirements for 2 days and administered at a constant rate over 48 hours.

DISPOSITION

▶ All infants who appear toxic with signs of moderate or severe dehydration should be admitted.

▶ Infants with significant ongoing losses or who are unable to tolerate oral rehydration should also be admitted.

▶ Admission should be considered in infants who are even mildly dehydrated with ongoing losses who do not have parents reliable to perform rehydration therapy.

▶ The parents of all children who are discharged should be given explicit discharge instructions to monitor for worsening dehydration.

CHAPTER 65

PEDIATRIC URINARY TRACT INFECTIONS

Thomas J. Deegan

▶ Pyelonephritis can lead to renal scarring in 27–64% of children < 5 years of age.
▶ Complications of renal scarring:
  • 10–20% risk of HTN
  • 10% risk of ESRD
▶ UTI is often the presentation of significant urinary anomalies that will increase risk of recurrent infection and complications.
  • Vesicoureteral reflux most common anomaly
▶ Pathogens same as adults—enteric bacteria: *Escherichia coli*, *Proteus*, *Klebsiella*, *Enterococcus*, *Enterobacter*, *Pseudomonas*, *Serratia*.
  • Neonates: enteric bacteria and group B streptococcus (GBS)
  • Viral hemorrhagic cystitis: adenovirus

CLINICAL PRESENTATION

▶ Young children do not manifest classic symptoms of UTI/ pyelonephritis.
▶ ~5% of children between 2 months and 2 years presenting with fever and no focus of infection on exam have a UTI as the source of infection.
  • URI and OM are not considered a focus.
▶ Risk factors: fever and no focus of infection in girls < 2 years, boys ≤ 1 year
  • Sex: girls 4.3%, boys 1.8%
  • Race: white 10.7%, African-American 2.1%, white girls 16.1%
  • Circumcision: yes 1.2%, no 8.0%
▶ Infants may present with fever, poor feeding, irritability, vomiting, or diarrhea.
▶ Febrile infants ≤ 2 months are at much higher risk.
  • UA and urine culture are routine part of septic work-up.

▶ All children with febrile UTI should be considered for pyelonephritis.

EMERGENCY DEPARTMENT MANAGEMENT
Obtaining a Urine Specimen

▶ "Bag" urine [pediatric urine collector (PUC)]: 85% false-positive rate
  • Only for immunocompromised patient, bladder catheterization contraindicated
▶ Supra-pubic aspiration (SPA): gold standard, but low success rate
▶ Bladder catheterization: most common method in non–toilet-trained child
▶ Midstream clean catch specimen in toilet-trained child

Making the Diagnosis

▶ UA and urine culture and sensitivities.
  • **Always** send urine culture and sensitivities if suspect UTI.
▶ CBC and blood cultures in child 2 months–2 years if clinically looks sick (occult bacteremia) or if suspect pyelonephritis.
▶ Consider CBC, ESR, CRP, and blood cultures if suspect pyelonephritis in older children.

Urinalysis

▶ Leukocyte esterase (LE) only: 83% sensitivity, 84% specificity
▶ Nitrite only: 50% sensitivity, 98% specificity
▶ LE or nitrite: 88% sensitivity, 93% specificity
▶ ≥ 10 WBC: 77% sensitivity, 89% specificity
▶ Gram's stain positive for bacteria: 93% sensitivity, 95% specificity

Urine Culture

▶ SPA: > 99% probability of infection if
  • Gram-negative bacilli: any growth
  • Gram-positive cocci: > few thousand colonies
▶ Bladder catheter
  • > 100,000 colonies: 95% probability of infection
  • 10–100,000 colonies: suspicious, repeat culture
▶ Clean catch
  • Male: > 10,000 colonies
  • Female: > 100,000 colonies, 80% probability of infection

Treatment

Uncomplicated Cystitis
▶ *E. coli* most common pathogen, ampicillin resistance common
▶ SMX-TMP, 8–12 mg/kg/day divided dose bid
▶ Cephalexin, 50–100 mg/kg/day divided dose tid
▶ Duration: 5–7 days, 3 days in adolescents

Febrile UTI/Pyelonephritis
▶ Admit
  • Any infant < 2 months
  • 2 months–2 years and > 2 years if
    ○ Toxic, vomiting, poor oral intake, dehydration, unable to take PO antibiotics
    ○ Failure to improve, still febrile after 24–48 hours oral antibiotics
  • Parenteral antibiotics
    ○ Ampicillin, 50 mg/kg q6h, **plus**
    ○ Gentamicin, 2–2.5 mg/kg q8h, **or**
    ○ Ceftriaxone, 50 mg/kg q24h or cefotaxime, 50 mg/kg q6h
    ○ Cefazolin, 50–100 mg/kg divided dose q8h
  • IV until afebrile for 24 hours then PO antibiotics for 10–14 days more
▶ Outpatient treatment
  • Cefixime, 8 mg/kg/day divided dose bid.
  • Cefprozil, 30 mg/kg/day divided dose bid.
  • Duration: 10–14 days.
  • Initial dose of ceftriaxone, 50 mg/kg IM/IV, is likely no more effective than PO, but is still often given.
▶ Prophylaxis
  • Consider prophylaxis until outpatient work-up complete.
  • SMX-TMP, single dose 4–6 mg/kg qhs.
  • Amoxicillin, 20 mg/kg qhs, if sulfa allergic.
▶ Outpatient work-up
  • Renal ultrasound plus VCUG or radionuclide VCUG (girls only).
  • All children < 5 years with a UTI.
  • Any child with a febrile UTI/pyelonephritis.
  • School-aged girls who have had two or more UTIs.
  • Any male with a UTI, regardless of age.

- Most common finding is vesicoureteral reflux in 40% of patients.

◐ **PEARLS AND PITFALLS**

- Diagnosis and treatment of UTI in infants and young children are aimed at prevention of renal scarring and long-term complications (HTN, renal failure/ESRD).
- All infants ≤ 2 months with fever: bladder catheterization or supra-pubic tap for UA and culture and sensitivities always part of the sepsis evaluation.
- Suspect (and look for) UTI in febrile girls < 2 years, boys ≤ 6–12 months without a focus of infection.
- A URI or OM does not constitute a focus of infection.
- A "bag" urine specimen is inadequate for culture.
- Strongly consider sending a urine culture and sensitivities if you catheterize, regardless of the UA result. UA may be negative in up to 20% of infants/children with UTI.
- **Never** treat presumptively at **any** age without sending a urine culture and sensitivities.

CHAPTER 66

OTITIS MEDIA

Michele Nypaver

- Most common infection for which antibiotics are prescribed in children in U.S.
- Relatively benign disease in industrialized nations where antibiotics are **not** routinely prescribed acutely without increased incidence of complication rate

DEFINITIONS

- **Acute OM (AOM):** *symptomatic* middle ear disease includes both symptoms and signs of inflammation in the presence of middle ear effusion (MEE).
- **OM with effusion (OME):** *asymptomatic* middle ear disease with signs of MEE without inflammation.
- Risk factors for AOM: respiratory viral illness, nasopharyngeal carriage of pathogens, attendance in day care, multiple siblings, absence of breast-feeding, tobacco smoke exposure.
- Risk factors for resistant bacterial AOM pathogens: recent antibiotic use, attendance in day care, and age < 2 years.

CLINICAL PRESENTATION

- Most children present with ear pain with or without fever or signs of respiratory illness.
- Pre- and non-verbal children may demonstrate irritability with or without above signs.

EMERGENCY DEPARTMENT MANAGEMENT

Diagnosis

- Clinical presentation and clear visualization of TM with otoscopy (otoscope **and** insufflator) for accurate diagnosis are key.

▶ **AOM diagnosis** (requires all three):
  • Recent onset of signs and symptoms of middle ear inflammation and effusion, **and**
  • Presence of MEE demonstrated by bulging TM, limited or absent TM mobility, air fluid level behind TM, or otorrhea, **and**
  • Signs and symptoms of middle ear inflammation: erythema of TM **or** otalgia [discomfort clearly referable to the ear(s) precluding normal activity or sleep]
▶ **OME diagnosis:** Patient has no specific ear symptoms!
  • Presence of MEE without TM inflammation (not red or bulging).
  • Insufflation shows reduced or absent TM movement.
  • Residual effusions after AOM may be present for weeks.
  • Persistent MEEs are defined as those present > 16 weeks after AOM.

Treatment

▶ Goals: Eradicate pathogen, relieve symptoms (treat pain), prevent OME, and avoid complications.
▶ Pain and fever relief:
  • Tylenol, 15 mg/kg/dose q4h.
  • Ibuprofen, 10 mg/kg/dose q6h.
  • Topicals (benzocaine): Topical drops may provide brief, effective pain relief.
▶ Criteria for initial antibiotic treatment vs. observation*. Observation option depends on age, certainty of diagnosis, and severity of illness.
  • Age < 6 months, certain or uncertain diagnosis: antibiotics
  • Age 6 months to 2 years:
    ○ Certain diagnosis: antibiotics
    ○ Uncertain diagnosis (severe illness†): antibiotics
    ○ Uncertain diagnosis (non-severe illness†): observation option
  • Age ≥ 2 years:
    ○ Certain diagnosis (severe illness): antibiotics

---

*Observation: delay of antibiotic treatment 48–72 hours, treat supportively only. Requires patient access to repeat medical evaluation during observation period if symptoms worsen or do not improve **and** convenient access to medications if needed. Antibiotics are indicated if child has not improved by 48–72 hours.
†Severe illness: moderate to severe otalgia or fever ≥ 39° C.

- ○ Certain diagnosis (non-severe illness): observation option
- ○ Uncertain diagnosis (non-severe illness): observation option
▶ Antibiotic regimen:
  - • First choice: amoxicillin, 80–90 mg/kg/day divided in two doses daily for 10 days (children > 6 years with mild to moderate disease may be treated for 5–7 days).
  - • Alternate therapy (for patients with severe illness or for whom better beta-lactamase organism coverage is desired):
    - ○ Augmentin, 80–90 mg/kg/day (or amoxicillin component) with 6.4 mg/kg/day (clavulanate component) in two divided doses for penicillin-allergic patients
    - ○ Type 1 allergy (urticaria or anaphylaxis):
      - ■ Azithromycin (Zithromax), 10 mg/kg/day on day one, 5 mg/kg/day once daily on days 2–5 (maximum 1 g/24 hours)
      - ■ Clarithromycin (Biaxin), 15 mg/kg/day divided in two doses daily
      - ■ Erythromycin ethylsuccinate/sulfisoxazole (Pediazole), 50 mg/kg/day erythromycin in three doses (maximum 2 g/24 hours)
      - ■ SMX-TMP (Bactrim), 6–10 mg/kg/day, TMP component
    - ○ Non–type 1 allergy:
      - ■ Cefdinir, 14 mg/kg/day divided once or twice daily (maximum 600 mg/24 hours)
      - ■ Cefpodoxime, 10 mg/kg/day once daily (maximum 400 mg/24 hours)
      - ■ Cefuroxime, 30 mg/kg/day divided in two doses daily (maximum 6 g/24 hours)
    - ○ Patients who cannot tolerate PO medications or are vomiting:
      - ■ Ceftriaxone, 50 mg/kg single IM dose
▶ Complications: treatment failure, mastoiditis, chronic OME, and meningitis.

Disposition

▶ Outpatient treatment with follow-up for worsening or non-improvement of symptoms
▶ Follow-up for responsive patients in 3–4 weeks for effusion evaluation

CHAPTER 67

BRONCHIOLITIS

Hadar Tucker

▶ Expiratory wheezing associated with a URI in children < 1 year

PATHOPHYSIOLOGY AND EPIDEMIOLOGY

▶ Predominantly caused by RSV.
▶ Epidemics each winter between the months of October and April.
▶ Upper respiratory viruses travel down the respiratory tract where dead epithelial cells cause mucous plugging.

CLINICAL FINDINGS

▶ Upper respiratory symptoms (cough, rhinorrhea, fever)
▶ Increased RR
▶ Expiratory wheezing
▶ Intercostal retractions

DIFFERENTIAL DIAGNOSIS

▶ Asthma: prior history of wheezing, children > 1–2 years, atopy, FH.
▶ Pneumonia: may coexist with bronchiolitis; most are viral. May be difficult to distinguish from chlamydial pneumonia in infants, unless have positive chlamydial serology.
▶ FB aspiration: sudden onset, no predominant URI symptoms.
▶ CHF: may mimic respiratory disease in infants. Cardiac murmurs on exam or evidence of cardiac enlargement on CXR favors diagnosis of CHF.

DIAGNOSTIC STUDIES

▶ Pulse oximetry.
▶ Consider CXR in first time wheezing patients or in less classic presentations.
▶ Other studies (CBC, electrolytes, blood gas, testing for RSV, blood culture) only in severely ill children, or when diagnosis is not clear by history and physical.

TREATMENT IS SUPPORTIVE

▶ O_2 and IVF are the only consistently useful supportive therapy if needed.

OTHER NON-PROVEN THERAPIES

▶ Albuterol: clinical improvement in minority of cases, most often those with history of atopy or FH of asthma. Discontinue if not effective (side effects).
▶ Racemic epinephrine (nebulized) may temporarily improve symptoms in minority of cases.
▶ Steroids: still controversial unless strong suspicion that patient has asthma.
▶ Ribavirin not useful in ED setting and infrequently used in PICU because of risk-benefit ratio.

PREVENTION

▶ Palivizumab (Synagis): monoclonal antibody that inhibits RSV replication. Indicated for prevention of RSV lower respiratory tract disease in high-risk patients. Monthly IM doses throughout RSV season.

ADMISSION CRITERIA

▶ Ill-appearing
▶ Hypoxia (O_2 saturation < 93% while patient awake)
▶ Dehydration
▶ Persistent tachypnea (> 60), concern about infant tiring out
▶ Most very young children (< 8 weeks or premature) and children with coexisting pneumonia, especially if no primary care provider or no follow-up available

CHAPTER 68

NEONATAL JAUNDICE

Michelle Macy

▶ Jaundice is yellowing of the skin and sclera associated with hyperbilirubinemia.

▶ Present in 65% of term infants in the first week of life.

▶ Clinically apparent at total bilirubin levels ≥ 5 mg/dl.

▶ Levels roughly correlate with degree of jaundice increasing from head to toe:
   • Face ~5 mg/dl
   • Mid-abdomen ~15 mg/dl
   • Soles ~20 mg/dl

DIFFERENTIAL DIAGNOSIS BASED ON ONSET OF JAUNDICE
First 24 Hours of Life

▶ Increased production of indirect/unconjugated bilirubin
   • Coombs'-positive hemolysis
     ○ ABO, Rh, minor blood type incompatibility
   • Coombs'-negative hemolysis
     ○ Hereditary spherocytosis, G6PD deficiency
   • Hemorrhage
     ○ Cephalohematoma, extensive skin bruising
   • Polycythemia (HCT > 60)
     ○ Infant of diabetic mother, delayed cord clamping
   • Increased enterohepatic circulation
     ○ Paralytic ileus or bowel obstruction
   • Infectious
     ○ Sepsis, cytomegalic inclusion disease, rubella, toxoplasmosis

24–72 Hours of Life

▶ Physiologic jaundice
   • Starts after 24 hours of life, rises < 5 mg/dl/day, peaks at day 3–5 with total bilirubin < 15 mg/dl.

- Clinical jaundice resolved by 1 week in term infants, 2 weeks in preterm.
- Due to increased destruction of RBCs with immature conjugation and excretion.
▶ Breast-feeding
  - Decreased intake, increased enterohepatic circulation
  - Without increased bilirubin production
▶ Decreased conjugation
  - Familial non-hemolytic icterus, Crigler-Najjar, Gilbert's syndrome

From 72 Hours through 7 Days of Life

▶ Breast-feeding, sepsis, UTI, congenital infections (syphilis, toxoplasmosis, CMV, enterovirus, rubella, HSV)

After 7 Days of Life

▶ Sepsis, hepatitis
▶ Metabolic: galactosemia, hypothyroid, and cystic fibrosis
▶ Anatomic: biliary atresia
▶ Breast milk jaundice
  - Diagnosis of exclusion
    ○ Hold breast milk 1–2 days, formula supplement
    ○ Then resume breast milk

CLINICAL PRESENTATION

▶ Mild: sleepiness and decreased feeding
▶ Severe: lethargy and loss of Moro reflex
▶ Presentation can be consistent with
  - Sepsis, asphyxia, hypoglycemia, and intracranial hemorrhage
▶ Bilirubin encephalopathy
  - Describes the acute changes in the setting of hyperbilirubinemia
▶ Kernicterus
  - Term for permanent sequelae of deposition of free unconjugated bilirubin in basal ganglia and brainstem nuclei
  - Increased risk if bilirubin levels > 20 in Rh-isoimmunized infant

TABLE 68-1.
BILIRUBIN RANGES FOR NEWBORNS

Age	Total bilirubin (mg/dl)
Birth	> 4–6
12 hours	> 6–9
24 hours	> 8–12
48 hours	> 11–15
72 hours	> 13–18
96 hours	> 15–20

EMERGENCY DEPARTMENT MANAGEMENT

▶ History including birth weight, feeding, elimination.
  - Average weight loss by day three is 5–10% in exclusively breast-fed infants.
  - 4–6 wet diapers.
  - 3–4 stools transitioning from meconium to mustard yellow, mushy.
  - Dark urine, acholic stools clue to obstructive jaundice.
▶ Measure total bilirubin.
▶ Interpret levels in terms of age in hours.
▶ Threshold for phototherapy is higher with increasing age.
▶ Consider phototherapy in well-appearing infants > 35 weeks' gestation using ranges listed in Table 68-1.
▶ Urine for reducing substances, newborn galactosemia, hypothyroid screen, especially if jaundice beyond 3 weeks or sick infant.
▶ Sepsis evaluation as clinically indicated.
▶ If bilirubin rising rapidly and unexplained by history and physical exam:
  - Blood type, Coombs' testing, CBC, smear for RBC morphology.
  - Measure direct/conjugated bilirubin.
▶ Approaching exchange transfusion level or not responding:
  - Consider reticulocyte count, G6PD, albumin.
  - $ETCO_2$ can confirm presence or absence of hemolysis.
▶ If elevated direct/conjugated bilirubin:
  - UA and urine culture, assess for sepsis.

TREATMENT

▶ Goal: Prevent concentration of indirect bilirubin from reaching neurotoxic levels.

▶ Continue breast-feeding, nursing 8–12 times per day, or bottle feed every 2–3 hours.

▶ IVF to correct dehydration but does not appear to impact bilirubin levels.

▶ If exchange transfusion level is reached or if > 25 at any time, admit directly to the hospital and begin intensive phototherapy.

▶ Phototherapy:
  • Expect decrease of 1–2 mg/dl in 4–6 hours.
  • Cover eyes when using overhead lights.
  • Converts toxic native unconjugated bilirubin to a water-soluble isomer.
  • If > 25 mg/dl, repeat within 2–3 hours.
  • If 20–25 mg/dl, repeat within 3–4 hours.
  • If < 20 mg/dl, repeat in 4–6 hours.
  • If continues to fall, repeat in 8–12 hours.
  • When < 13–14 mg/dl, discontinue phototherapy (check for rebound in 24 hours).

▶ Bronze baby syndrome: accumulation of porphyrins and other metabolites in plasma of infants who develop cholestasis and are treated with phototherapy.

▶ Exchange transfusion:
  • Bilirubin > 25 mg/dl, or > 20 mg/dl if sick, or < 38 weeks' gestation
    ◦ Type and cross-match and prepare for exchange transfusion.
  • If the total bilirubin level is above the exchange level
    ◦ Repeat measurement every 2–3 hours.
    ◦ Consider exchange if the total bilirubin remains above levels indicated.

CHAPTER 69

METABOLIC DISORDERS IN CHILDREN

Rachel Stanley

- ▶ Diverse group of enzyme or transport system disorders.
- ▶ Metabolites accumulate in the body causing serious CNS toxicity.
- ▶ Consider in the differential diagnosis of any patient with unexplained neurologic findings.

HISTORICAL CLUES

- ▶ Episodic nature (vomiting, lethargy)
- ▶ Preceding infection or high protein intake
- ▶ Multiple admissions to hospital with recovery after IVF and glucose
- ▶ Psychomotor retardation or growth failure

TYPES OF DISORDERS

Urea Cycle Defects

- ▶ Ammonia is converted to urea via the urea cycle. Accumulation of ammonia occurs in primary urea cycle defects or hepatic amino acid transport defects.

Organic Acidurias

- ▶ Excessive accumulation of one or more organic acids in body fluids; may be secondary to lactic acidosis (tissue hypoxia) or ketoacidosis (diabetes mellitus)

Galactosemia

- ▶ Failure to metabolize galactose to glucose.
- ▶ Most cases inherited deficiency of galactose-1-phosphate uridyltransferase.
- ▶ Accumulation of galactose in the body affects brain, liver, eyes, and kidneys.

CLINICAL PRESENTATION
Neonatal

▶ Appears well at birth, then progressive deterioration after protein ingestion in formula.

▶ Vomiting, poor feeding, hypotonia, decreased level of consciousness, coma.

▶ Organic acidurias may also have hepatomegaly and a bizarre odor to urine, breath, saliva, or cerumen. Maple syrup smell: maple syrup urine disease. Sweaty socks smell: isovaleric acidemia.

▶ Galactosemia can present within 1 week of life with jaundice, hepatomegaly, vomiting, lethargy, cataracts, or *Escherichia coli* sepsis.

Post-Neonatal Period

▶ Recurrent coma with retarded psychomotor development.

▶ Undiagnosed patients often have diagnosis of cerebral palsy or developmental delay of unknown etiology.

▶ Vomiting or lethargy after ingestion of protein-rich foods, recurrent vomiting, or ataxia.

▶ Minor infections precipitate hyperammonemia, recurrent hospitalizations.

▶ Organic acidurias/galactosemia may not present with hyperammonemia.

▶ Galactosemia may not present until older (2–3 years), with hepatomegaly, growth failure, cataracts, and mental retardation.

LAB DIAGNOSIS

▶ Urea cycle defects: routine electrolytes, pH, CBC, UA, and CSF testing usually normal. OTC deficiency: orotic acid crystals in urine. CSF enzymes may be high. Check ammonia and blood amino acids.

▶ Organic acidurias: may present with unexplained high anion gap, hyperchloremic metabolic acidosis, ketonuria, hypoglycemia, hyperammonemia, neutropenia, thrombocytopenia, elevated lactate, and pyruvate in primary lactic acidosis. Urine organic acid analysis points to the specific disorder.

▶ Galactosemia: presence of reducing substances in the urine. Assay of blood and urine for galactose. Abnormal LFTs, jaundice with initial elevated indirect bilirubin followed by elevated direct bilirubin 1–2 weeks later. Renal tubular dysfunction manifest by hyperchloremic metabolic acidosis.

▶ Many states screen for the most common inborn errors at birth.

MANAGEMENT
Urea Cycle Defects

▶ Lower ammonia, minimize production, increase removal
- IV D10 0.5NS at twice maintenance (beware cerebral edema)
- Dialysis and exchange transfusion

▶ Antidotes
- Carbamyl phosphate synthetase deficiency or OTC deficiency: give sodium benzoate, 250–500 mg/kg/day as a 10% solution
- Citrullinemia or argininosuccinicaciduria: give arginine parenterally, 1–3 mmol/kg/day

▶ Mainstay of treatment
- Low-protein diet, 1–2 g/kg/day

Organic Acidurias

▶ Correction of metabolic abnormalities (acidosis)
- Bicarbonate, 1–2 mEq/kg, titrate to acidosis.
- Treat hypoglycemia with D10 infusion.

▶ Reduction of organic acid production
- Reduce protein intake and give adequate glucose to prevent endogenous protein catabolism.

▶ Enhancement of organic acid disposal
- Vitamins that stimulate the defective metabolic pathway
- Administration of L-carnitine, a cofactor for fatty acid oxidation, which may alleviate the toxicity associated with organic acidurias

Galactosemia

▶ Complete exclusion of dietary galactose by feeding infant lactose-free formula such as Nutramigen or Pregestimil. Appropriate cultures obtained if septic and antibiotic therapy promptly started.

FACTORS LEADING TO FALSELY ELEVATED SERUM AMMONIA

▶ Capillary blood specimen
▶ Prolonged standing of specimen at room temperature
▶ Specimen collected in ammonium heparin tube
▶ Mixed with air bubbles during collection
▶ Ammonia contaminated reagent water
▶ Improper lab standardization according to patient's age

CHAPTER 70

CHILD ABUSE

Elaine Pomeranz

▶ Child abuse is all too common and crosses all demographic lines. It should always be in the differential diagnosis of unwitnessed or unexplained injury.

CLINICAL PRESENTATION
Red Flags in History

▶ Lack of explanation for injury or story that changes over time
▶ History that does not fit pattern or severity of injury
▶ History that does not match developmental level of child
▶ Person caring for child at time of injury not present in the ED
▶ Delay in seeking medical care for injury
▶ Unusually large number of past ED visits for unexplained medical problems or injuries

Red Flags on Physical Exam

▶ Bruises in non-ambulatory infants, especially on the face
▶ Bruises in areas of the body that are usually protected
▶ Loop marks or parallel linear marks
▶ Sharply delineated pattern injury
  • Look for recognizable pattern such as finger marks or bite.
▶ Bilaterally symmetric or sharply demarcated burn injuries (e.g., stocking-glove distribution)
  • Check that pattern of sparing fits alleged mechanism.
▶ Long bone fractures in non-ambulatory infants
▶ Frenulum tears in infants
▶ Retinal hemorrhages in infants
▶ Genital injury in the absence of injury to labia majora, groin, and/or medial thighs

EMERGENCY DEPARTMENT MANAGEMENT

▶ Obtain history from verbal child without parent in the room when possible.

▶ Skeletal survey (without casts or splints) in children < 2 years; suspicious findings include
  • Posterior rib fractures
  • Multiple fractures in different stages of healing
  • Long bone fractures in non-ambulatory infants
  • Scapula fractures
  • Metaphyseal avulsion ("corner" or "bucket handle") fractures
  • Any fracture or healing pattern that does not fit history provided

▶ Head CT and dilated eye exam (by ophthalmologist if possible) if head trauma suspected in infant or toddler; this should include cases of infants with altered mental status and apparent life-threatening events (ALTEs).

▶ Documenting color of sclerae in cases with suspicious fractures.

▶ If sexual abuse is suspected, STD testing (when indicated based on history or physical exam) should include cultures (not just PCR or DNA amplification testing) for GC and chlamydia.

▶ Consider deferring exam to outpatient setting experienced in child sexual abuse evaluations if suspected abuse occurred > 72 hours previously.

▶ Consider using sedation, if indicated, to do genital exam in traumatized child.

▶ **Order lab tests** needed to exclude medical conditions that mimic abuse such as
  • PT/PTT and platelet count with worrisome bruising or intracranial hemorrhage
  • Calcium, phosphorus, alkaline phosphatase, copper, and PTH in cases with suspicious fractures
  • Toxicology testing with cases of altered mental status
  • Group A streptococcus rapid test and culture for cases of vulvovaginitis or anitis

▶ **Documentation** should include
  • Recording the sources for history given and details of what child says happened
  • Who lives in household with child; list all caregivers, custody arrangements, etc.

- Photos (digital or 35 mm) of any skin findings when possible; drawings (skin maps) if camera not available
- Description of demeanor of patient and all parties with patient
- Legible recording

❶ **PEARLS AND PITFALLS**
- Physicians are mandated reporters of suspected, not proven, abuse and neglect.
  - ○ Call your hospital's child abuse team, if available; **if not:**
  - ○ Call Protective Services in your county.
  - ○ Also call law enforcement if child needs to be hospitalized for injury thought to be the result of abuse.
  - ○ You do not need to report someone else's suspicions if you do not share them. Anyone can report their own suspicions.
- Do not assume you know who the perpetrator is; avoid making allegations in the ED setting.
- Do not suggest a plausible mechanism of injury to the caretakers if one has not been offered.
- A normal genital exam does not rule out sexual abuse.
- Consider the possibility of Münchhausen by proxy (MBP) if
  - ○ There is a discrepancy between history given and benign physical exam findings.
  - ○ Child is repeatedly brought for medical evaluation for problems only witnessed by one care provider, and increasingly invasive testing is sought.
  - ○ Usual treatments repeatedly fail.
  - ○ Rare diseases are frequently suspected or diagnosed.
  - ○ Child has had multiple health care providers at multiple medical institutions.
- If you suspect MBP:
  - ○ Do not confront the family in the ED with your suspicion.
  - ○ Carefully document what you observe vs. what you are told.
- Be safe. Ask for security to be present if you feel it is necessary before telling family that you are reporting the possibility of abuse.

CHAPTER 71

PHARYNGITIS

Athina Sikavitsas

- ► Pharyngitis (sore throat) common presentation.
- ► Majority of cases are infectious.
- ► The main bacterial cause is group A beta-hemolytic streptococcus (GABHS).
- ► GABHS is most common in 5- to 15-year-olds; less common < 5 years and in adults.
- ► Transmission of infectious cases is primarily by hand contact of nasal discharge.

CLINICAL PRESENTATION

- ► It is important to identify and treat GABHS so as to prevent acute rheumatic fever, suppurative complications, and to reduce transmission, along with improving clinical symptoms.
- ► GABHS usually presents with fever, headache, anterior cervical lymphadenopathy, sore throat, inflammation of pharynx and tonsils, erythema and exudates, nausea, vomiting, abdominal pain, and history of recent exposure.
- ► Symptoms of sore throat along with fever, coryza, cough, conjunctivitis, and diarrhea are suggestive of a viral etiology. EBV is most common.
- ► A sudden onset of severe sore throat, muffled voice, excessive drooling, and toxic appearance should raise the suspicion for epiglottitis, retropharyngeal abscesses, and peritonsillar abscess. Exam may reveal unequal tonsillar hypertrophy with uvular deviation.
- ► Exam should focus on oral and pharyngeal areas for any ulcers, bleeding gums, FBs, dental abscesses.

DIFFERENTIAL DIAGNOSIS

- ► Bacterial vs. viral etiologies

▸ Other causes include
  - FB, epiglottitis, peritonsillar abscess, retropharyngeal or lateral abscess, Kawasaki disease

EMERGENCY DEPARTMENT MANAGEMENT

▸ If GABHS is suspected by clinical exam, it should be confirmed by throat culture (gold standard) or rapid antigen detection test (RADT). RADTs have excellent specificity (> 90%) but lower sensitivity (< 80%).

▸ A positive culture or RADT confirms the diagnosis of GABHS. Negative RADT tests should be confirmed by culture in pediatric and adolescent patients. You have up to 9 days post-initiation of symptoms to treat.

Treatment

▸ Amoxicillin, 10 mg/kg/dose PO tid for 10 days.
▸ Alternative is single shot of IM penicillin G benzathine.
  - 600,000 units if < 27 kg
  - 1,200,000 units if > 27 kg
▸ For penicillin-allergic patients, erythromycin is acceptable, as are first-generation cephalosporins.
▸ Viral pharyngitis: symptomatic treatment, no antibiotics are indicated.
▸ Pain management of pharyngitis: analgesics, NSAIDs, oral dexamethasone (studies still underway in pediatrics, some pain relief in GABHS, good results in adults).
▸ Consider admission if unable to tolerate oral fluids, airway compromise.

CHAPTER 72

PEDIATRIC VIRAL EXANTHEMS

Nicole S. Sroufe

ERYTHEMA INFECTIOSUM (FIFTH'S DISEASE)— PARVOVIRUS B19

▶ Cases of erythema infectiosum (EI) occur sporadically or in outbreaks during late winter and early spring.

▶ Parvovirus B19 is spread via direct contact with respiratory secretions, percutaneous exposure to blood/blood products, and vertical transmission.

▶ Incubation period from acquisition of the virus to onset of initial symptoms is typically 4–14 days but may be as long as 21 days. Rash typically develops 2–3 weeks after infection.

▶ Patients with EI are most infectious prior to the onset of rash and are unlikely to shed virus after the rash develops.

Clinical Presentation

▶ EI is characterized by mild systemic symptoms, fever (15–30%), and a distinctive rash.

▶ Fever, malaise, myalgias, and headache often precede the characteristic rash by 7–10 days.

▶ The rash of EI is intensely red with a "slapped cheek" appearance, with circumoral pallor.

▶ Patients often develop a symmetric, maculopapular, lace-like rash on the trunk, which spreads peripherally to the arms, thighs, and buttocks, and is occasionally pruritic.

▶ The rash of EI fluctuates and may recur for weeks to months with exposure to sunlight or extremes of temperature.

▶ Transient aplastic crisis may develop in patients with hemolytic anemias and persists for 7–10 days. In these patients, rash is usually absent.

▶ Parvovirus B19 infection during pregnancy can cause fetal hydrops and death.

Management

▶ Diagnosis is primarily clinical.

▶ Detection of serum parvovirus B19–specific IgM antibody is the preferred diagnostic test in immunocompetent patients.

▶ No specific therapy is indicated. Treat supportively.

▶ Patients with aplastic crisis may require transfusion of PRBCs.

ERYTHEMA SUBITUM (ROSEOLA)—HUMAN HERPESVIRUS 6

▶ Human herpesvirus 6 (HHV-6) is a virus belonging to the Herpesviridae family.

▶ Infections occur throughout the year, with no seasonal variation.

▶ Rate of infection peaks between 6 and 24 months of age.

▶ Transmission of the virus occurs secondary to asymptomatic shedding of persistent virus in secretions.

▶ Mean incubation period is 9–10 days.

Clinical Presentation

▶ 20% of children infected with HHV-6 develop roseola.

▶ Infection manifests as high fever (> 39.5° C) persisting 3–7 days, followed by an erythematous maculopapular rash that lasts hours to days.

▶ Rash typically consists of small rose-pink macules and maculopapules that are most prominent on the neck and trunk.

▶ Rash lasts from a few hours to 2 days.

▶ Children often develop cervical and post-occipital lymphadenopathy, GI or respiratory tract signs, and inflamed TMs.

▶ Febrile seizures occur in 10–15% of all primary infections.

Management

▶ Diagnosis is primarily clinical.

▶ Commercial assays for detecting HHV-6 are under development.

▶ No specific therapy is indicated. Treat supportively.

▶ Immunocompromised patients may benefit from the administration of ganciclovir.

▶ Hospitalized patients with roseola require standard precautions only.

HAND-FOOT-MOUTH SYNDROME—COXSACKIE A16 VIRUS

▶ Transmission of coxsackie A16 occurs via fecal-oral and respiratory spread, as well as from mother to infant in the peripartum period.

▶ Mean incubation period is 3–6 days.

▶ Viral shedding occurs in asymptomatic patients, and fecal viral shedding can persist for several weeks after onset of infection. Respiratory viral shedding is limited to ≤ 7 days.

Clinical Presentation

▶ A brief prodrome of low-grade fever, anorexia, malaise, and pharyngitis is present prior to the development of a characteristic enanthem.

▶ Vesicular lesions develop in the mouth, quickly eroding to develop sharply marginated ulcers varying in size from a few millimeters to 2 cm.

▶ Lesions are commonly found on the buccal mucosa, tongue, palate, uvula, and anterior tonsillar pillars.

▶ The classic exanthema of hand-foot-mouth syndrome consists of gray-white angulated or round vesicles ranging from 3–7 mm in diameter.

▶ Lesions are most common on the dorsum of the hands and feet but may be present on the palms and soles, as well as the diaper region in infants.

▶ Lesions may be painful or pruritic.

Management

▶ Diagnosis is primarily clinical.

▶ No specific therapy is available. Treat supportively.

▶ In hospitalized patients with hand-foot-mouth syndrome, contact precautions are indicated in addition to standard precautions.

MEASLES (RUBEOLA)

▶ Measles virus is a paramyxovirus, an RNA virus with one serotype.

▶ Transmitted by direct contact with infectious droplets or by airborne spread. Humans are the only known natural host for the virus.

▶ Incubation period is generally 8–12 days from exposure to onset of symptoms.

▶ Patients are contagious from 1–2 days before onset of symptoms (3–5 days before the rash) to 4 days after appearance of the rash.

Clinical Presentation

▶ Onset of illness is characterized by high fever, cough, coryza, and conjunctivitis, lasting 2–4 days.

▶ Patients are often ill-appearing during the prodromal phase, and fever persists several days after onset of rash.

▶ Koplik's spots, tiny white or blue-gray specks superimposed on an erythematous base, located on the buccal mucosa, are pathognomonic of measles.

▶ 1–3 days after prodromal symptoms develop, patients develop an erythematous maculopapular rash that begins behind the ears and at the scalp margin with rapid spread caudally to involve the entire body.

▶ Measles rash is non-pruritic. Lesions gradually become confluent, persisting for 4–7 days.

▶ Most common complications: OM, bronchopneumonia, laryngotracheobronchitis (croup), diarrhea.

▶ Less common, but severe, complications: acute encephalitis (1/1000 cases), death (1–3/1000 cases), and subacute sclerosing panencephalitis (virtually non-existent in immunized populations).

Management

▶ All suspected and confirmed cases of measles should be reported to the local health department.

▶ Efforts should be made to confirm the diagnosis and to prevent transmission to susceptible individuals.

▶ Diagnosis is primarily clinical. However, it can be confirmed by several methods: positive serologic test for measles IgM antibody, significant increase in measles IgG antibody concentration in paired acute and convalescent serum samples, and isolation of the virus from blood, urine, or nasopharyngeal secretions.

▶ No specific antiviral therapy is available. Treat with supportive care.

▶ Hospitalized patients require standard precautions, with airborne transmission precautions from 4 days after onset of rash (if healthy child), or for the duration of the illness (immunocompromised patients).

RUBELLA

▶ Rubella virus is an enveloped, positive-stranded RNA virus.
▶ Postnatal transmission occurs primarily through direct or droplet contact from nasopharyngeal secretions.
▶ Incubation period for postnatally acquired rubella ranges from 14–23 days.
▶ Patients with postnatally acquired rubella are contagious from a few days before to 7 days after onset of rash.
▶ Patients with congenital rubella may shed virus in nasopharyngeal secretions and urine for over a year, with transmission to susceptible contacts possible.

Clinical Presentation

▶ 25–50% of infections are asymptomatic.
▶ Postnatal rubella:
  • Characterized by mild constitutional symptoms with low-grade fever, generalized lymphadenopathy, and a generalized erythematous maculopapular rash.
  • Rash consists of pink macules and papules, begins on the face with cephalocaudal spread to involve the trunk and extremities, and resolves within 72 hours.
  • Forschheimer's spots, pinpoint rose-colored and petechial macules on the soft palate, may be present.
  • Adolescents and adults may experience polyarthralgia and polyarthritis.
  • Encephalitis and thrombocytopenia are rare complications.
  • Maternal infections with rubella during pregnancy can result in miscarriage, fetal death, or congenital rubella syndrome.
▶ Congenital rubella:
  • Risk of congenital rubella with maternal infection: 85% if in first 4 weeks, 20–30% if in the second month, 5% in the third or fourth month
  • Most common anomalies: ophthalmologic, cardiac, auditory, neurologic

- May have growth retardation, radiolucent bone disease, hepatosplenomegaly, thrombocytopenia, and purpuric skin lesions (blueberry muffin spots)

Management

▶ Diagnosis of postnatal rubella is confirmed by detection of rubella-specific IgM antibody.

▶ Congenital rubella is confirmed by stable or increasing serum concentrations of rubella-specific IgG over several months; isolation of the virus from nasal specimens, blood, urine, CSF, and throat cultures; or via a 4-fold or greater rise in antibody titer or seroconversion between acute and convalescent serum titers.

▶ No specific therapy is available. Treat with supportive care.

▶ If patients with postnatal rubella are hospitalized, droplet precautions should be instituted for 7 days after the onset of the rash, in addition to standard precautions.

▶ Children with congenital rubella require contact isolation until they are at least 1 year of age, unless nasopharyngeal and urine culture results after 3 months of age are repeatedly negative.

VARICELLA-ZOSTER INFECTIONS

▶ VZV is a member of the Herpesviridae family.

▶ Varicella is highly contagious. Person to person transmission occurs primarily by direct contact with patients with varicella or zoster, occasionally occurs by airborne spread from respiratory tract secretions, and rarely from zoster lesions.

▶ Transplacental passage of the virus during maternal varicella infection results in *in utero* infection.

▶ Incubation period is generally from 14–16 days but has a range of 10–21 days after contact.

▶ Patients are most contagious from 1–2 days before to shortly after onset of rash.

▶ Contagiousness persists until all lesions are crusted over.

Clinical Presentation

▶ Primary infection with the virus results in varicella (chickenpox).

▶ Varicella manifests as a generalized, intensely pruritic, vesicular rash consisting of 250–500 lesions.

▶ Lesions begin as red macules that progress to papules, ultimately forming crops of discrete vesicles, each with a 1–2 mm surrounding area of erythema.

▶ Lesions begin on the scalp, face, and trunk and spread peripherally to the extremities over a period of several days.

▶ New crops of lesions develop over 3–5 days, with the presence of lesions in many stages of evolution characteristic of varicella.

▶ Mild fever and other systemic symptoms often accompany the rash.

▶ Immunocompromised patients are at risk of developing progressive severe varicella with continued eruption of vesicles and high fever persisting into a second week of illness, encephalitis, hepatitis, and pneumonia.

▶ Children taking corticosteroids are at high risk of invasive disease.

▶ Maternal varicella during the first or early second trimester resulting in fetal infection occasionally results in varicella embryopathy (limb atrophy, scarring of the skin of the extremities).

▶ Maternal infection 5 days prior to delivery to 2 days post-delivery can be fatal for an infant.

▶ Reactivation of virus after primary infection results in herpes zoster (shingles).

▶ Shingles manifests as grouped vesicular lesions distributed in one to three sensory dermatomes, with acute pain localized to the dermatome. Systemic symptoms are rare.

▶ Immunocompromised patients may develop disseminated zoster with visceral complications.

▶ Patients may develop pain after resolution of herpes zoster (postherpetic neuralgia).

Management

▶ Diagnosis is primarily clinical; however, it can be confirmed by isolating VZV from scrapings of vesicle bases during the first 3–4 days of the eruption (tissue cultures, Tzanck smear, DFA).

▶ Diagnosis can also be confirmed retrospectively by a significant increase in serum varicella IgG antibody.

▶ Oral acyclovir is not recommended for routine use in healthy children.

▶ Oral acyclovir should be considered for immunocompetent individuals at risk for developing moderate or severe disease (patients > 12 years of age, patients with chronic cutaneous or pulmonary disorders, patients receiving long-term salicylate therapy, and patients receiving short, intermittent, or aerosolized courses of steroids).

▶ IV acyclovir should be administered to pregnant patients with severe disease.

▶ IV acyclovir is recommended for immunocompromised patients, with maximal efficacy if given in the first 24 hours of illness.

▶ Salicylates should be avoided given the increased risk of developing Reye's syndrome with varicella infections.

▶ Airborne, contact, and standard precautions are necessary in the hospitalized patient for a minimum of 5 days after onset of rash, and as long as vesicular lesions are present.

▶ Neonates delivered by mothers with varicella require airborne and contact precautions until 21 days of age (28 days of age if they received VZIG).

▶ Airborne and contact precautions are required for immunocompromised patients with localized or disseminated zoster, and for immunocompetent patients with disseminated zoster.

▶ Post-exposure prophylaxis (VZIG and/or varicella vaccine) is available for susceptible contacts meeting specified criteria.

CHAPTER 73

PEDIATRIC BACTERIAL EXANTHEMS

Nicole S. Sroufe

MENINGOCOCCEMIA

- ▶ Meningococcemia is caused by *Neisseria meningitides*, a gram-negative diplococcus with at least 13 serogroups.
- ▶ Meningococcemia is most common in children < 5 years of age; however, about half of infections occur in adolescents and adults > 16 years of age.
- ▶ Transmission from person to person occurs via respiratory tract droplets.
- ▶ Incubation period is from 1–10 days, most commonly < 4 days.
- ▶ Patients with meningococcemia may transmit the organism for up to 24 hours post-initiation of effective treatment.

Clinical Presentation

- ▶ Invasive infection may result in meningococcemia, meningitis, or both.
- ▶ Patients with meningococcemia have an abrupt onset of fever, chills, malaise, and rash.
- ▶ Rash may be macular, maculopapular, or petechial.
- ▶ In fulminant meningococcemia, purpura, disseminated intravascular coagulation, shock, coma, and death can occur over a span of hours despite appropriate treatment.

Management

- ▶ Blood, urine, and CSF cultures should be obtained in patients suspected of having meningococcemia.
- ▶ Gram stains of CSF can be helpful in making the diagnosis.
- ▶ Isolation of *N. meningitides* from the nasopharynx is not diagnostic, as many individuals carry *N. meningitides* as nasopharyngeal flora.

- ▶ IV penicillin G, 250,000 U/kg/day (maximum dose of 12 million U/day) divided every 4–6 hours, is recommended therapy.
- ▶ Alternative antimicrobials include cefotaxime, ceftriaxone, and ampicillin.
- ▶ Penicillin-allergic patients (characterized by anaphylaxis) should be treated with chloramphenicol.
- ▶ Droplet precautions, in addition to standard precautions, are recommended for hospitalized patients until 24 hours after initiation of effective antimicrobial therapy.
- ▶ Prophylactic therapy is indicated for high-risk contacts.

STAPHYLOCOCCAL SCALDED SKIN

- ▶ SSSS is a *Staphylococcus aureus* toxin–mediated disease caused by the circulation of exfoliative toxins A and B.
- ▶ Most cases of SSSS develop prior to age 5 years.
- ▶ Incubation period is 1–10 days.

Clinical Presentation

- ▶ The hallmark of SSSS is cleavage of the stratum granulosum layer of the epidermis.
- ▶ The syndrome may be heralded by sudden onset of fever, irritability, cutaneous tenderness, and scarlatiniform erythema.
- ▶ In the neonate, SSSS results in generalized exfoliation (Ritter disease) with flaccid blister formation within 24–48 hours.
- ▶ Older children develop a tender scarlatiniform eruption and localized bullous impetigo.
- ▶ Infants and toddlers develop a combination of these lesions in addition to thick, white/brown, flaky desquamation of the entire skin.
- ▶ In patients with extensive exfoliation, dehydration and superinfection may occur.
- ▶ The mucous membranes are spared, with no involvement.
- ▶ Healing occurs without scarring.

Management

- ▶ Diagnosis is primarily clinical but can be confirmed via skin biopsy or with an exfoliated skin sample.
- ▶ SSSS in infants should be treated with a parenteral beta-lactamase–resistant beta-lactam antimicrobial agent.

▶ SSSS in older children may be treated with oral agents if their disease is not severe.

▶ Hospitalized patients with SSSS require contact precautions in addition to standard precautions for the duration of illness.

STREPTOCOCCAL SCARLET FEVER

▶ Scarlet fever is caused by one or more erythrogenic exotoxins produced by group A *Streptococcus pyogenes* strains.

▶ Infection is most common in school-aged children and adolescents.

▶ Transmission occurs via contact with a person with streptococcal pharyngitis (primarily contact with respiratory secretions).

▶ Incubation period is 2–5 days.

▶ Infection is most contagious during acute infection, diminishing over a period of weeks in untreated patients.

▶ Patients receiving appropriate antimicrobial therapy are not contagious after 24 hours of treatment.

Clinical Presentation

▶ Scarlet fever occurs most commonly with pharyngitis, rarely with pyoderma or an infected wound.

▶ Scarlet fever is characterized by a confluent, erythematous, sandpaper-like rash.

▶ Illness usually presents with abrupt onset of fever, headache, vomiting, malaise, and pharyngitis.

▶ Early in illness, bright red mucous membranes.

▶ The exanthema of scarlet fever develops 12–48 hours after onset of the fever, starting as a blanchable fine punctuate eruption.

▶ Acute glomerulonephritis can occur secondary to scarlet fever; however, rheumatic fever is not a sequela of streptococcal skin infection.

Management

▶ Diagnosis is primarily clinical.

▶ Confirmation of group A streptococcal pharyngitis can be made via throat culture or rapid testing (a positive culture will not differentiate between patients with true infection and those who are carriers).

▶ Rising antistreptolysin-O titers also provide support for the diagnosis.

▶ Penicillin V is the drug of choice for treatment of scarlet fever, except in patients allergic to penicillins.

▶ Treatment should be for 10 days.

▶ Penicillin-allergic patients should be treated for 10 days with orally administered erythromycin (other macrolides are also effective in the treatment of scarlet fever).

▶ Hospitalized patients with pharyngitis or pneumonia secondary to group A streptococcus require droplet precautions in addition to standard precautions until 24 hours after initiation of therapy.

TOXIC SHOCK SYNDROME

▶ *S. aureus* and *S. pyogenes* (group A streptococci) can produce TSS via toxin production.

Clinical Presentation

▶ Acute illness characterized by fever, rapid-onset hypotension, rapidly accelerated renal failure, and multisystem organ involvement.

▶ In staphylococcal mediated TSS, profuse watery diarrhea, vomiting, generalized erythroderma, conjunctival injection, and severe myalgias are common.

▶ Erythroderma associated with TSS is diffuse, generalized, and macular, with desquamation of palms, soles, fingers, and toes 1–2 weeks after onset of illness.

▶ The rash of TSS is flexurally accentuated, initially developing on the trunk, spreading to involve the arms and legs.

▶ Erythema and edema of the palms and soles are common, but it is uncommon for patients to develop petechiae, vesicles, and bullae.

▶ TSS associated with streptococcal infection is often characterized by local soft tissue infection associated with severe increasing pain.

▶ TSS may be associated with invasive infections, such as pneumonia, osteomyelitis, bacteremia, pyarthrosis, or endocarditis.

Management

▶ TSS is a clinical diagnosis. Lab studies may reflect multisystem organ involvement and disseminated intravascular coagulation.

▶ In patients with *S. aureus*–mediated illness, blood cultures are positive in < 5% of all patients.

▶ In patients with *S. pyogenes*–mediated illness, blood cultures have a higher yield, positive in > 50% of all patients.

▶ Treatment for TSS is first directed at resuscitation, with aggressive fluid therapy and management of respiratory and cardiac failure, if present.

▶ Initial empiric antimicrobial therapy should include a beta-lactamase–resistant antistaphylococcal antimicrobial agent and a protein synthesis–inhibiting antimicrobial drug (clindamycin).

▶ In patients with staphylococcal disease, treatment should be continued for a minimum of 10–14 days to eradicate the organism.

▶ In patients with streptococcal disease, parenteral therapy should continue until the patient is hemodynamically stable, afebrile, and has negative blood cultures.

▶ IVIG may be considered for treatment of either form of TSS.

▶ Hospitalized patients with TSS secondary to infection with streptococcus require droplet, contact, and standard precautions, whereas patients with staphylococcal infection require standard precautions only.

CHAPTER 74

PEDIATRIC FRACTURES

Thomas J. Deegan

▶ The types of pediatric fractures differ from those of adults due to the unique anatomy and physiology of a child's growing bones.

▶ The "weak" cartilaginous growth centers predispose to unique fracture patterns [Salter-Harris (S-H) classification] and make ligamentous sprains less likely.

▶ The plasticity of a child's bones allows for incomplete diaphyseal and metaphyseal fractures: greenstick fractures, torus fractures, buckle fractures.

▶ The thick periosteum allows for most displaced fractures to be managed with closed reduction without internal fixation.

▶ The osteogenic periosteum allows for faster healing and efficient remodeling that will straighten many mildly displaced diaphyseal fractures.

SALTER-HARRIS CLASSIFICATION OF FRACTURES

▶ See Figure 74-1.

▶ S-H type I
  • Fracture through the physis or growth plate
  • Non-displaced fractures have normal X-ray

▶ S-H type II
  • Fracture through the metaphysis exiting the physis
  • May be subtle if the metaphyseal fragment is small and may have the appearance of an avulsion fracture

▶ S-H type III
  • Fracture through the physis exiting the epiphysis
  • Intra-articular fracture

▶ S-H type IV
  • Fracture through the metaphysis exiting the epiphysis
  • Very unstable intra-articular fracture

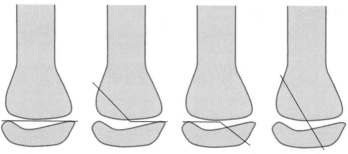

FIGURE 74-1.

Salter-Harris classification of fractures.

- High risk for growth abnormalities
- Usually requires operative management
▶ S-H type V
  - Complete crush of the physis
  - Difficult to distinguish from type I
▶ May result in impaired growth; risk highest with type III–V.
▶ All represent potentially unstable fractures requiring immobilization.
▶ Treat all injuries as presumptive S-H I fractures even if X-rays are negative if there is any tenderness or swelling over the growth center (Figure 74-1).

OTHER PEDIATRIC FRACTURE PATTERNS
▶ Greenstick fractures
  - Bending deformation of the diaphysis until the bone begins to "fray," causing an incomplete, often angulated fracture
  - If require reduction, usually can be done with procedural sedation analgesia
▶ Torus and buckle fractures
  - Compression force causing metaphysis to buckle and impact upon itself.
  - Fall on outstretched arm is common mechanism for distal radius/ulna fractures.
  - Buckle fracture may be very subtle on X-ray, seen only as slight change in the normal flare of the metaphysis.

IMAGING

▶ Because sprains are much less likely than fractures, must have a low threshold for obtaining X-rays

▶ With upper-extremity injuries resulting from a **fall on an outstretched arm,** X-rays should include both the elbow and wrist, easily accomplished by an AP and lateral forearm.

▶ Comparison views are usually **not** necessary.

▶ A good "true" lateral is absolutely necessary for evaluation of elbow injuries.

▶ Ottawa ankle rules can be applied to children, though X-rays often obtained because of refusal to ambulate and pain over the distal fibular physis.

▶ With obvious displacement, make NPO, place IV, and provide IV analgesia prior to X-ray for better quality images and patient comfort.

NURSEMAID'S ELBOW (RADIAL HEAD SUBLUXATION)

▶ Slip of the annular ligament from the radial head into the joint, resulting from a pulling mechanism, usually in children < 6 years old.

▶ Presents with refusal to use arm, holding it slightly flexed at the elbow and pronated as though it is "limp."

▶ **Never** swollen or ecchymotic. If it is, it is a fracture.

▶ X-ray imaging not necessary if mechanism and exam consistent with nursemaid's elbow.

▶ Classic method of reduction:
  • Hold as though shaking hands with your other hand at elbow with thumb over the radial head.
  • Supination with full extension, then full flexion at elbow.
  • Pop felt over radial head signifies success followed by spontaneous movement by the child.

▶ Hyperpronation method of reduction:
  • Same hand positions
  • Forearm hyperpronated until pop felt over radial head

SUPRACONDYLAR FRACTURES

▶ Mechanism is often a fall on outstretched arm.

▶ Very high risk for neurovascular compromise; serial exams especially after X-ray.

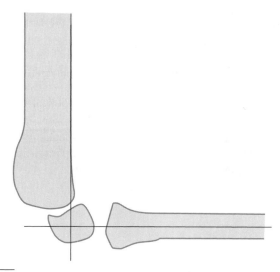

FIGURE 74-2.
Anterior humeral line can be used to detect posterior displacement of a supracondylar fracture.

▶ Present with tender, swollen elbow.
▶ Even mildly displaced fractures require operative management.
   • Make patient NPO with IV analgesia prior to X-ray.
   • Consider splinting prior to X-ray if large amount of swelling.
▶ X-ray findings:
   • Often obvious
   • Non-displaced fractures suggested by anterior and posterior fat pad sign
     ○ Anterior fat pad closely adherent to bone is normal.
     ○ Any visible posterior fat pad is abnormal.
   • Anterior humeral line (Figure 74-2)
     ○ Detects posterior displacement of the fracture.
     ○ Line drawn along anterior of the humerus should intersect the middle third of the capitellum.
   • Mid-radial line
     ○ Detects radius malposition.
     ○ Line drawn though the mid shaft of the radius perpendicular to the proximal radial physis should intersect with the middle third of the capitellum (Figure 74-2).

TODDLER'S FRACTURE

▶ Spiral fracture of the tibia in young ambulating child usually < 3 years old.

▶ May present without history of trauma—only refusal to bear weight.

▶ Accidental if able to ambulate even slightly (cruising toddler).

▶ Non-displaced fractures may be difficult to see on X-ray and may require bone scan or follow-up X-rays looking for signs of healing/periosteal new bone formation. Splint with long-leg posterior splint if suspect and normal X-ray.

CHAPTER 75

PEDIATRIC PROCEDURAL SEDATION AND ANALGESIA

Heather S. McLean

▶ Goal is to gain cooperation (e.g., radiologic studies) and/or provide analgesia for painful procedures (e.g., orthopedic procedures, lacerations).

▶ Sedation risks: hypoventilation, apnea, airway obstruction, and cardiopulmonary impairment ($\uparrow$ risk in those < 6 years old).

▶ Use of structured sedation guidelines decreases risks.

▶ Continuum of sedation: anxiolysis $\rightarrow$ moderate sedation $\rightarrow$ deep sedation.

DEFINITIONS

▶ Moderate sedation: responds to verbal commands, protective airway reflexes remain, patient maintains airway independently.

▶ Deep sedation: unconscious, partial or complete loss of airway reflexes, may not maintain airway independently (Table 75-1 and Table 75-2).

TABLE 75-1.
SEDATION CHECKLIST

Pre-sedation: informed consent, past history, length of fasting time, medications, allergies, vital signs, physical exam (including airway assessment, heart and lung exam)

Sedation: age/size-appropriate equipment checked and available, sedate in presence of person skilled in airway management/ CPR, continuous pulse oximetry ± cardiac monitoring, reversal agents calculated and available, specific person assigned to monitor cardiovascular status and sedation level (vitals q5min for deep sedation)

Discharge: easily aroused, protective reflexes intact, talks, sits up unaided, hydration adequate; NPO 2 hours after giving ketamine because of nausea and vomiting

TABLE 75-2.
DRUGS USED FOR SEDATION

Drug	Indication	Dose	Onset (minutes)	Duration (minutes)	Reversal agent	Adverse effects
Midazolam (Versed)	Sedation/anxiolysis	IV: 0.05–0.15 mg/kg (0.5–5 years); IV: 0.025–0.05 mg/kg (6–12 years); max 0.4 mg/kg	2–3	45–60	Flumazenil IV: 0.02 mg/kg, may give q1min to max of 1 mg	Respiratory depression, paradoxical reaction, hypotension, nausea, and vomiting
		IM: 0.1–0.15 mg/kg PO: 0.5–0.75 mg/kg IN: 0.2–0.5 mg/kg PR: 0.25–0.5 mg/kg	10–20 15–30 10–15 10–30	60–120 60–90 60 60–90		
Pentobarbital (Nembutal)	Diagnostic imaging	IV:1–6 mg/kg IM: 2–6 mg/kg PO/PR (< 4 years): 3–6 mg/kg; PO/PR (≥ 4 years): 1.5–3 mg/kg; max 100 mg	3–5 10–15 15–60	15–45 60–120 60–240	None	Respiratory depression, hypotension, emergence reaction, paradoxical reaction, nausea, and vomiting
Methohexital (Brevital)	Diagnostic imaging	PR: 25 mg/kg	10–15	60	None	Respiratory depression, hypotension, nausea, and vomiting
Thiopental (Pentothal)	Diagnostic imaging	PR: 25–50 mg/kg	10–15	60–120	None	Respiratory depression, hypotension, nausea, and vomiting

Drug	Indication	Dose			Reversal	Adverse effects
Fentanyl (Sublimaze)	Moderate to severe pain	IV: 1.0 mcg/kg q3min	2–3	30–60	Naloxone IV/IM: 0.1 mg/kg; max 2 mg/dose	Respiratory depression, *chest wall rigidity* (large/fast bolus), nausea, and vomiting
Ketamine (Ketalar)	Moderate to severe pain or immobilization	IV: 1–2 mg/kg over 1–2 minutes, may repeat ½ dose q10min IM: 4–5 mg/kg	1 / 3–5	Dissoc: 15; recovery: 60 / Dissoc:15–30; recovery: 90–150	None	Respiratory depression, *laryngospasm*, HTN, emergence reaction, nausea, and vomiting
Etomidate (Amidate)	Sedation/ hypnotic	IV: 0.15–0.2 mg/kg. Have 0.075–0.1 mg/kg up to 10 mg drawn up if more needed. Max 20 mg	1	10–15	None	Respiratory depression, *myoclonus*, hypotension, nausea, vomiting, injection site pain
Propofol (Diprivan)	Sedation/ hypnotic	IV: 1 mg/kg bolus, followed by 67–100 mcg/kg/minute infusion or 0.5 mg/kg boluses q1min PRN	< 1	5–15	None	Respiratory depression, hypotension, ↓ nausea, vomiting, injection site pain, allergic reaction (eggs)

◑ **PEARLS AND PITFALLS**

- Use a sedative-hypnotic agent alone for radiologic studies. Methohexital or thiopental given per rectum is safely used and very efficacious. Use of chloral hydrate is not recommended.

- Use an analgesic with sedative-hypnotic agents for painful procedures. Ketamine is a popular choice for orthopedic procedures and lacerations—very efficacious and safe. Midazolam used with ketamine does not decrease emergence reactions as previously thought; it may decrease emesis, however. Atropine or glycopyrrolate is often given with ketamine to reduce excess salivation; however, this has not been proven to decrease the risk of adverse events. Midazolam/fentanyl may cause more respiratory depression and are less effective when compared to ketamine/midazolam for orthopedic procedures. Ketamine is contraindicated in patients with intracranial HTN, wheezing, upper airway abnormalities, seizures, or psychosis, and in those < 3 months old. Caution is advised in patients with colds or cardiovascular disease or during intraoral procedures.

- There is limited pediatric research with etomidate, an ultra-short-acting sedative/hypnotic drug, but it is promising given its rapid onset/recovery and ability to titrate. A small number of studies have shown that it is safe and effective, though it is not licensed for children < 10 years of age. Consider pre-treatment with lidocaine because of painful infusion.

- Preliminary studies show that propofol with fentanyl may be a safe and efficacious alternative regimen for painful procedures. This agent is not available in all EDs nor is it universally recommended at this time. Consider lidocaine pre-treatment of vein prior to infusion and concomitant use of rapid NS infusion to reduce pain of infusion.

- Fasting guidelines are idealized, and shorter fasting times are often used in the ED because many procedures are considered non-elective. The hypothesis of pre-procedural fasting reducing adverse outcomes has not been tested in the literature.

CHAPTER 76

APPROACH TO THE TRAUMA PATIENT

Terry Kowalenko and Gregory Kowalenko

- ▶ Trauma is the leading cause of death between ages 1 and 44 years.
- ▶ There is a trimodal death distribution: The first peak occurs within seconds to minutes of injury (lacerations of brain, heart, major vessels); second peak is within minutes to several hours (epi- or subdural hematomas, liver, lung, spleen, pelvic injuries); third peak is several days to weeks (multi-organ system failure).

PRE-HOSPITAL CARE

- ▶ Attention to airway maintenance, control of bleeding and shock, patient immobilization, and immediate transport to the closest appropriate facility, preferably a trauma center, is paramount.
- ▶ EMS notification of arrival allows preparation ± activation of trauma team if available. Trauma team should be in universal precautions (gown, mask/eye shield, gloves, shoe covers).

PRIMARY SURVEY

- ▶ Airway, Breathing, Circulation, Disability, Expose.
- ▶ Life-threatening conditions are identified and managed simultaneously.

Airway (and Cervical Spine Immobilization)

- ▶ Assess for patency and inspect for FBs and facial fractures and abnormalities of the larynx and trachea.
- ▶ If the patient is able to speak clearly, the airway is not likely to be an immediate problem, but repeated assessment is necessary.
- ▶ Indications to secure airway with intubation include severe head injury with altered mental status or a GCS of 8 or less and patient can tolerate an oral airway.
- ▶ Remember to keep the C-spine immobilized throughout the survey.

Breathing

▶ Expose the chest and inspect, auscultate, and palpate for abnormalities such as tracheal deviation, crepitus, flail chest, sucking chest wound, fractured sternum, and absence of breath sounds.

▶ Interventions may include a three-sided occlusive dressing for a sucking chest wound, withdrawal of the ETT from the right mainstem bronchus, insertion of a 38Fr chest tube for hemopneumothorax, or needle decompression for tension PTX.

▶ All patients should have supplemental O_2.

Circulation

▶ Hemorrhagic shock is a common cause of post-injury death in the trauma patient and is considered present in any hypotensive trauma patient.

▶ If hypotensive → two large-bore IVs, infuse 2 L NS or LR and check for response. If there is not marked improvement, infusion of type O blood (O– for women of child-bearing age) should be initiated.

▶ Assess breath sounds, heart sounds, and the neck veins for evidence of cardiac tamponade (hypotension, agitation, distended neck veins, and muffled heart sounds).

▶ Apply direct pressure to any bleeding wounds.

▶ Hemorrhage:
  • Class I: 750 cc blood loss (15%), HR < 100, BP normal or elevated
  • Class II: 750–1500 cc loss (15–30%), HR > 100, BP normal
  • Class III: 1500–2000 cc loss (30–40%), HR > 120, BP decreased
  • Class IV: > 2000 cc loss (> 40%), HR > 140, BP decreased considerably

Disability

▶ Brief neurologic exam to evaluate level of consciousness, pupillary size and reactivity, and motor function

Exposure

▶ Remove all clothing and examine the entire body surface. Be careful not to cause hypothermia.

SECONDARY SURVEY

▶ Head to toe evaluation that should include a complete history and physical exam. Vital signs should be reassessed at this time.

▶ Inquire about mechanism and timing of accident, past medical history, medications, and allergies.

▶ Inspect the scalp for lacerations, nasopharynx for bleeding or septal hematoma, TMs for blood. An NG tube should be placed to empty stomach contents and check for blood. Palpate the face for crepitus or instability (place an orogastric tube if suspected facial fractures).

▶ Palpate C-spine for bony tenderness.

▶ Inspect, palpate, and auscultate chest for focal lung findings.

▶ Inspect and palpate abdomen for tenderness. Perform a rectal exam, noting sphincter tone and whether the prostate is boggy or displaced, and check for rectal blood. Look for blood at the urethral meatus; if present, perform a retrograde urethrogram prior to placement of a Foley catheter.

▶ A bimanual exam should be performed; if blood is present, perform a speculum exam to identify any vaginal lacerations; inspect for minor injuries.

▶ Extremities—inspect, palpate, and test range of movement. Remember to document neurovascular status.

▶ Patient should be log rolled to inspect and palpate back.

▶ Detailed neurologic exam should be performed at this time.

LABS

▶ CBC: Hgb/HCT may be normal initially, even in the face of significant hemorrhage, because fluid shifts may not have occurred to an appreciable extent early in hemorrhage.

▶ WBC and platelets may be elevated initially as a stress reaction.

▶ Chem-7 may show acidosis if in shock.

▶ LFTs may be normal initially even with significant liver injuries.

▶ Serum amylase/lipase may be normal even with pancreatic injury; amylase may be elevated with significant facial, salivary gland, or bowel injury.

▶ ABG: Assess oxygenation, pH, and base deficit.

▶ T&S is necessary in all trauma patients. Type and cross early if you suspect significant hemorrhage.

▶ UA: Microscopic hematuria is not uncommon and usually clinically insignificant. > 50 RBCs/hpf may indicate a more significant injury; however, renal avulsion may occur without hematuria. Gross hematuria requires further evaluation.

▶ ETOH and urine toxicology screens are often performed as trauma screening labs to evaluate for intoxication.

RADIOGRAPHIC STUDIES

▶ CXR: pneumo/hemothorax, widened mediastinum (> 8 cm), lung contusion, fractures

▶ Lateral C-spine X-ray: fracture/dislocations

▶ Pelvis X-ray: fractures/dislocations

▶ Fast ultrasound: evaluate for free intraperitoneal fluid, cardiac tamponade

▶ CT: may be necessary for evaluation of patients with head injury, blunt thoraco-abdominal trauma, or more precise evaluation of specific skeletal structures (pelvis, knee)

▶ Arteriography: may be necessary for further evaluation of vascular structures following penetrating and blunt trauma (aorta, pelvis, elbow/knee dislocations)

TREATMENT

▶ IV: two large-bore (≥ 16-gauge) IVs. 2 L NS or LR in hypotensive patients. Consider limited volume resuscitation in face of uncontrolled hemorrhage.

▶ Pulse oximeter: assess oxygenation.

▶ O_2: supplemental O_2 to maintain O_2 saturation ≥ 97%.

▶ Monitor: assess heart rate and rhythm.

▶ BP: assess volume status (may be normal in compensated hemorrhagic shock).

▶ Update tetanus immunization.

▶ Blood: PRBCs required if continued evidence of hemorrhagic shock despite 2 L of crystalloid in average adult (70 kg).

▶ Pediatric fluid resuscitation: 20 cc/kg of NS initially. If continued hypotension, repeat, then PRBCs 10 cc/kg.

▶ FFP: to be given if evidence of coagulopathy or if transfusing > 4 units PRBCs initially.

▶ With significant head injuries and evidence of mass effect, consider intubation, adequate oxygenation, elevation (30 degrees),

mild hyperventilation (P_{CO_2} = 35 mmHg), adequate fluid resuscitation, IV Mannitol, neurosurgical consultation.
▶ Spinal cord injury with deficit: consider high dose of methylprednisolone.
▶ Long bone fractures require splinting and traction.
▶ Hip and knee dislocations require immediate reduction.

DISPOSITION
▶ Minor injury, clinically stable: home
▶ Major trauma, clinically unstable despite initial resuscitation: OR, ICU
▶ Major trauma, clinically stable without evidence of surgical injury: home or brief inpatient observation
▶ Major trauma, clinically stable with potential surgically amenable injury (grade 1–3 hepatic/splenic lacerations, pelvic fracture with hemorrhage): admission to ICU

◑ **PITFALLS**
• Deterioration of patient at any time requires return to the primary survey.
• Do not allow patient to leave resuscitation bay if unstable unless it is to the OR or ICU.
• Be cognizant of the power of distracting injuries.
• Stroke-like symptoms in the setting of trauma, even minor: consider vertebral/carotid artery dissection.
• Decreasing level of consciousness or evidence of soot/singed hair in airway: intubate early due to the potential for airway edema.
• Early initiation of transfer protocol is imperative if at a less than level II facility. Stabilize and transfer.

CHAPTER 77

CARDIAC ARREST IN TRAUMA

Steven Schmidt

▶ Half of all trauma deaths occur in the first seconds to minutes after injury and are usually caused by lacerations to the aorta, heart, brainstem, and spinal cord.

▶ The remaining trauma deaths occur at later time periods (minutes to months) and represent potentially salvageable victims.

▶ Overall, traumatic arrests have very poor survival rates.

▶ Factors involved in differentiating potentially salvageable vs. unsalvageable patients:

- Presenting cardiac rhythm (pre-hospital or ED)
  - Asystole, severe bradycardia, or idioventricular rhythm is indicative of an unsalvageable patient.
  - VT, VF, and PEA (especially if sinus-based PEA) may have slight chance of survival.
- Resuscitation duration
  - Arrest for longer than 15 minutes has no chance of meaningful survival.

PRE-HOSPITAL

▶ All trauma (both blunt and penetrating)

- May withhold or cease resuscitation efforts in any patient with
  - Evidence of significant time lapse since pulselessness (such as dependent lividity, rigor mortis, and decomposition)
  - Unsuccessful CPR > 15 minutes
  - Estimated transport time to ED > 15 minutes and unsuccessful resuscitative time measures for > 15 minutes

▶ Blunt trauma

- May withhold resuscitation efforts in patients without vital signs or organized ECG activity

► Penetrating trauma
- May withhold resuscitation efforts in patients without vital signs or other significant signs of life (pupillary response, motor activity, or organized ECG activity)
- If in cardiac arrest but signs of life present, consider transport provided that
  ○ < 15 minutes transport time
  ○ No injuries incompatible with survival (i.e., decapitation, hemicorporectomy)

EMERGENCY DEPARTMENT

► Blunt trauma
- Standard resuscitation (ACLS protocols).
- No indication for thoracotomy in blunt trauma, unless clear evidence (DPL or ultrasound) of intraperitoneal hemorrhage.
- Cease resuscitation if CPR > 5 minutes with no signs of life.

► Penetrating trauma
- Standard resuscitation (ACLS protocols)
- Consideration of ED thoracotomy
  ○ Arrest while in ED or vital signs present in the field.
  ○ Especially in isolated thoracic trauma.
  ○ Stab wounds to chest have highest chance of recovery.
- Termination of resuscitation
  ○ Pre-hospital CPR > 15 minutes with no signs of life
  ○ Asystole without a penetrating wound that could result in tamponade

CHAPTER 78

HEAD INJURY

Sara Chakel

▶ The annual incidence of head injury in the U.S. is 600–900/ 100,000. Around 50% present to the hospital for evaluation and treatment.

GENERAL APPROACH TO HEAD INJURY IN THE EMERGENCY DEPARTMENT

▶ Emergency physicians must be able to use history and physical exam findings to determine which patients need further diagnostic studies, which patients require admission to the hospital, and which patients can be observed and discharged home.

▶ **Initial assessment:** C-spine collar and spine immobilization if appropriate. Intubation if unable to protect airway or for GCS ≤ 8. Immediate treatment of hypoxia, hypotension, and hypothermia.

▶ **History:** mechanism of injury, mental status before and after injury, LOC, vomiting, seizure activity, past medical history, medications including anticoagulants, recent alcohol or drug use.

▶ **Physical exam:** vital signs, mental status, GCS, pupillary size and responsiveness, motor strength and symmetry, sensation in extremities.

▶ **Radiology:** Obtain non-contrast head CT on all patients with GCS < 15 or abnormal neurologic exam and those patients with GCS of 15 with LOC, amnesia to the event, vomiting, headache, seizure, age > 60 years, evidence of injury above the clavicles, or drug/alcohol intoxication.

▶ **Observation/discharge:** Patients with GCS of 15, a normal neurologic exam, and a negative non-contrast head CT who are > 6 hours from time of injury may be discharged; if patient is < 6 hours from time of injury, may be discharged to the observation of a reliable third party.

TABLE 78-1.
GLASGOW COMA SCALE

	Eye opening	Verbal response	Motor response
1	None	None	None
2	To pain	Incomprehensible	Decerebrate extension
3	To speech	Inappropriate	Decorticate flexion
4	Spontaneously	Confused	Withdraws to pain
5		Oriented	Localizes pain
6			Obeys commands

► GCS: uses score of eye opening (1–4), verbal response (1–5), and motor response (1–6) to classify impaired consciousness; scores range from 3 to 15 (Table 78-1).
  • Mild traumatic brain injury: GCS 14–15
  • Moderate traumatic brain injury: GCS 9–13
  • Severe traumatic brain injury: GCS 3–8

SCALP LACERATION

► Rich blood supply may lead to hemodynamically significant blood loss.

Management

► Direct pressure to immediately control bleeding; if ineffective, use local infiltration of lidocaine with epinephrine or surgically clamp bleeding vessels.
► Careful exploration to identify underlying skull fractures.
► Closure of laceration with sutures or staples.
► Galea should be closed separately if also involved.

SKULL FRACTURE

► Categorized by location (basilar vs. cranial vault), pattern of fracture (linear vs. comminuted), and whether fracture is open or closed

Clinical Presentation

► Skull fractures (other than basilar) frequently herald underlying intracranial pathology.
► Signs of basilar skull fracture include hemotympanum, mastoid ecchymosis (Battle's sign), periorbital ecchymosis (raccoon

eyes), CSF rhinorrhea or otorrhea, hearing loss, and cranial nerve deficits.

Management

▶ All patients with suspected or demonstrated skull fracture require non-contrast head CT to evaluate for intracranial abnormality.

▶ Admit all patients with skull fracture for observation or surgical management.
  • Patients with linear or simple comminuted skull fracture should be observed overnight.
  • Obtain neurosurgical consultation for patients with depressed, open, or basilar skull fracture.

▶ Initiate antibiotics for open skull fracture: third-generation cephalosporin.

INTRACRANIAL BLEED

▶ Includes epidural hematoma, subdural hematoma, traumatic SAH, and intraparenchymal hemorrhage

Pathophysiology

▶ Epidural hematoma
  • Blood fills the potential space between the skull and the dura mater.
  • Most commonly follows blunt trauma with fracture of temporal bone and injury to the middle meningeal artery.

▶ Subdural hematoma
  • Blood accumulates in the subdural space.
  • Results from tearing of cortical bridging veins between dural venous sinus and cerebral cortex.
  • Frequently associated with underlying cerebral contusion or hemorrhage.
  • More common in the elderly.

▶ Traumatic SAH
  • Blood seen in the CSF caused by subarachnoid vessel disruption.
  • May occur with mild to moderate head injury.

▶ Intraparenchymal hemorrhage
  • Includes intracerebral hematoma and cerebral contusion.

- Occurs following angular acceleration in which cerebral tissue impacts the overlying skull.
- Most hematomas occur in the frontal and temporal lobes.

Clinical Presentation

▶ Epidural hematoma
  - Classic presentation: LOC followed by period of lucency and subsequent neurologic deterioration
  - Appears hyperdense and lenticular on CT scan
▶ Subdural hematoma
  - Variable presentation depending upon location, size, and mass effect of the hematoma as well as injury to the underlying brain tissue.
  - May present unconscious or may present conscious with subtle focal neurologic deficits, seizures, pupillary abnormalities.
  - Acute subdural hematoma appears crescent-shaped on CT scan.
▶ Traumatic SAH
  - Isolated injury may present similar to non-traumatic SAH, with headache, stiff neck, photophobia, and vomiting.
  - More severe injury has variable presentation depending upon constellation and location of other intracranial abnormalities.
  - Initial CT scan frequently demonstrates blood in cisterns and ventricles, but in some cases, blood is only seen on repeat CT scans 6–8 hours later.
▶ Intraparenchymal hemorrhage
  - Variable presentation depending upon location, size, and mass effect of the lesion.
  - Appear as hyperdense regions of the brain tissue on CT scan; often surrounded by cerebral edema.
    ○ May not be seen on CT scan until > 24 hours after injury.
    ○ Multiple contusions may coalesce to form one larger hematoma.

Management

▶ Admit all patients for serial neurologic exams and/or surgery.
▶ Neurosurgical consultation for all intracranial bleeding.
  - Size, location, and mass effect on CT scan as well as neurologic exam determine which patients need surgery.

▶ Initiate anticonvulsants for all patients with intracranial bleed.
  • Phenytoin most commonly used; loading dose 18 mg/kg
▶ Elevated ICP may be heralded by neurologic deterioration, HTN, and bradycardia.
  • Repeat CT scan on all patients with clinical deterioration.
  • Elevate head of bed to 30 degrees.
  • Hyperventilation to P_{CO_2} 30–35 mmHg.
  • Osmotic diuresis using mannitol 0.25–1 g/kg bolus.
  • Emergency decompressive trephination ("burr hole") only if acute rapid decompensation in the face of epidural or subdural hematoma and neurosurgery is unavailable.

DIFFUSE AXONAL INJURY

▶ Shearing forces disrupt axons in the brainstem and white matter.
▶ Often results from acceleration/deceleration mechanism of injury.
▶ Injury is irreversible; patients have high morbidity and mortality.

Clinical Presentation

▶ Immediate and prolonged unconsciousness
▶ May appear as cerebral edema, blurring of gray-white differentiation, and punctate hemorrhages in deep white matter on CT scan

Management

▶ Admission to ICU.
▶ Obtain neurosurgical consultation to assist with management and prognosis.
▶ Supportive treatment aimed at reduction/prevention of cerebral edema; ventriculostomy may be indicated.

PENETRATING TRAUMA

Clinical Presentation

▶ Initial GCS predicts survivability.
  • GCS < 5: mortality > 92%
  • GCS > 8: mortality < 10%
▶ CT scan findings consistent with high mortality: SAH, intracerebral hematoma, ventricular injury, bihemispheric involvement,

missile passing through geographic center of brain, fragmentation of missile, midline shift > 10 mm.

Management

▶ All patients with penetrating intracranial trauma should be intubated.

▶ Prophylactic antibiotics and anticonvulsants should be initiated.

▶ Obtain neurosurgical consultation to assist with management and prognosis.

NON-ACCIDENTAL HEAD TRAUMA
Clinical Presentation

▶ History inconsistent with injury pattern.

▶ Infants may be irritable, lethargic, or comatose; seizure activity may be present.

▶ Retinal hemorrhages present in 65–90% of children with intentional head trauma.

▶ Injuries resulting from intentional head trauma tend to be more severe than non-intentional trauma.

Management

▶ In addition to CT scan and funduscopic exam, all patients with suspected abuse must have a skeletal survey or bone scan to evaluate for occult fractures.

▶ Obtain coagulation studies to rule out coagulopathy.

▶ Mandatory reporting of suspected abuse to appropriate authorities.

CHAPTER 79

MAXILLOFACIAL TRAUMA

J. Jeff Downie and Stephen P. R. MacLeod

▶ Approximately 3 million facial injuries occur annually in the U.S.
▶ Motor vehicle collisions account for more injuries in rural areas, and interpersonal violence–related injuries are more frequent in inner cities.
▶ Male:female ratio is 3:1.

CLINICAL PRESENTATION OF COMMON FACIAL INJURIES

Nasal Bone Fracture

▶ Most common facial bone fractured.
▶ Diagnosed by a history of trauma with swelling, flattening or deviation, and crepitus over the nasal bridge. The patient may have epistaxis.
▶ Check for septal deviation and a septal hematoma by inspecting the nasal airways.
▶ Leakage of CSF indicates a fracture through the cribriform plate of the ethmoid bone (basilar skull fracture).

Naso-Orbital-Ethmoidal (NOE) Fractures

▶ Usually the result of a significant impact. Suspect an NOE fracture if the patient has evidence of flattening of the nasal bridge with telecanthus or widening of the nasal bridge with detached medial canthus, and epistaxis.
▶ Other features include circumorbital edema, ecchymosis, and CSF rhinorrhea.

Zygomatic Complex (ZMC) Fracture

▶ Physical findings of flattened cheek prominence with tenderness and numbness in the distribution of the infra-orbital nerve suggest a ZMC fracture. Often edema is marked, which can obscure the depression of the prominence.

▶ The patient may complain of pain in the cheek on movement of the jaw or trismus. Other features include peri-orbital ecchymosis, subconjunctival hemorrhage, and epistaxis.

▶ Eye injuries may be associated with these fractures, thus a thorough eye exam is essential. Early documentation of visual acuity is important.

Orbital Blow-Out Fracture

▶ This results from a direct blow to the globe, where the resulting force is transferred to the thin orbital bones resulting in a fracture or "blow out."

▶ Periorbital fat tends to herniate through the defect, along with the inferior rectus and inferior oblique muscles. These muscles may become entrapped, preventing upward movement and outward rotation of the eye. The patient may experience diplopia on upward gaze.

▶ Other clinical features include peri-orbital edema, infra-orbital anesthesia, enophthalmos, and restriction of eye movements. Complete eye exam is vital.

Dento-Alveolar Fractures

▶ Injuries involve teeth and their supporting bone. Clinically, there is a mobile segment of teeth and malocclusion. These injuries are often associated with mucosal tears and intra-oral hematomas.

Mandibular Fractures

▶ Usually the result of a blunt force applied to the lower face.

▶ Anatomical classification: condylar neck (36%), angle (20%), body (21%), symphysis (14%). Multiple fractures are common because of ring structure.

▶ Clinical features: swelling, tenderness, malocclusion, SL hematoma, and anesthesia of the lower lip. Tongue blade test: Ask patient to bite down on a tongue depressor. Tongue depressor is then twisted and should break. If patient is unable to do this, suspect fracture.

Le Fort Fractures

▶ Result from a significant impact to the mid-face.
▶ Le Fort I fracture: transverse fracture of the maxilla above the roots of the teeth and the palate.
▶ Le Fort II fracture: pyramidal fracture of the mid-face that extends from the bridge of the nose laterally and inferiorly through the infra-orbital rims.
▶ Le Fort III fractures: a high-level fracture where the facial bones are disconnected from the base of the skull.
▶ Physical exam findings include marked facial edema and mobility of the maxilla and other facial bones. Epistaxis or CSF rhinorrhea may be noted.

EMERGENCY DEPARTMENT MANAGEMENT

▶ ABCs take priority. The airway is reassessed frequently. With severe facial injury, early intubation should always be considered before edema increases.
▶ Evaluation of facial fractures is part of the secondary survey. Examination should include
  • Inspect face for asymmetry or swelling. This is often best assessed from an overhead view.
  • Thoroughly examine eyes and document visual acuity.
  • Inspect nasal septum for septal hematoma and clear rhinorrhea, which may suggest a CSF leak.
  • Assess facial stability and palpate facial bones for tenderness.
  • Examine for malocclusion of teeth.
  • Cranial nerves should be tested.

Imaging

▶ CT scan with thin cuts (coronal and axial for orbital fracture) is the imaging modality of choice for most facial fractures.
▶ The following are exceptions:
  • Nasal bone fracture is a clinical diagnosis that does not require imaging unless other injuries are suspected.
  • Mandibular fractures: panoramic (most helpful), AP, and lateral X-rays.

Other Studies

▶ CSF rhinorrhea
  • Place a drop of fluid onto filter paper—CSF migrates farther than blood, forming a target shape with blood in the center and blood-tinged CSF on the outer ring.
  • Check the glucose content of the fluid—CSF generally contains 60% of the glucose of serum.
▶ Maintain high suspicion for spinal injuries with facial fractures.

Treatment

▶ Other than simple nasal bone fractures, consultation should take place with the on-call maxillofacial or ENT surgeon to assist with work-up and disposition.
▶ Avoid placement of NGT in maxillofacial trauma until cribriform plate fracture is excluded.
▶ Nasal septal hematomas must be drained in ED to avoid septal necrosis.
▶ Always consider injury to parotid gland or Stensen's duct with facial trauma, particularly if it involves lacerations.
▶ Antibiotics and tetanus should be considered for all open fractures.

Disposition

▶ After excluding other injuries, many of these fractures can be managed as an outpatient. Consultation, however, is required with either a maxillofacial surgeon or ENT to ensure appropriate follow-up.

CHAPTER 80

NECK TRAUMA

Nathan Goymerac and Rahul K. Khare

▶ Multiple organ systems (airway, vascular, neurologic, GI) in compact area
▶ Divided into anterior and posterior triangles by sternocleido-mastoid:
  • Anterior triangle contains majority of vascular and visceral organs.
  • Posterior triangle contains few vital structures.
▶ Divided into three anatomic zones:
  • Zone I (base of neck): from clavicles to cricoid cartilage
  • Zone II (mid-neck): from cricoid cartilage to angle of mandible
  • Zone III (upper neck): from angle of mandible to base of skull

PENETRATING NECK TRAUMA

▶ Blood vessel damage most common injury (25–40% penetrating wounds).
  • Internal jugular vein (9%) and carotid artery (7%) most commonly injured vessels.
▶ Tracheobronchial injury occurs in 10–20%, pharynx/esophageal injury in 5–10%, and major nerve injury in 3–5%.

Pathophysiology

▶ Zone I: injuries to subclavian artery and vein, jugular vein, proximal common carotid artery, vertebral artery, aortic arch, trachea, esophagus, lung apices, C-spine, spinal cord
▶ Zone II: injuries to carotid and vertebral arteries, jugular veins, pharynx, larynx, trachea, esophagus, C-spine, spinal cord, vagus, and recurrent laryngeal nerve
▶ Zone III: injuries to distal carotid arteries and jugular veins, salivary and parotid glands, esophagus, trachea, C-spine, cranial nerves IX–XII

Clinical Presentation

▶ Presence or absence of symptoms misleading, serve as poor predictor of clinical outcome

▶ Zone I injuries often hidden from inspection in chest/mediastinum—worst prognosis

▶ Zone II injuries most apparent on clinical exam—best prognosis

▶ Spinal cord injury
  - Complete cord transection: absence of motor, sensory, reflex function below level of injury
  - Brown-Séquard's syndrome (hemisection of spinal cord): ipsilateral motor paralysis with contralateral sensory deficits

▶ Larynx injury
  - Voice alteration, hoarseness, stridor, hemoptysis, subcutaneous emphysema, bubbling neck wound

▶ Tracheobronchial injury
  - Subcutaneous emphysema, cough, respiratory distress, hemoptysis, PTX, continuous air leak after chest tube placement

▶ Carotid artery injury
  - Decreased consciousness, contralateral hemiparesis, hemorrhage, hematoma, thrill, bruit, distal pulse deficit

▶ Pharynx/esophageal injury
  - Dysphagia, bloody saliva, bloody NG aspirate, pain and tenderness in neck, crepitus

▶ Cranial nerve injury
  - Glossopharyngeal nerve (IX): dysphagia, altered gag reflex
  - Vagus nerve (X): hoarseness
  - Spinal accessory nerve (XI): inability to shrug shoulder
  - Hypoglossal nerve (XII): deviation of tongue with protrusion

Emergency Department Management

▶ ABCs and follow ATLS guidelines for primary and secondary survey.

▶ Airway likely to be bloody or distorted by swelling.
  - Have suction, multiple sized ETTs, and surgical airway supplies prepared.
  - Secure airway early before swelling makes intubation impossible.

▶ If respiratory distress in zone I injury, consider chest tube placement due to frequent association with intrathoracic injury.

- ▶ Active bleeding should be controlled with direct pressure.
- ▶ Never blindly clamp bleeding vessels—may damage surrounding structures.
- ▶ Never remove impaled objects in ED—may cause hemorrhage.
- ▶ Secondary survey should include determination of any platysma violation.
    - • If platysma not penetrated, little risk of significant injury.
    - • If platysma violated, requires trauma surgery consultation.
- ▶ Do not probe wound in ED—may dislodge clot and cause hemorrhage.
- ▶ C-spine X-rays: evaluate for bony injury, FBs, wound tract.
- ▶ CXR: for all zone I injuries to rule out associated intrathoracic injury.
- ▶ CT of neck: better delineation of bony and soft tissue injury, good at detecting laryngeal injury.
- ▶ Angiography: gold standard to evaluate for arterial injury.
    - • Four-vessel study (bilateral carotid and vertebral arteries)
    - • Employed to evaluate penetrating wounds in zone I and zone III
    - • Allows embolization of bleeding vessels not accessible surgically
- ▶ CT angiogram: screening test for arterial injury.
- ▶ Duplex ultrasound: screening test for low-risk vascular injury in zone II
- ▶ Esophagram/esophagoscopy: nearly 100% sensitive for esophageal injury.
- ▶ Laryngoscopy/bronchoscopy: tests of choice to rule out injury to airway.
- ▶ Hemodynamic instability with continuous hemorrhage from neck wound mandates surgical exploration in the OR.
- ▶ Signs of arterial injury that mandate surgical exploration or angiogram:
    - • Expanding hematoma, severe active or pulsatile bleeding, shock unresponsive to fluids, signs of cerebral infarction, new bruit or thrill, diminished distal pulses
- ▶ Stable penetrating wounds to zone I and III evaluated with angiogram (difficult to gain access to vessels and control bleeding surgically).
- ▶ Stable penetrating wounds to zone II surgically explored or evaluated with screening tests (selective surgical approach) dependent on institution.

▶ Any injury to major vessels, nerves, airway, or esophagus must be surgically repaired.

BLUNT NECK TRAUMA

▶ C-spine injuries more common than in penetrating injury.
▶ Clinical findings more subtle than with penetrating injuries.
▶ Vascular injuries have a worse outcome compared with penetrating injuries.
▶ Esophageal injury rare due to protected location.

Clinical Presentation

▶ Delay between vascular injury and onset of symptoms
  • 10% have neurologic deficits within 1 hour.
  • 75% have neurologic deficits between 1 and 24 hours.
  • 15% have neurologic deficits after 24 hours.
▶ Carotid artery injury: hematoma over lateral neck, bruit, Horner's syndrome, stroke-like syndrome.
▶ Vertebral artery injury: ataxia, vertigo/nystagmus, hemiparesis, dysarthria/diplopia.
▶ 50% of vascular injuries have no external signs of trauma.
▶ Brachial plexus injuries tend to affect upper nerve roots (C5–C7)—diminishes capacity of upper arm but spares lower arm.
▶ Complete avulsion of brachial plexus results in flaccid, numb extremity.

Emergency Department Management

▶ ABCs and follow ATLS guidelines.
▶ Maintain C-spine immobilization until spinal injury excluded by X-ray and/or CT imaging.
▶ MRI/MRA for otherwise stable patients with neurologic deficits.
▶ Four-vessel angiogram, CT angiography, or duplex ultrasound to evaluate for vascular injury.
▶ Laryngoscopy, bronchoscopy to rule out airway injury.
▶ Esophagoscopy, esophagram to rule out esophageal injury.
▶ Any injury to major vessels, nerves, airway, or esophagus must be surgically repaired.
▶ If spinal cord injury suspected, Solu-Medrol, 30 mg/kg IV bolus, followed by 5.4 mg/kg/hour for 24 hours.

CHAPTER 81

CERVICAL SPINE INJURY

Robert M. Domeier

▶ C-spine fracture occurs in 1–3% of patients with a significant traumatic mechanism of injury.

▶ Spinal cord injury occurs in 25–40% of patients with C-spine fracture.

▶ Additional fracture in thoracic or lumbar spine occurs in 10–15% of those with C-spine fracture.

▶ Mechanisms of injury involve flexion, extension, rotational, or compression forces.

▶ Spinal cord injury generally occurs at the time of initial injury.

▶ Spinal cord injury as a secondary insult after cervical fracture without immediate cord injury is extremely rare without a secondary insult.

▶ SCIWORA is rare, approximately 10%, and usually occurs in cases with pre-existing spinal stenosis or isolated ligamentous or intervertebral disk injury.

▶ Incidence of isolated ligamentous injury is unknown and considered rare.

▶ In the elderly patient, physical findings of injury may not be as evident as in younger patients, so a high index of suspicion in the elderly is important.

CLINICAL PRESENTATION

▶ Presenting symptoms include any of the following: altered mental status, intoxication (alcohol or drugs), distracting painful injury, neurologic deficit, midline neck pain or tenderness, pain or tenderness with ROM of the neck.

▶ Complete cord injury results in distal paralysis and sensory loss. Spinal shock may be a complication.

▶ Neurologic deficit will not always be obvious. Presenting neurologic symptoms of a partial cord injury may include vague weakness, numbness or sensory loss, persistent shooting pains ("stingers"), or unexplained hypotension.

PRE-HOSPITAL MANAGEMENT

▶ Spine immobilization is indicated in the pre-hospital trauma patient who has sustained an injury with a mechanism of injury having the potential for causing spine injury and who has at least one of the following:
- Altered mental status
- Evidence of intoxication
- A distracting painful injury (e.g., long bone extremity fracture)
- Neurologic deficit
- Spinal pain or palpation tenderness

EMERGENCY DEPARTMENT MANAGEMENT
Diagnosis

▶ Assessment for C-spine injury should be performed in any patient with a mechanism of injury judged sufficient to potentially cause a C-spine injury.
▶ Assessment for C-spine injury may be performed on any patient, age < 65, independent of the mechanism of injury.
▶ Evaluate for findings consistent with a potential C-spine injury (C-spine injury assessment).
▶ Alert, awake, not intoxicated, neurologically normal, no midline neck pain or tenderness even with full ROM of neck and palpation of C-spine:
- C-spine X-rays are not necessary.
▶ Alert, awake, complains of neck pain:
- Three-view C-spine X-rays are obtained.
- Axial CT images at 3-mm intervals obtained through suspicious areas identified on three-view C-spine X-rays.
- If lower C-spine is not adequately visualized on lateral C-spine X-ray:
  ◦ Swimmer's view: if inadequate, axial CT images at 3-mm intervals through lower C-spine
- If the patient has persistent significant neck pain, obtain voluntary flexion/extension lateral C-spine X-rays to evaluate for potential ligamentous injury. If voluntary excursion

326 PART IX / TRAUMATIC EMERGENCIES

      is < 30 degrees or produces significant pain, consider cervical collar and repeat flexion/extension lateral C-spine X-rays in 2 weeks.

▶ Neurologic deficit referable to a C-spine injury:
  • Plain films and CT images as described above
  • MRI of the C-spine

▶ Altered mental status, intoxication, or distracting injury making C-spine assessment unreliable:
  • Plain films and CT images as described above.
  • Axial CT images at 3-mm intervals from the base of the occiput through C2.
  • If patient's mental status changes persist, inpatient management may include fluoroscopic flexion/extension C-spine evaluation.

▶ Elderly patients (age > 65) with mechanisms of concern for C-spine risk (e.g., falls with a head strike on a fixed object, any significant head injury, major trauma):
  • Plain films and CT images as described above
  • Axial CT images at 3-mm intervals from the base of the occiput through C2

Treatment

▶ Hard cervical collar with log-roll precautions for patients who have a significant mechanism and have not been assessed or have a positive C-spine injury assessment.

▶ Cervical collar may be removed from those who are cleared of C-spine injury by clinical or radiographic assessment.

▶ Maintain collar and log-roll precautions in those with an injury identified.

▶ Obtain spine specialist evaluation.

Disposition

▶ Spine specialist evaluation and condition of the patient will determine the disposition. Many patients with C-spine injuries may be treated as outpatients with cervical collar; others require surgical or other rigid stabilization.

CHAPTER 82

SPINAL CORD INJURY

J. Jeremy Thomas and Diamond Vrocher III

▶ 82% of spinal cord injury victims are male with mean age of 31.
▶ Usually, patients are left with permanent and often devastating neurologic deficits.

CLINICAL PRESENTATION

▶ Complete cord lesion:
  • Loss of motor and sensory function distal to the injury site.
  • Poor prognosis: minimal improvement expected even with ideal treatment.
▶ Incomplete cord lesions often demonstrate gradual improvement over time.
  • Central cord syndrome: ischemic injury to the central area of the cervical cord after hyperextension injury
    ○ Decreased strength: upper extremities > lower extremities and distal strength decreased > proximal
    ○ Variable sensory deficits
  • Anterior cord syndrome: following damage or ischemic injury to the anterior two-thirds of the spinal cord
    ○ Involves the corticospinal and spinothalamic tracts
    ○ Loss of motor function distal to the injury
    ○ Sensory deficit distal to the injury with sparing of proprioception and vibratory sense
  • Brown-Séquard's syndrome: caused by injury to one side of the spinal cord with interruption of the lateral corticospinal and spinothalamic tracts as well as the posterior column
    ○ Ipsilateral findings: Babinski sign with spastic paralysis, loss of tactile discrimination, vibratory, and proprioception below the level of the lesion
    ○ Contralateral findings: loss of pain and temperature sensation

- Cauda equina syndrome: compression of nerve roots in the lumbar spine
  - Loss of bowel or bladder function (incontinence or inability to void)
  - Decreased sensation in the saddle area distribution
  - Pain or weakness in the lower extremities
- SCIWORA
  - Significant neurologic finding with normal radiographic evaluation (X-ray, CT, MRI).
  - Seen in children < 9 years of age.
  - Hypermobility and ligamentous laxity of the pediatric cervical and thoracic spine predispose children to these injuries.

EMERGENCY DEPARTMENT MANAGEMENT
Diagnosis

▶ Consider spinal cord injury:
  - In all patients with significant trauma (especially high-speed MVA, falls, and diving accidents)
  - When altered mental status is present or patient is unresponsive and there is definite or possible history of head or neck trauma
▶ Clues on physical exam
  - Weakness or sensory deficits, loss of rectal tone and perianal sensation, areflexia, and priapism
▶ Imaging
  - X-ray (fractures, listhesis) of cervical, thoracic, and lumbar spine
  - CT (fractures, listhesis): increased sensitivity and specificity. Indication: inability to visualize all vertebrae, conspicuous findings, or to further delineate extent of fracture and other injuries
  - MRI: able to visualize cord. Indication: all suspected cord lesions
  - CT myelogram: for visualization of cord if MRI is not available

Treatment

▶ C-spine immobilization and address ABCs.

▶ Evaluation that proceeds with ATLS guidelines, with complete primary and secondary survey.
  • Breathing: Assess respiratory/ventilatory status.
▶ Steroids: Current recommendation is to treat all acute spinal cord injuries with steroids; however, some debate certainly still remains regarding the efficacy.
  • Methylprednisolone, 30 mg/kg IV over 15 minutes, then infuse at 5.4 mg/kg/hour for 23 hours.

CHAPTER 83

THORACIC TRAUMA

Nathan Goymerac

▶ Accounts for 20–25% of trauma-related deaths.
▶ Specific injuries differ based on blunt vs. penetrating mechanism.
▶ Penetrating wounds that enter the "box" (medial to nipples or medial scapular borders) require ancillary studies to rule out injury to heart, great vessels, esophagus, trachea/bronchi.
▶ Penetrating thoracic wounds that traverse inferior to nipples or below the scapula require ancillary studies to rule out intra-abdominal injuries.

RIB FRACTURES

▶ Most common blunt thoracic injury.
▶ CXR to rule out underlying thoracic injury (misses 50% of rib fractures).
▶ Rib X-rays unnecessary as they do not alter management.
▶ Management includes analgesia and deep breathing exercises.

FLAIL CHEST

▶ Three or more adjacent rib fractures in two or more places
▶ Creates free-floating segment of chest that moves paradoxically (in with inspiration, out with expiration)
▶ Judicious use of IVF to prevent blossoming of underlying pulmonary contusion (inpatient observation)

PULMONARY CONTUSION

▶ Bruise of lung parenchyma followed by hemorrhage into alveoli.
▶ Tachypnea, dyspnea, decreased breath sounds over affected area.
▶ CXR shows alveolar infiltrate by 4–6 hours (CT shows contusion earlier).
▶ Avoid over-aggressive fluid resuscitation.

SIMPLE PNEUMOTHORAX

▶ Accumulation of air in pleural space
▶ Varying degrees of lung collapse and respiratory compromise
▶ Dyspnea, pleuritic pain, decreased breath sounds, hyper-resonance
▶ CXR: decreased lung markings peripherally (expiratory films more sensitive)
▶ Small PTX (< 20%): observation with repeat CXR in 6 hours
▶ Large PTX (> 20%): large-bore (36–40 Fr) chest tube in fourth/fifth intercostal space anterior/mid-axillary line

TENSION PNEUMOTHORAX

▶ PTX with air leaking into pleural space, but unable to escape.
▶ Causes increased pleural pressure, mediastinal shift, decreased venous return to heart, and subsequent reduction in cardiac output.
▶ Dyspnea, agitation, altered consciousness, tachycardia, cyanosis, absent breath sounds, hyper-resonance, JVD, tracheal deviation.
▶ Diagnosis is clinical (should not require a CXR).
▶ Immediate needle decompression with 14-gauge Angiocath through second intercostal space in mid-clavicular line, followed by chest tube.

COMMUNICATING PNEUMOTHORAX "SUCKING CHEST WOUND"

▶ PTX with large chest wall defect allowing air to enter through defect rather than trachea.
▶ Involved lung collapses on inspiration and expands on expiration.
▶ Occlude defect with three-way flutter valve, followed by chest tube.

HEMOTHORAX

▶ Accumulation of blood in pleural space.
▶ Bleeding from lung parenchyma, hilar/great vessels, intercostals, or internal mammary vessels of the chest wall.
▶ Dyspnea, pleuritic pain, decreased breath sounds, dull to percussion.
▶ Upright CXR: blunting of costophrenic angle (requires 300 cc).
▶ FAST scan may also demonstrate hemothorax.
▶ Treatment is with large-bore chest tube.

▶ Thoracotomy if initial chest tube output > 1500 cc, output > 200 cc/ hour for several hours, persistent instability despite resuscitation.

CARDIAC TAMPONADE

▶ Accumulation of blood in pericardial sac with decreased ventricular filling and subsequent decrease in cardiac output.
▶ Beck's triad: hypotension, JVD, muffled heart sounds (all three in < 30%).
▶ Pulsus paradoxus: drop in SBP > 10 with inspiration—poor sensitivity and specificity.
▶ Other findings include tachycardia and elevated CVP (> 15 cm).
▶ Ultrasound shows pericardial fluid, diastolic collapse of R ventricle.
▶ ECG may show electrical alternans—rarely present.
▶ Aggressive fluid resuscitation in ED.
▶ Thoracotomy and operative repair of underlying cardiac injury.
▶ Pericardiocentesis if immediate surgery not available.
▶ ED thoracotomy if patient loses vitals in ED or en route if penetrating.

BLUNT CARDIAC INJURY

▶ Range from mild arrhythmias, to decreased contractility, to rupture of valves, septum, or myocardium.
▶ May be asymptomatic, have chest pain, CHF, or cardiogenic shock.
▶ Normal ECG essentially rules out clinically significant blunt cardiac injury (BCI).
▶ Cardiac markers do not correlate with clinical outcome.
▶ Telemetry monitoring for at least 12 hours if abnormal ECG.
▶ Echocardiogram for those with hemodynamic instability.
▶ Arrhythmias and cardiogenic shock as per ACLS guidelines.

TRAUMATIC AORTIC INJURY

▶ Usually immediately lethal (85% die at scene).
▶ Chest pain radiating to back, hypotension, upper-extremity BP differential, decreased lower-extremity pulses, harsh inter-scapular murmur.

▶ Upright CXR: widened mediastinum, tracheal deviation to right, left mainstem bronchus depression, loss of aortic knob, apical cap.

▶ CT chest: test of choice if injury to great vessels suspected (sensitivity near 100%).

▶ TEE: sensitivity of 90–100% for aortic injury.

▶ Angiogram is still gold standard.

▶ BP control with beta-blockers (MAP of 60) to reduce shearing forces.

▶ Thoracotomy (some centers use endovascular stents to repair).

TRACHEAL/BRONCHIAL INJURY

▶ Most blunt injuries occur within 2.5 cm of carina.

▶ Most penetrating injuries occur in cervical trachea.

▶ Dyspnea, stridor, hoarseness, subcutaneous emphysema, massive persistent air leak.

▶ ET intubation (preferably fiberoptically to prevent passage of tube into false lumen).

▶ Bronchoscopy if injury suspected, with surgical repair if found.

ESOPHAGEAL INJURY

▶ Blunt injuries rare due to location in posterior mediastinum.

▶ Injuries often missed due to subtle clinical findings.

▶ Missed diagnosis often leads to mediastinitis (50% mortality).

▶ Upper chest pain out of proportion of findings, dyspnea, hematemesis, subcutaneous emphysema, pneumomediastinum.

▶ If any suspicion, require esophagoscopy and esophagram—together near 100% sensitive.

▶ Broad-spectrum antibiotics and surgical repair and drainage.

CHAPTER 84

ABDOMINAL TRAUMA

Victoria L. Hogan and Diamond Vrocher III

▶ Preventable trauma deaths are frequently due to missed abdominal injuries.

▶ A high index of suspicion is needed to diagnose abdominal injuries (Table 84-1).

CLINICAL PRESENTATION

▶ Patients may present as hemodynamically unstable with or without obvious visible injuries. Emergent surgical consultation is necessary in these patients.

▶ Signs of abdominal injury may be obvious, such as evisceration, open pelvic fracture, or penetrating injury. Signs suggestive of abdominal injury include an abrasion on the abdominal wall from the seatbelt or flank ecchymosis.

▶ The physical exam is considered unreliable if the patient has painful distracting injuries or has decreased level of consciousness secondary to neurologic injury or alcohol/drug intoxication.

▶ The physical exam should include an examination of the perineum and a digital rectal exam.

EMERGENCY DEPARTMENT MANAGEMENT

▶ The primary goal while beginning aggressive resuscitation is to determine the need for early surgical intervention, especially in the hemodynamically unstable patient.

▶ Immediate surgical consultation/intervention should be considered for hemodynamically unstable patients with suspected intra-abdominal bleeding. Early surgical involvement is also necessary for evisceration, peritonitis, ruptured diaphragm, or gross hematuria.

▶ The diagnostic modalities chosen depend on mechanism of injury, patient's clinical status, and the institution-specific guidelines.

TABLE 84-1.
MOST FREQUENTLY INJURED ORGANS IN ABDOMINAL TRAUMA

Blunt injury	Stab wound	Gunshot wound
Spleen	Liver	Small bowel
Liver	Small bowel	Colon
Retroperitoneum	Diaphragm	Liver
	Colon	Abdominal vascular structures

Diagnostic Studies

▶ Chest radiograph
  • Inferior rib fractures are suggestive of abdominal injury (liver or splenic lacerations).
  • Preferably completed after orogastric or NG tube placement to help diagnose diaphragm injuries. CXR is diagnostic in about 27% and is abnormal in about 85% of those with diaphragm injuries.
▶ Abdominal radiograph
  • Helpful for localizing FBs in penetrating injuries.
▶ DPL
  • Advantages: rapid, inexpensive, used on unstable patients.
  • Disadvantages: invasive, complications possible, may lead to a non-therapeutic laparotomy for injuries that could otherwise have been managed non-operatively, pregnancy and prior surgery are relative contraindications.
  • A positive DPL in blunt abdominal trauma requires at least one of the following:
    ○ 10 cc gross blood aspiration
    ○ > 100,000 RBC/mm^3
    ○ ≥ 500 WBC/mm^3
    ○ Bowel or bladder contents
    ○ Positive Gram's stain
  • In a hemodynamically unstable patient with a positive DPL, urgent laparotomy should be considered.
  • In a hemodynamically stable patient with a positive DPL, management is controversial.
▶ CT
  • Advantages: images the retroperitoneum and pelvis, allows for grading of solid organ injuries and possible non-operative management.
  • Disadvantages: requires 10–20 minutes to complete; IV contrast needed for optimal study; reserved for relatively stable

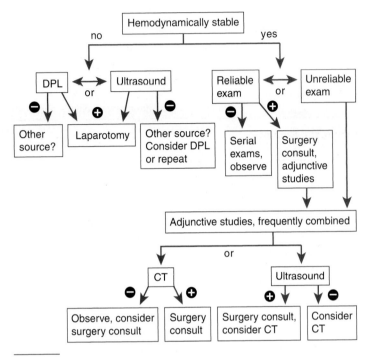

FIGURE 84-1.

Algorithm for the management of abdominal injuries.

patients; may miss hollow viscus, mesenteric, pancreatic, or diaphragmatic injuries.
- If intraperitoneal free fluid is visualized on CT without solid organ injury, bowel or mesenteric injuries should be considered.
- CT has only a very limited role in the evaluation of penetrating abdominal injuries.

▶ Ultrasound
- Advantages: fast, non-invasive, can be used in unstable patients, done in the resuscitation area
- Disadvantages: operator dependent, visualization difficult in the obese patient or patient with SC emphysema, may miss hollow viscus or retroperitoneal injuries

▶ Retrograde urethrogram, cystogram, and CT (Figure 84-1)
- These studies may be useful for further evaluation of gross hematuria.

- Indicated if gross blood at the penile meatus or boggy prostate on rectal exam.
▶ Local wound exploration of the penetrating abdominal injury
  - Penetrating wounds to the anterior abdomen inferior to the costal margins are an indication for local wound exploration. If the wound penetrates the peritoneum (or it is unclear if the peritoneum has been penetrated), the patient should be further evaluated. DPL, laparoscopy, and laparotomy are further diagnostic possibilities with surgical consultation.
  - Wounds superior to the inferior costal margin, but inferior to the fourth intercostal space anteriorly or seventh intercostal space posteriorly (the thoracoabdominal region) should not be explored locally. Surgical consultation is necessary for this type of wound. Further evaluation with laparoscopy, thoracoscopy, or laparotomy may be indicated.
  - Local exploration of flank or back wounds is not indicated. A triple contrast CT (IV, oral, and rectal contrast) may be considered.

CHAPTER 85

GENITOURINARY TRAUMA

Sanjeev Malik

▶ GU trauma is divided into three distinct categories:
  • Upper GU tract: kidney and ureters
  • Lower GU tract: bladder and urethra
  • External genitalia: scrotum, testes, and penis
▶ Upper GU injuries: blunt trauma or deceleration mechanism
▶ Bladder and posterior urethral injuries: pelvic fractures
▶ Anterior urethral injuries: straddle injuries or penetrating trauma

CLINICAL PRESENTATION

▶ History
  • Gross hematuria
  • Inability to urinate
  • Flank, suprapubic, or genital pain
▶ Physical exam
  • Tachycardia, hypotension may be present secondary to associated injuries
  • Abdominal tenderness (bladder rupture)
  • Flank or scrotal ecchymosis
  • Pelvic bone instability or crepitus
  • Blood at urethral meatus (urethral injury until proven otherwise)
  • High-riding prostate on rectal exam
  • Blood at vaginal introitus

EMERGENCY DEPARTMENT MANAGEMENT
Diagnosis

▶ ABCs, initial evaluation as per ATLS protocol
▶ CBC, coags, BUN, creatinine, UA
▶ AP pelvic X-ray

▶ Retrograde urethrogram (RUG)
  • Indications: blood at urethral meatus, high-riding prostate, or high index of suspicion
  • Technique:
    ○ Since many of these patients are on a back board, patients are supine, penis is raised perpendicular to the legs.
    ○ Inject 20–30 cc of 30% diluted water-soluble contrast using a Tumey syringe inserted into the tip of the penis or place Foley catheter 1 inch into the tip of penis and inject.
    ○ During injection, shoot an AP image.
  • Extravasation of contrast indicates urethral injury.
  • Place Foley catheter if negative urethrogram.
▶ Retrograde cystogram
  • Indications: hematuria or suspicion of GU injury with negative urethrogram
  • Technique:
    ○ Sterile placement of Foley catheter.
    ○ Pre-injection KUB.
    ○ Inject 300–400 cc of 30% diluted water-soluble contrast through catheter and then clamp catheter (higher incidence of false negative with insufficient contrast).
    ○ AP and lateral KUB then post-void KUB.
  • Intra-peritoneal bladder rupture: extravasation of contrast outlining intra-peritoneal structures (bowel, spleen)
  • Extra-peritoneal bladder rupture: extravasation of contrast near pubic symphysis
▶ CT retrograde cystogram
  • Technique is the same for plain film retrograde cystogram, but instead of doing a KUB, you take them to the CT scanner and do 1-cm cuts through the bladder.
▶ CT abdomen/pelvis with contrast
  • Test of choice for evaluation of upper GU tract injuries
  • Indications:
    ○ Gross hematuria
    ○ Microscopic hematuria with shock
    ○ Mechanism of sudden deceleration without hematuria or shock
    ○ Pediatrics: microscopic hematuria > 50 RBC/hpf
▶ Testicular ultrasound with color flow Doppler
  • Indication: significant testicular trauma or pain

Treatment

▶ Urethral injury
- Supra-pubic catheter placement or Foley placement by cystoscopy by urology
▶ Extra-peritoneal bladder rupture
- Foley catheter placement 7–14 days
- Prophylactic antibiotics
▶ Intra-peritoneal bladder rupture
- Operative repair
- Prophylactic antibiotics
▶ Renal lacerations and pedicle injuries
- Trauma surgery and urology consultation
- Conservative vs. operative therapy
▶ External genital trauma
- Penile fractures
  - Ice packs, pressure dressing, analgesia
  - Urologic consultation for typically operative repair
- Hair tourniquets (pediatrics) and other constricting devices
  - Removal of constricting agent and observe in ED
▶ Testicular injuries
- Ultrasound, rest, ice, analgesia, urologic follow-up
- Operative repair of lacerations, hematomas

Disposition

▶ Significant urologic injury requires admission and urologic evaluation for definitive therapy.
▶ Microscopic hematuria with normal vital signs can be safely discharged from ED with outpatient follow-up for clearance of hematuria.

CHAPTER 86

THERMAL BURNS AND SMOKE INHALATION

Erich C. Kickland and James Mattimore

▶ Burns result in approximately 2 million injuries, 80,000 hospitalizations, and 6500 deaths annually.

▶ Definitive treatment for large burns is at regional burn centers with dedicated resources and personnel.

THERMAL BURNS

▶ Three main types of thermal burns are scald, contact, and flame burns.

▶ Burn severity is related to rate of heat transfer to skin (which is dependent upon temperature of the agent, duration of contact, and heat conductivity of local tissues, etc.).

Clinical Presentation

▶ **First degree:** minor epithelial damage characterized by erythema, pain, and tenderness, but no blistering (e.g., sunburn); heals completely.

▶ **Second degree:** partial-thickness burns (only epidermal involvement). Subdivided into superficial (erythematous, moist, blistering, very tender; usually heals without scarring), and deep (red/blanched, blistered, decreased sensation; heals with variable degree of scarring).

▶ **Third degree:** full-thickness burns (dermis involved). White or brown, leathery, insensate; requires skin grafting to heal.

▶ **Fourth degree:** involves underlying tissue such as fascia, muscle, or bone.

▶ Estimate TBSA involved using the rule of nines:
  • Adults
    ○ 9% to head, each upper extremity
    ○ 18% each to front and back of torso, each lower extremity
    ○ 1% to perineum, genitals

- Infants
  - 18% each to front and back of torso, head
  - 9% to each upper extremity
  - 13.5% to each lower extremity
  - 1% to perineum, genitals
▶ "Hand rule" for quick estimate of smaller burns: area of hand (palm + fingers) is 1% of TBSA.

Management

▶ Rapidly assess for signs of airway involvement—signs of airway involvement warrant early intubation. Difficult airway should be expected and preparations made for rescue device if unable to perform orotracheal intubation.
▶ Fiberoptic laryngoscopy may facilitate airway placement in burns.
▶ Facial or closed space burns have high incidence of airway involvement.
▶ Indications for securing airway in the setting of burns:
  - Decreased level of consciousness found in enclosed space
  - Respiratory distress: increased RR, stridor, or labored breathing
  - Mild distress with evidence of inhalational injury
    - Singed facial hairs, facial burns, erythema of oropharynx, and carbonaceous sputum
▶ 100% O_2 by face mask and pulse oximetry monitor.
▶ Third- and fourth-degree burns of thorax and neck can cause respiratory/ventilatory compromise due to restrictive and compressive effects; escharotomy of thorax or neck may be required.
▶ Patients with burns > 20% TBSA require fluid resuscitation.
▶ Fluid resuscitation in adults is guided by the Parkland formula:
  - LR 4 ml/kg × % BSA with second- and third-degree burns given in the first 24 hours from burn time
  - One-half of total administered in the first 8 hours, the other half over the next 16 hours
▶ Fluid resuscitation in pediatric patients is guided by the Galveston formula:
  - 5% dextrose with LR 5 L/m^2 BSA with second- and third-degree burns plus 2 L/m^2 TBSA given in the first 24 hours from burn time
  - One-half of total administered in the first 8 hours, the other half over the next 16 hours

▶ Fluid resuscitation is best monitored by urinary output (UOP)
- < 2 years old: 1 cc/kg/hour
- Children: 0.5 cc/kg/hour
- Adults: 30 cc/hour

▶ Control pain with liberal amounts of narcotic analgesia.

▶ Wound care considerations for major burns:
- **Extremity escharotomy:** must be considered with circumferential burns, when compartment pressures > 40 mmHg or loss of distal pulse by Doppler.
- **Wound dressing:** covering with clean sheet is sufficient if transport immediately available; if transport is not immediately available, initial wound care consists of cleansing/irrigation, debridement, and topical antimicrobial ointment.

▶ Wound care considerations for minor burns:
- **Cleansing:** irrigation and debridement required (do not debride blisters on palms and soles).
- **Wound dressing:** various ointments and synthetic dressings available; agents of choice vary widely. Use caution with Silvadene and facial burns, as there is concern it may cause permanent pigment change.

▶ Provide tetanus prophylaxis. Prophylactic antibiotics are not indicated in most cases.

▶ Disposition per American Burn Association criteria (Table 86-1).

SMOKE INHALATION
Clinical Presentation

▶ Carbonaceous sputum, singed nasal hairs, mental status, and decreased level of consciousness are all clues to the possibility of smoke exposure.

▶ The onset of respiratory symptoms is often delayed, and initial ABG can be deceptively normal.

▶ Respiratory tract injury is the leading cause of morbidity/mortality in smoke inhalation; inflammation cascade produces so-called smoke lung injury, which leads to eventual gas exchange impairment.

▶ Metabolic poisoning by gaseous components, such as CO, cyanide, plastics, and acids or aldehydes is the other major cause of mortality in smoke inhalation.

TABLE 86-1.
AMERICAN BURN ASSOCIATION DISPOSITION CRITERIA

	Partial-thickness involvement (% TBSA)	Full-thickness involvement (% TBSA)	Other considerations	Disposition recommended by American Burn Association
Major burn injury	25% age 10–50 years; 20% < 10 years or > 50 years	> 10%	Partial/full thickness burns on face, hands, feet, genitals, perineum, major joints; electrical (including lightning) or chemical burns; inhalation injury; trauma or pre-existing comorbidities	Immediate transfer to specialized burn center.
Moderate burn injury	15–25% adults; 10–20% children/older adults	2–10%	Must not have any of above criteria	Consider transfer to burn center; may possibly be managed at tertiary care facility.
Minor burn injury	< 15% adults; < 10% children/older adults	< 2%	Must not have any of above criteria	May usually be managed as outpatient.

▶ Metabolic poisoning can compound morbidity/mortality caused by airway injury or can be the predominant process in exposures to filtered smoke (source in another room or on another floor) or relatively smokeless combustion (exhaust).

Management

▶ As with most forms of inhalation injury, treatment is supportive.

▶ Airway must be assessed rapidly and managed aggressively: intubation with large-diameter ET tube to allow for clearance of copious, thick secretions should take place early. Expect and prepare for a difficult airway.

▶ Use NMT with bronchodilators for bronchospasm in acute phase.

▶ Supportive care with suctioning, pulmonary toilet, and maintenance of oxygenation using PEEP as appropriate are mainstays.

▶ Antibiotics indicated only for infections diagnosed by serial sputum cultures.

▶ Corticosteroids are not indicated and actually increase mortality in the presence of cutaneous burns.

▶ Other treatment modalities (surfactant, antioxidants) are under investigation.

▶ Disposition requires ICU admission for evidence of major exposure, such as sooty sputum, hoarseness, or history of exposure in a confined space.

▶ Remember to consider CO and cyanide poisoning in any patients with enclosed-space burns or with decreased level of consciousness.

CHAPTER 87

CHEMICAL, ELECTRICAL, AND LIGHTNING INJURIES

Erich C. Kickland and James Mattimore

CHEMICAL BURNS

▶ Potentially harmful chemicals can be categorized by the reactions they produce and include acids and alkalis, oxidizers and reducers, desiccants and vesicants, protoplasmic poisons, and corrosives.

▶ Exposure leads to disintegration of the protective keratin layer and direct exposure of dermal layers to the damaging effects of the agent.

▶ Injury severity is a direct function of concentration of the offending agent, length of exposure, and penetration rate.

▶ Many agents can produce systemic toxicity through absorption.

Clinical Presentation

▶ Presentation is variable, making a detailed history and physical exam the most valuable diagnostic tools.

▶ Thorough history should include the agent and concentration, if known. If this information is not known, ask about cleaners, solvents, or other household products that may contain harmful agents.

▶ Other critical history points are physical form of agent, route, volume, and timing of exposure.

▶ On physical exam, note size and depth of burns.

▶ Look for signs of ocular involvement, such as periorbital or scleral lesions, vitreous humor leak, or decrease in visual acuity.

▶ Signs of ingestion include oral burns, edema, drooling, dysphagia, stridor, dyspnea, abdominal tenderness, crepitus, or SC air.

Management

▶ Vigilant airway management—any signs of ingestion or inhalation injury due to fumes warrant consideration of definitive airway.

▶ Removal of the agent is crucial first step.

▶ The mainstay of treatment in chemical injury is hydrotherapy, or flushing of the area with copious amounts of low-pressure water (major exception to this is lime that must be removed prior to flushing with water).

▶ Attempts to neutralize the agent can exacerbate injury by creating an exothermic reaction that can worsen burns and incite fumes.

▶ Ocular involvement requires low-pressure irrigation with a large volume of 0.9% NS, topical anesthetic, slit lamp exam (SLE)—see Chap. 152.

▶ For ingestions, lavage is contraindicated. Symptomatic patients should all have GI consult to determine if endoscopy is needed.

▶ Wound care is similar to thermal burns with a few notable exceptions:

  • **Hydrofluoric acid (HF)** (rust removers): Skin contamination causes progressive destruction and, therefore, progressive pain. Classically presents with delayed onset of symptoms, especially when exposed to household products containing HF. Treat fluoride toxicity with calcium, which can be delivered via topical, direct infiltrative, or intra-arterial routes.

    ◦ Calcium gluconate gel 2.5–10% with Surgilube applied directly in surgical glove

    ◦ Subcutaneous/intradermal infection: 5% calcium gluconate solution via 30 G needle into HF burned skin (maximum dose 1 ml of calcium gluconate per square centimeter of burned skin)

  • **Formic acid:** used in industry and agriculture. Systemic toxicity caused by hemolysis and hemoglobinuria. This may require mannitol as plasma volume expander and for initiation of osmotic diuresis. Exchange transfusions may be necessary in severe cases.

  • **Phenol:** used in manufacturing, agriculture, cosmetics, medicine. Systemic toxicity is manifested as CNS depression, which may be severe enough to cause respiratory arrest and death. Skin exposure must be decontaminated as quickly as possible to prevent absorption. Polyethylene glycol or isopropyl alcohol applied directly is the most effective decontamination agent. Contaminated hair must be removed as hair traps phenol.

  • **Nitrates:** lead to methemoglobinemia. Treat with IV methylene blue, 2 mg/kg.

▶ Disposition for cutaneous injury is per American Burn Association criteria (see Chap. 86).

▶ Disposition for systemic manifestations dictated by degree of exposure and severity of symptoms.

ELECTRICAL INJURY

▶ Electrocution is the fourth leading cause of work-related deaths.
▶ Most home-related electrical injury results from malfunction or misuse of household appliances.
▶ For characterization, electrical injury is described as a voltage phenomenon and is divided into low and high voltage, usually by a 500 V or 1000 V cutoff.
▶ Variables that affect the degree of injury are
  • **Type of circuit:** Alternating current (AC) circuits are more dangerous, because they cause tetanic muscle contraction, prolonging victim contact with the source. DC circuit causes one muscle spasm, which usually throws the victim clear from the source. AC most commonly results in VF arrest. DC results in asystole.
  • **Resistance:** depending on area of body contact, different tissues have different inherent resistance properties. Nerves, blood vessels, and muscles have least resistance and, therefore, are good conductors. Bone, tendons, and fat have high resistance and are poor conductors.
  • **Voltage:** product of resistance × current (Ohm's law V = IR). Higher voltages usually result in a more significant injury.
  • **Duration of contact** of victim with source.

Clinical Presentation

▶ Two mechanisms of injury: direct effect of electricity and indirect effect via trauma caused by falls, anoxia caused by cardiac arrest, etc.
▶ Head and neck injuries include neurologic damage, cataract formation (acute or chronic), and TM rupture (up to 50% of patients).
▶ Cardiac effects are twofold, including direct myocardial necrosis and dysrhythmias. VF is most common in both high- and low-voltage injury.
▶ Cutaneous involvement, if present, is usually in the form of burns and follows the principles of thermal burn assessment and management. Besides cardiac arrest, burns are the most acutely devastating injury. Pay special attention to source and ground contact points, often where burns are worst, but every

▶ square inch of body must be examined as electricity can have an unpredictable course.

▶ Acute CNS manifestations vary widely, including LOC, confusion, impaired recall, seizure, hypoxic brain injury, and spinal cord injury. Peripheral nervous system deficits range from transient paresthesias to permanent loss of function. Autonomic instability is also possible.

▶ Respiratory arrest can be due to CNS dysfunction or respiratory muscle paralysis.

▶ Muscular necrosis is caused by vasospasm-induced ischemia and can lead to compartment syndromes.

▶ Kidneys are particularly susceptible, incurring either hypoxic injury or renal tubular damage secondary to myoglobin and Hgb release by damaged skeletal muscle.

▶ Skeletal damage can occur via muscle contractions or falls. Commonly affected are upper-extremity long bones and vertebrae (potential for spinal cord injury).

Management

▶ ABCs, IV, O_2, monitor.

▶ Clinician must have a high index of suspicion for occult injuries.

▶ Serial evaluation of cardiac, hepatic, renal, and pancreatic function is recommended, especially when there is possibility of ischemic injury.

▶ Head CT for any persistent neurologic deficits or history of fall.

▶ Evaluation for rhabdomyolysis, myoglobinuria, and compartment syndrome is essential in all but minor injuries.

▶ Rhabdomyolysis should be treated with fluids with a goal to maintain urinary output (UOP) at 1.5–2 cc/kg/hour. Alkalinization of urine may also be helpful.

▶ In the presence of burns, disposition is per American Burn Association criteria.

▶ Criteria for admission include all high-voltage injuries and low-voltage injuries with LOC, ECG changes, persistent dysrhythmias, history of heart disease, or significant risk factors, associated conditions, or injuries warranting admission.

▶ Low-voltage injury patients without burns, neurologic deficits, or LOC, and a normal ECG may be safely discharged.

▶ Children with lip burns after biting an electric cord need close follow-up. They may have delayed hemorrhage from the labial artery at 3–5 days. These injuries should not be debrided.

LIGHTNING INJURY

▶ The exact incidence of lightning-related injury and death is unknown.

▶ Lightning is a massive unidirectional current impulse.

▶ Current flows internally for an extremely short time and can interrupt the body's electrical systems, such as heart, respiratory centers, CNS, and autonomic nervous system.

Clinical Presentation

▶ Asystole is much more common than VF. Intrinsic pacing may resume spontaneously.

▶ Respiratory arrest is frequently caused by paralysis of medullary respiratory centers and may last longer than initial cardiac arrest. This can lead to a secondary arrest due to hypoxia.

▶ Skin involvement may include burns. Feathering burns are considered pathognomonic. May also get thermal burns related to super-heating of clothes or if clothes ignite.

▶ CNS injury is varied and can include coagulation of brain matter, intracranial hemorrhages, respiratory center paralysis, seizures, LOC for variable periods of time, confusion, and amnesia. Peripheral nerve damage is common with poor prognosis for recovery of function. Autonomic instability can also occur.

▶ Keraunoparalysis is a unique temporary paralysis with blue, cold, pulseless extremities caused by vascular spasm and autonomic dysfunction. Usually persists a few hours.

▶ Ruptured TM present in > 50%.

▶ Delayed cataract formation commonly observed.

Management

▶ ABCs.

▶ IV/O_2/monitor.

▶ Combined ACLS/ATLS protocols should be followed in an attempt to identify all injuries.

▶ Extensive burns are uncommon, so usually do not require large-volume fluid resuscitation.

▶ As in electrical burns, obtain ECG for arrhythmia. Assess for evidence of rhabdomyolysis and treat per guidelines in Electrical Injury section above.

▶ Almost all are admitted for 24 hours of cardiac monitoring.

CHAPTER 88

APPROACH TO TOXIC INGESTION

Daniel R. Wachter and Laura Roff Hopson

► > 2 million toxic exposures per year in the U.S. reported to poison control centers—most of which have good outcomes.

► Toxic ingestions account for 5–10% of ED visits and > 5% of admissions to adult ICUs.

► Approximately 1100 annual deaths in the U.S. related to poisonings (majority of these are related to suicide attempts and drug abuse).

DIFFERENTIAL DIAGNOSIS

► The differential diagnosis is very broad and should be narrowed based upon presenting signs and symptoms. Specific considerations include
  • Known/expected drug effect or drug-drug interaction
  • Drug/alcohol withdrawal states
  • Metabolic/endocrine disorders
  • Trauma
  • Infection, including meningitis and sepsis
  • Psychiatric disease

CLINICAL PRESENTATION

► See Chapters 89–116 for details of presentations.
► See Table 88-1.

DIAGNOSIS

► Obtain a careful history of the toxic exposure from the patient (may be unreliable, particularly if a suicide attempt), accompanying family, friends, pre-hospital personnel, and/or police. When appropriate, these people may be sent to the patient's home or workplace to look for pill bottles, prescriptions, over-

TABLE 88-1.
CLINICAL PRESENTATION OF TOXIC INGESTION

	Opioid	Anticholinergic	Cholinergic	Sympathomimetic
Mental status	Depressed	Agitated/depressed	Depressed	Agitated
Pupil size	Miosis	Mydriasis	Miosis/mydriasis	Mydriasis
Pulse	↓	↑	↔	↑
BP	↓	↔	↔	↑
RR	↓	↔	↔	↑
Temperature	↓	↑	No effect	↑
Bowel sounds	↓	↓	↑↑	↑
Skin	Dry	Dry, red, hot	Diaphoretic	Diaphoretic

the-counter medications, occupational hazardous materials, or a suicide note. May need to contact patient's pharmacy or physician to determine recently filled prescriptions or purchases.

► Relevant historical information to collect includes the type and amount of toxins involved, the timing and route of exposure, symptoms, and any home or pre-hospital interventions; relevant medical and surgical history, along with other prescribed or over-the-counter medications and allergies, should also be elicited.

► After initial ABCs including close attention to respiratory status, complete a thorough toxicologic physical exam. Be attentive for the characteristic toxidromes as well as abnormal odors and remaining toxic substances or drug paraphernalia in patient's clothes/belongings. Examine skin for "track marks" and stigmata of chronic alcohol and drug abuse. Perform a complete neurologic exam, and note bowel sounds and degree of skin moisture.

► Maintain a high index of suspicion for a toxic ingestion/exposure in a patient who does not have another complete explanation for altered mental status or metabolic abnormalities.

Laboratory Testing

► Bedside glucose.

► Basic metabolic panel.

► CBC.

► ABG: if concerned for metabolic acid-base disorder or respiratory compromise.

► UA: may detect crystals or clues regarding complicating rhabdomyolysis.

► Urine drug screen: typically only detects drugs of abuse but may provide clues if history is unclear.

► Blood alcohol level: common coingestant, particularly in suicide attempts.

► Urine pregnancy test (for all women of childbearing age).

► Specific drug level [e.g., acetaminophen (APAP), salicylate, lithium] if needed to guide further treatment. Due to the ubiquitous nature of APAP in readily available medications, it is wise to routinely obtain a level.

► Unreliable (suicidal) patients or those whose histories are unclear should have more liberal use of diagnostic lab testing to exclude presence of significant toxic ingestion.

Imaging

▶ CXR: may show evidence of non-cardiogenic pulmonary edema or aspiration. Use when warranted by clinical presentation.

▶ Abdominal X-ray: may show bezoar, radio-opaque pill fragments, or "body packing/stuffing."

▶ Head CT: indicated if concern of trauma or if history of toxic exposure does not account for altered mental status.

Ancillary Testing

▶ ECG: on every suicidal ingestion and/or if concern for block, arrhythmia, or occult MI. Some ingestants cause characteristic ECG findings (e.g., tricyclic antidepressants and widened QRS).

▶ Pulse oximetry.

▶ Cardiac monitor.

Consults

▶ Contact poison control center or medical toxicologist early for significant, unusual, or complicated exposures.

▶ Early communication with ICU personnel and/or nephrologist as indicated for admission and hemodialysis (HD)/hemoperfusion, respectively.

TREATMENT/DISPOSITION

▶ Should occur along with and not be delayed by diagnostic work-up.

▶ **Skin decontamination:** if exposed to biological or chemical substance that may place health care workers or other patients at risk—all clothing/jewelry should be removed and gross decontamination should be performed prior to entering ED.

▶ *A*irway, *B*reathing, *C*irculation, *D*isability, *E*xposure.

▶ IV, O_2, cardiac monitor.

▶ Consider early ET intubation for

- Airway compromise—existing or impending respiratory failure
- Depressed mental status and risk for aspiration
- Need for gastric lavage
- Significant acid-base disturbance
- Poor or unstable hemodynamic status

▶ Consider specific antidote if ingested substance is identified, but beware polysubstance ingestion and be aware of risks and contraindications to standard antidotes (see Chapters 89–116 specific to individual toxins for more information).

▶ "Coma cocktail": thiamine, 100 mg IV (if suspect significant malnutrition); dextrose, 25 g given as 50 ml of D50 (unless hypoglycemia can be rapidly excluded); naloxone (for suspected acute opioid toxicity), 0.1–2 mg IV, repeat if needed.

▶ **Gastric decontamination:**
- Orogastric/NG lavage
  - May be considered only for potentially life-threatening exposures that present within 60 minutes of ingestion
  - Contraindications: altered mental status or concern for loss of airway protection, caustic ingestions (acid, alkali), hydrocarbon ingestions, patients at high risk for GI hemorrhage or perforation
  - Should be followed by placement of activated charcoal per tube
  - Potential complications: hypoxia, aspiration, esophageal or gastric injury, PTX, placement of tube in trachea
- Syrup of ipecac (to induce emesis)
  - Almost never indicated in the hospital setting
  - Risk of aspiration, especially with decreased mental status
  - One potential use: toxic substance exposure that is not associated with altered mental status, has been consumed within the last hour, with patient who will be significantly delayed in reaching hospital
- Activated charcoal, 1 g/kg (with or without single dose of a cathartic such as sorbitol or magnesium citrate)
  - Reported to reduce substance bioavailability by 69% when given within 30 minutes of toxic ingestion.
  - Does not bind/remove alcohols, heavy metals, hydrocarbons, organophosphates, or corrosives.
  - Major risk of gastric decontamination with activated charcoal is aspiration pneumonitis and subsequent respiratory complications (hypoxia, pneumonia, ARDS, etc.).
  - Prophylactic intubation in patient with significantly depressed mental status is necessary due to increased risk of aspiration.

- ○ Multi-dose activated charcoal may be helpful if drug absorption already occurred, ingested substance undergoes significant enterohepatic recirculation, or a very large dose/bezoar is present.
- Whole bowel irrigation (polyethylene glycol or similar lavage solution) may be of benefit for
  - ○ Patients who ingest large amount of toxic substances (especially enteric-coated or sustained-release formulations)
  - ○ Patients with bezoars or who are "body packers/stuffers"
- Depending on suspected ingested substance, may consider urine alkalinization, HD, or hemoperfusion

► Supportive care should continue with frequent reevaluations for changing vital signs and mental status.

► After 4–6 hours of observation, a patient with no to mild symptoms and a low predicted toxicity may be a candidate for discharge from the ED with close observation and follow-up.

► Moderate to severe symptoms in the ED or a high risk for toxicity is an indication for admission to an ICU or general care floor.

► Intentional toxic ingestion is an indication for a psychiatric evaluation prior to discharge from the ED or inpatient setting.

CHAPTER 89

ACETAMINOPHEN

David Moyer-Diener

▶ Acetaminophen (APAP; N-acetyl-p-aminophenol) is a common drug, present in hundreds of over-the-counter preparations and prescribed medications.

▶ It is the most frequently taken drug in overdose given its wide availability.

▶ Most commonly reported drug in fatal ingestions (implicated in over 230 deaths in 2003).

PATHOPHYSIOLOGY

▶ At therapeutic doses, APAP is metabolized primarily through conjugation with hepatic glutathione.

▶ At toxic doses, saturation of the glutathione pathway leads to increased metabolism by the cytochrome p450 system.

▶ This alternate pathway leads to the accumulation of toxic metabolite, named unconjugated NAPQI.

▶ NAPQI covalently bonds to cell proteins in hepatocytes, leading to oxidative damage, inflammatory changes, impaired cell defense, and cell lysis.

CLINICAL PRESENTATION

▶ A single dose of > 150 mg/kg (child) or 7.5 g (adult) of APAP is considered potentially toxic.

▶ As little as 60 mg/kg/day or 4 g/day has been reported to produce liver failure in the setting of chronic ingestions.

▶ Special situations that may affect toxicity include multiple-dose or chronic ingestions, ingestions of extended-release preparations, alcoholics, and malnourished individuals, as well as individuals taking p450-inducing medications.

▶ The four stages of clinical disease (assumes a single acute ingestion):
  • Stage 1 (0.5–24 hours): diaphoresis, anorexia, nausea, and vomiting (these symptoms are frequently absent, and this is not indicative of the severity of intoxication).
  • Stage 2 (24–48 hours): resolution of stage 1 symptoms, RUQ pain/tenderness, and elevated angiotensin sensitivity test (AST) and ALT; bilirubin and PT/INR may start to elevate.
  • Stage 3 (48–96 hours): recurrence of anorexia, nausea, and vomiting, peak of AST/ALT, coagulopathy, encephalopathy, renal failure, hypoglycemia, and acidosis.
  • Stage 4 (after 96 hours): complete recovery or progressive liver failure and death.

DIFFERENTIAL DIAGNOSIS

▶ Viral hepatitis
▶ Alcoholic hepatitis
▶ Other medications including barbiturates, phenytoin, methyldopa, sulfa-containing compounds, and others
▶ Mushroom ingestion (*Amanita* sp.)
▶ Hepatobiliary disease

EMERGENCY DEPARTMENT MANAGEMENT

Diagnosis

▶ Clinicians should check APAP level on all suspected intoxications (including any patient presenting with suicidal ingestion).
▶ APAP level should be sent immediately if time of last dose is unknown; otherwise send at 4 hours and correlate with Rumack-Matthew nomogram (Figure 89-1). (Level will not be useful for treatment or risk stratification if sent before 4 hours post-ingestion.)
▶ High-risk ingestions include
  • Patients with history of APAP ingestion of > 150 mg/kg or 7.5 g in a 24-hour period
  • Serum APAP level above the possible toxic range on the Rumack-Matthew nomogram after known ingestion time
  • Unknown time of ingestion and a APAP level > 10 mcg/ml
  • Patients with lab evidence of hepatotoxicity and history of any potentially toxic APAP ingestion

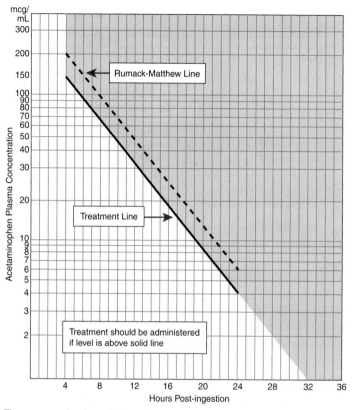

The nomogram has been developed to estimate the probability of whether a plasma acetaminophen concentration in relation to the interval post-ingestion will result in hepatotoxicity and, therefore, whether acetylcysteine therapy should be administered.

CAUTIONS FOR USE OF THIS CHART:
1. Time coordinates refer to time post-ingestion.
2. Graph relates only to plasma concentrations following a single, acute overdose ingestion.
3. The Treatment Line is plotted 25% below the Rumack-Matthew line to allow for potential errors in plasma acetaminophen assays and estimated time from ingestion of an overdose.

FIGURE 89-1.

Rumack-Matthew nomogram.

- Patients with risk factors for APAP-induced hepatotoxicity (alcoholics, p450-inducing medications) and a serum APAP level > 10 mcg/ml

▶ Electrolytes, creatinine, AST, ALT, bilirubin, and PT should be checked on suspected APAP intoxication.

Treatment

▶ ABCs
▶ GI decontamination
  • Consider gastric lavage if within 1 hour of potentially lethal dose, ingestion of extended-release formulations, or if co-ingestants slow GI motility (APAP is quickly absorbed).
  • Activated charcoal, 1 g/kg single dose, if patient seen within 4 hours; consider single dose up to 8 hours if co-ingestants slow GI motility or if extended-release APAP tablets were taken; there is no evidence that activated charcoal decreases bioavailability of N-acetylcysteine (NAC).
  • Consider whole bowel irrigation if a large number of extended-release tablets were ingested.
▶ NAC (Mucomyst), 140 mg PO/NG, then 70 mg PO/NG q4h
  • NAC acts as glutathione precursor as well as a substrate, preventing the build up of NAPQI in the cells.
  • Duration of NAC therapy is controversial: traditional length of therapy is 18 total doses (72 hours); consultation with a poison center is recommended.
  • Indications for IV NAC administration include fulminant hepatic failure, inability to tolerate PO/NG NAC (after aggressive trial of antiemetics), and possibly pregnancy (controversial).
▶ Vitamin K and FFP as necessary for prolonged PT/INR and significant bleeding.
▶ Antiemetics as needed for symptomatic relief and to keep charcoal and NAC in the GI tract.
▶ Early consultation with a toxicologist or regional poison center is recommended for significant intoxications.
▶ Consider early transfer to a liver transplantation center if INR > 5, creatinine > 2.3 mg/dl, pH < 7.35, bicarbonate < 18 mEq/L, hypotension, encephalopathy, or significant hypoglycemia is present.

Disposition

▶ Single ingestions of < 100 mg/kg: no treatment is necessary.

- ► Single ingestions of 100–150 mg/kg or 4–7.5 g: GI decontamination with activated charcoal; if 4 hour level < 150 mcg/ml, discharge with arranged visit with primary care provider within 24 hours may be adequate.
- ► Single dose of > 140 mg/kg or 7.5 g or a level above the "possible hepatic toxicity" line on the Rumack-Matthew nomogram should receive appropriate GI decontamination, NAC, supportive treatment, and hospitalization.
- ► Chronic ingestions with signs of hepatotoxicity and APAP levels > 10 mcg/ml should receive NAC, supportive treatment, and hospitalization.

CHAPTER 90

SALICYLATES

David Moyer-Diener

▶ Salicylates are a common class of drugs that are present in hundreds of medication preparations including: ASA, bismuth subsalicylate (Pepto-Bismol®), methyl salicylate (oil of wintergreen), and topical pain preparations.
▶ Chronic ingestions are associated with a mortality rate of 25%, in part due to delayed diagnosis in many cases.
▶ Clinicians should consider salicylism in individuals with anion-gap acidosis and/or mental status changes.

PATHOPHYSIOLOGY

▶ Salicylates directly stimulate the respiratory centers, increasing depth and rate of respirations, causing a respiratory alkalosis.
▶ Salicylates block the Krebs cycle and uncouple oxidative phosphorylation, which arrests ATP production and leads to accumulation of pyruvic acid, lactic acid, and ketones; a wide anion-gap acidosis results.
▶ Hyperthermia may develop secondary to catabolism and increased metabolic rate.
▶ Direct irritation to the GI tract leads to slowed GI motility, pyloric spasm, and gastritis (though significant GI bleeds are rare in the acute ingestion).
▶ Increase in insulin production and glucose consumption in the tissues may lead to hypoglycemia (tissue and CNS hypoglycemia may be present even if serum glucose is normal).
▶ Hyperglycemia may result as well from stimulation of gluconeogenesis and catecholamine release.

CLINICAL PRESENTATION

▶ Nausea, vomiting, and anorexia.
▶ Diaphoresis and hyperpyrexia.

▶ Tachypnea or "panting dog" respiration, tachycardia, and hypotension.

▶ Dehydration is common and may be severe, due to tachypnea, diaphoresis, and vomiting; renal failure may result.

▶ Tinnitus, hearing loss, alterations in consciousness, hallucinations, seizures, and cerebral edema.

▶ Respiratory alkalosis followed by progressive metabolic acidosis (mixed acid-base disturbance varies depending on the age and nutritional status of the individual as well as the severity, timing, and chronicity of the intoxication).

▶ Hypokalemia and hypocalcemia.

▶ Hypo- or hyperglycemia.

▶ Non-cardiogenic pulmonary edema can develop due to increases in pulmonary capillary permeability and hypoxia.

▶ Chronic toxicity (more common in the elderly) has many of the same symptoms but a more insidious onset, and misdiagnosis is frequent.

DIFFERENTIAL DIAGNOSIS

▶ Theophylline, caffeine, and other stimulant intoxications

▶ Acute iron ingestion

▶ Alcohol, methanol, and ethylene glycol

▶ Diabetic, alcoholic, and starvation ketoacidosis

▶ Urosepsis, meningitis, encephalitis, pneumonia, and sepsis

EMERGENCY DEPARTMENT MANAGEMENT
Diagnosis

▶ Salicylate levels should be drawn on any suspected overdose, given the wide availability of these products and mortality associated with intoxication.

▶ Maintain a high degree of clinical suspicion in any patient presenting with an unexplained acid-base disturbance (especially if mixed).

▶ Estimate ingested dose: 150–300 mg/kg may produce moderate toxicity, > 300 mg/kg severe toxicity in acute ingestions; > 100 mg/kg/day is toxic for chronic ingestions.

▶ Serum salicylate levels correlate poorly with toxicity; more important are the patient's clinical course and acid-base status.

▶ As a general rule, > 40 mg/dl correlates with *moderate* and > 100 mg/dl with *severe* toxicity in an acute ingestion.

▶ The Done nomogram (once applied widely) has very little applicability and generally should not be used.

▶ A bedside ferric chloride test (2–3 drops of 10% ferric chloride in a 1-ml sample of urine will produce a purple color) can demonstrate the presence of salicylates in the urine.

Treatment

▶ Administer dextrose if hypoglycemia is present.

▶ Administer crystalloid fluid to correct dehydration and hypotension; however, excess fluid and forced diuresis are unnecessary and can worsen cerebral and pulmonary edema.

▶ GI decontamination:
  • Consider gastric lavage within 1–2 hours of large single dose, as salicylates slow GI motility and cause pylorospasm.
  • Single dose activated charcoal, 1 g/kg; multiple doses (0.5 mg/kg every 2–4 hours) may be helpful for large ingestions.
  • Consider whole bowel irrigation if a large number of extended-release tablets were ingested or if concretion is present.
  • Endoscopy may be required to remove concretions.

▶ Blood and urine alkalinization is indicated in acute ingestions with blood levels > 35 mg/dl.
  • Sodium bicarbonate IV boluses of 1 mEq/kg (target arterial pH 7.5).
  • 2–3 ampules (88–132 mEq) of sodium bicarbonate in 1 L D5W, administered at 1.5–2 times maintenance (target urine pH 7–8).
  • Potassium chloride, 20–40 mEq/L, is required in IVF to alkalinize urine if hypokalemia is present.

▶ Indications for hemodialysis (HD) include blood levels > 100 mg/dl in acute ingestions, persistent acidosis, renal or hepatic failure, pulmonary edema, or severe CNS dysfunction; also consider in chronic ingestions with level > 60 mg/dl.

▶ Serial salicylate levels every 2–4 hours should be obtained until level is clearly decreasing.

▶ Vitamin K for treatment of coagulopathy.

▶ GI prophylaxis with an H_2 blocker or proton pump inhibitor given propensity for GI irritation.

Disposition

▶ Mild intoxications following a second *clearly* decreasing salicylate level of < 30 mg/dl may be discharged if patients are asymptomatic and a follow-up visit with a primary care provider within 24 hours can be arranged.

▶ Patients who overdosed with enteric-coated preparations or have suspicion for concretions should be admitted for observation and serial salicylate levels.

▶ Patients with pulmonary edema, persistent acidosis, renal failure, or mental status changes should be admitted to the ICU with consideration of HD.

CHAPTER 91

DIGOXIN

Jacques W. Kobersy

▶ Digoxin is used most commonly in the U.S.; less common glycosides are digitoxin and ouabain; plants with similar properties include oleander, foxglove, lily of the valley, and red squill.

▶ Narrow toxic to therapeutic window; 14 deaths attributed to digoxin toxicity in the U.S. in 2003 (most of these therapeutic errors).

▶ Digoxin used commonly today in CHF and for control of ventricular rate in atrial tachydysrhythmias.

PATHOPHYSIOLOGY

▶ Digoxin inhibits the myocardial Na^+-K^+-ATPase pump $\rightarrow$ increases intracellular Na^+ $\rightarrow$ increases Na^+-Ca^{2+} exchange $\rightarrow$ increases intracellular Ca^{2+} $\rightarrow$ augments myocyte contractile performance and LV systolic function.

▶ Digoxin slows conduction through SA and AV nodes; it also decreases levels of plasma vasoconstrictors—angiotensin II and norepinephrine—which decreases afterload.

▶ Hypokalemia can increase digoxin toxicity, especially if $K^+ < 2.5$ mEq/L (it also inhibits the Na^+-K^+-ATPase pump); hyperkalemia (> 5.0 mEq/L) may be associated with increased mortality in the setting of digoxin toxicity.

CLINICAL PRESENTATION

▶ Toxicity following acute overdose may develop within minutes to hours of exposure; chronic toxicity develops insidiously and may be difficult to diagnose because of the non-specificity of symptoms and therapeutic drug levels.

▶ Non-cardiac: headache, nausea/vomiting/diarrhea, blurred vision, disturbed color vision (yellow-green haze), dizziness, malaise, and altered mental status.

▶ Cardiac: virtually any ventricular or supraventricular dysrhythmia can occur; typical changes include increased PR, decreased QT, frequent ectopy, AV nodal blocks with increased ventricular automaticity, SVTs with AV nodal block, AV dissociation, and bidirectional VT.

DIFFERENTIAL DIAGNOSIS

▶ With significant cardiac toxicity, consider other intoxicants: CCBs, beta-blockers, antidysrhythmics (especially class Ia and Ib), clonidine, TCAs, sympathomimetics, organophosphates, plant exposures (monkshood, yew berry, false hellebore, and rhododendron, among others).

▶ Other systemic disease that can cause similar cardiac manifestations: myocardial ischemia/infarct, CHF, pericarditis/myocarditis, sick sinus syndrome, pre-excitation syndromes, electrolyte abnormalities, and thyroid dysfunction.

EMERGENCY DEPARTMENT MANAGEMENT

Diagnosis

▶ Clinical suspicion and history are paramount; especially with chronic toxicity, signs and symptoms can be insidious and non-specific.

▶ Therapeutic serum digoxin levels are 0.5–2.0 ng/ml, though there is considerable patient-to-patient variability; a patient may have significant digoxin toxicity with a serum level < 2 ng/ml.

▶ Levels should be measured 6 hours after last dose; drug distribution phase may lead to inaccurately elevated serum levels prior to 6 hours.

▶ Falsely elevated digoxin levels can be found in pregnancy, hepatobiliary disease, newborns, or cross-reactions with steroid derivatives like spironolactone or methylprednisolone.

▶ Serum digoxin levels > 3 ng/ml measured after drug distribution are generally considered toxic, if the clinical picture is consistent.

▶ Other mandatory diagnostic evaluation includes ECG, full electrolyte panel (including calcium, magnesium, and phosphorus), renal function studies, and other labs dictated by clinical presentation and suspicion of co-ingestants and/or complications.

Treatment

▸ ABCs, IV, O_2, monitor, and general supportive care.

▸ Gastric lavage is generally not helpful as GI absorption is rapid; additionally, vagal stimulation from procedure can potentially exacerbate conduction block.

▸ Activated charcoal (1 g/kg) should be given to acute ingestions; patients with chronic toxicity may benefit as well if they have taken a dose within 6 hours; consider multi-dose charcoal for those with significant toxicity (significant enterohepatic recirculation occurs).

▸ Correction of electrolyte abnormalities is indicated, especially hypokalemia and hypomagnesemia (use caution with potassium administration—close monitoring of serum potassium is necessary to avoid iatrogenic hyperkalemia).

- Hyperkalemia (> 5.5 mEq/L) should be treated with Digibind® (see below), insulin/glucose, $NaHCO_3$, and exchange resin sodium polystyrene sulfonate.

- Use of calcium is **not** recommended in digoxin toxicity with hyperkalemia, as it may exacerbate intracellular hypercalcemia, resulting in dysrhythmias or cardiac arrest.

▸ Treatment of cardiac arrhythmias: most will require Digibind® (see below); other agents to consider: atropine (0.5–2.0 mg IV) for severe bradycardia; lidocaine (1 mg/kg IV) or phenytoin (15 mg/kg IV) for ventricular arrhythmias; diltiazem (0.25 mg/kg IV) for SVT.

- Class Ia agents, such as quinidine and procainamide, are contraindicated, as they further depress AV-nodal activity.

- Cardioversion and defibrillation are indicated for unstable VT and VF, respectively, but should be avoided for supraventricular tachydysrhythmias (lethal ventricular dysrhythmias may be precipitated).

▸ Digoxin-specific antibody Fab fragments (Digibind®) indications include

- Ingestion of > 10 mg of digoxin in adults (or 4 mg in children)
- Serum digoxin levels > 10 ng/ml 6 hours post-ingestion or > 15 ng/ml at any time
- Hyperkalemia > 5.5 mEq/L (some experts recommend treatment for > 5.0 mEq/L)
- Any significant digoxin-related dysrhythmias including VT or VF, progressive bradycardia, high-degree AV nodal block, or any rhythm resulting in hypoperfusion

- Chronic digoxin poisoning with significant altered mental status, GI symptoms, or renal failure
▶ Dosing:
  - **Number of vials = [serum digoxin level (ng/ml) × weight in kg]/100, OR**
  - **Number of vials = amount ingested (mg)/0.5.**
  - If amount ingested and serum level unknown, give 10–20 vials for an acute overdose.
  - Chronic toxicity: give 3–6 vials to an adult, 1–2 vials to a child.
▶ Hemodialysis (HD) or hemoperfusion can be used for severe hyperkalemia, but both are largely ineffective for removal of digoxin itself due to large volume of distribution.

DISPOSITION

▶ All symptomatic patients with acute or chronic digoxin toxicity should be admitted to a monitored setting.
▶ Patients with hemodynamic instability or significant dysrhythmias should be in an ICU setting.

CHAPTER 92

CARBON MONOXIDE

Brian D. McBeth

▶ Leading cause of death due to poisoning in the U.S. (approximately 500/year).

▶ Often present in late fall/early winter when furnaces turned on.

▶ Exposure can come from house fires, car exhaust, furnaces, gas stoves, propane-powered tools—typically with inadequate ventilation.

▶ Most common misdiagnosis is viral illness or food poisoning with multiple family members ill.

PATHOPHYSIOLOGY

▶ CO binds avidly to Hgb, displacing O_2 and causing a functional hypoxia to cells.

▶ CO causes a leftward shift of the oxyhemoglobin dissociation curve, resulting in decreased offloading of O_2 as well.

▶ CO also inactivates cytochrome oxidase, leading to an accumulation of O_2 free radicals, lipid peroxidation, and neuronal damage/death.

▶ CO causes vasodilation, which can lead to hypotension, exacerbating hypoxia with decreased perfusion.

CLINICAL PRESENTATION

▶ Symptoms depend on level of intoxication and correlate generally with COHb level for an acute exposure (Table 92-1).

▶ However, with chronic exposure, delay in presentation, medical comorbidity, and treatment (EMS-administered O_2 en route), the correlation of COHb level with symptoms may vary widely.

▶ CO exposure can also present as an exacerbation of chronic disease, such as worsening symptoms of CAD or COPD due to ischemia.

TABLE 92-1.
SYMPTOMS ASSOCIATED WITH COHb LEVELS

COHb level (%)	Symptoms
10	Headache, mild dizziness (may be asymptomatic)
20	Dizziness, nausea, possible syncope
30	Confusion, weakness, blurred vision
40	Ataxia, disorientation, cognitive deficits
50	Seizures, coma, hypotension
≥ 60	Ventricular arrhythmias, severe ischemia, death

▶ Neuropsychiatric symptoms are also characteristic and may arise after a patient has otherwise seemed to recover from the exposure; visual disturbances, Parkinsonism, dementia, neuropathy, memory loss, and psychosis have all been reported.

EMERGENCY DEPARTMENT MANAGEMENT
Diagnosis

▶ Based on history of exposure and presentation.
▶ Check COHb level by CO-oximeter (normal 0–5%, but may be up to 10% in smokers).
▶ Expect a normal O_2 saturation (pulse oximeters cannot distinguish COHb and oxyhemoglobin) and normal PO_2.
▶ Other labs are dependent on symptoms and degree of toxicity: ABG and lactate (increasing acidosis correlates with more severe or prolonged exposure), CPK (rhabdomyolysis), ECG, cardiac enzymes.
▶ Head CT (non-contrast) indicated in any patients with neurologic symptoms as prognostic tool; low-attenuation lesions may be seen in globus pallidus, putamen, and caudate nucleus as soon as 12 hours after exposure and are associated with poor neurologic outcome.

Treatment

▶ Pre-hospital: immediate removal of patient from exposure and treatment with 100% O_2 by non-rebreather face mask or intubation if necessary.
▶ O_2 is the mainstay of treatment: half-life of COHb ranges from 4–5 hours in room air to 90 minutes with 100% FiO_2 (normobar-

ic) to 20–30 minutes with hyperbaric oxygen (HBO) treatment (2–3 atm).

▶ HBO therapy is controversial: it unquestionably reduces COHb levels more quickly but has not been shown consistently to improve neurologic function in clinical trials.

▶ Hyperbaric therapy is most likely to benefit severe intoxication including symptoms of syncope, seizures, coma; persistent neurologic symptoms despite 100% normobaric O_2 therapy; pregnant patients; symptoms of ongoing cardiac ischemia; and significantly elevated COHb levels (> 40%).

▶ In cases of significant exposure, a toxicologist and hyperbaric center should be contacted as early as possible to facilitate expedited therapy.

Disposition

▶ Patients with significant exposures, including any receiving hyperbaric therapy or having any persistent neurologic symptoms, should be admitted and monitored.

▶ Patients with minor exposures, whose symptoms have completely resolved with normobaric O_2 in the ED, may be discharged with primary care follow-up in 1–2 days.

▶ Patients and families should be educated about environmental safeguards to prevent recurrent exposure.

CHAPTER 93

TRICYCLIC ANTIDEPRESSANTS

James C. Mitchiner

▶ Patients with TCA overdose can initially appear non-toxic in the ED, before sudden clinical deterioration.
▶ Typical ECG findings that predict lethal ventricular arrhythmias include a wide QRS complex and/or a prominent terminal R wave in lead aVR.

PATHOPHYSIOLOGY

▶ TCAs act therapeutically by promoting release of CNS norepinephrine and by blocking reuptake of amines (norepinephrine, serotonin, dopamine) in the CNS.
▶ TCAs competitively antagonize muscarinic acetylcholine receptors leading to central and peripheral anticholinergic effects; they also antagonize peripheral alpha-adrenergic receptors, which can lead to hypotension; tachycardia results from anticholinergic effects and increased levels of norepinephrine.
▶ Seizures are likely due to increased levels of CNS norepinephrine and blockage of GABA receptors.

CLINICAL PRESENTATION

▶ Cardiac: sinus tachycardia (50%), hypotension (14–51%).
  • ECG changes include sinus tachycardia, wide QRS complex, prominent R wave in the terminal 40 milliseconds of the QRS complex of lead aVR, prolonged QT interval, AV blocks, nonspecific ST-T wave changes.
  • SVT and VT may result, as well as VF and torsades de pointes.
▶ Neurologic: confusion, ataxia, myoclonus, nystagmus, seizures (3–8%, usually seen within 6 hours of presentation, with greater

373

likelihood in patients with QRS > 100 milliseconds), obtundation, coma (~17%); multiple seizures may cause complications of rhabdomyolysis and renal failure, hyperthermia, severe acidosis.

▶ GI: abdominal pain, vomiting, diarrhea, prolonged ileus, decreased or absent bowel sounds; slowed gut motility results in increased absorption.

▶ Other: urinary retention, hypoxia, aspiration pneumonitis, ARDS, ischemic colitis; most of these are related to prolonged hypotension and decreased respiratory effort associated with significant ingestion.

▶ The muscle relaxant cyclobenzaprine is structurally similar to amitriptyline, and poisoning with this agent shares many of the features of TCA overdose (including induction of ventricular arrhythmias).

DIFFERENTIAL DIAGNOSIS

▶ Other toxicologic causes for tachycardia, hypotension, and/or seizures: anticholinergics, sympathomimetics, clonidine, sedative/hypnotics, toxic alcohols, antipsychotics, salicylates, MAOIs, CO (severe).

▶ Withdrawal states, such as ethanol or benzodiazepine withdrawal, should be considered.

▶ See Table 99-1 for differential diagnosis for altered mental status.

EMERGENCY DEPARTMENT MANAGEMENT

Diagnosis

▶ Diagnosis of TCA overdose may be obvious in a patient with a history of ingestion with tachycardia, hypotension, altered mental status, and seizures; remember to consider polysubstance intoxication.

▶ Serum TCA levels should be checked to confirm exposure, but treatment should not be delayed awaiting confirmation, nor should drug levels be used to guide treatment.

▶ Characteristic ECG changes (sinus tachycardia, wide QRS > 100 milliseconds, terminal R wave in aVR) are not diagnostic by themselves but help to confirm the clinical syndrome and predict risks for malignant arrhythmias and seizures.

▶ See Chap. 88 for other appropriate lab testing.

Treatment

▶ ABCs with particular attention to early airway intervention if altered mental status or suspicion of significant intoxication with predicted decline.

▶ IV access, O_2, and continuous cardiac monitoring are indicated.

▶ Consider gastric lavage with NS and large-bore orogastric tube for patients presenting 1–2 hours after a significant ingestion; airway protection is generally indicated, and discussion with a toxicologist/poison control center is recommended.

▶ Ipecac is contraindicated due to seizure and aspiration risk.

▶ Single dose activated charcoal (1 g/kg) should be given to all patients orally or by gastric tube; a cathartic (sorbitol) may be added.

▶ IV $NaHCO_3$ is indicated for patients with wide QRS complexes, prominent R waves in aVR, malignant arrhythmias, hypotension, or metabolic acidosis; some experts advocate treating sinus tachycardia with bicarbonate, even in the absence of widened QRS or hypotension.

▶ Dose of $NaHCO_3$:
  - 1–2 mEq/kg IV of 8.4% solution, by bolus or rapid infusion.
  - Continuous infusion (2–3 ampules or 100–150 ml of 8.4% $NaHCO_3$ added to 1 L D5/W) at 2–3 ml/kg/hour.
  - The endpoint is narrowing of QRS interval and patient improvement; blood pH should be maintained 7.5–7.55.

▶ Refractory hypotension is the most common cause of death in severely intoxicated patients.
  - Treat hypotension initially with isotonic IVF and bicarbonate.
  - Options for refractory hypotension include hypertonic saline and vasopressor therapy with norepinephrine, dopamine, or epinephrine.
  - If still refractory, consider aggressive extracorporeal support of BP with cardiopulmonary bypass or ECMO.

▶ Seizures can be treated with usual doses of benzodiazepines, along with bicarbonate; barbiturates and propofol are potential second-line agents for refractory seizures; avoid phenytoin as it can worsen cardiotoxicity.

▶ Physostigmine and flumazenil are contraindicated in mixed ingestions, as either can precipitate seizures.

▶ Several case reports have described successful use of high-dose glucagon (10 mg IV) for patients with refractory hypotension and cardiac arrhythmias.

▶ Certain antiarrhythmics are contraindicated: agents from classes 1A (quinidine, procainamide), 1C (flecainide), and III (amiodarone); also beta-blockers and CCBs.

▶ Therapy with TCA-specific antibody fragments (anti-TCA Fab) has been proposed based on experimental studies; clinical trials are ongoing, but this treatment modality is generally not readily available at this time.

Disposition

▶ Patients with symptoms and signs of toxicity, including sinus tachycardia, should be admitted to a monitored bed.

▶ ICU admission is appropriate for patients with altered mental status, respiratory depression, seizures, hypotension, QRS prolongation, or arrhythmias.

▶ Inpatient monitoring should continue until the ECG remains stable for at least 18–24 hours; sinus tachycardia can persist up to a week following ingestion. Consultation with a poison center is recommended for assistance with appropriate disposition.

▶ Patients with normal mental status, stable vital signs (without tachycardia), and a normal neurologic exam should be observed in the ED for a minimum of 6 hours prior to discharge or admission to a psychiatric unit.

CHAPTER 94

SELECTIVE SEROTONIN REUPTAKE INHIBITORS (SSRIs)

Brian D. McBeth

▶ Most commonly prescribed class of antidepressants today
▶ Frequently taken in overdose—more than 46,000 calls to poison centers in 2002 related to SSRI exposures

PATHOPHYSIOLOGY

▶ Inhibit reuptake of serotonin at the synapse level.
▶ Increased serotonin activity and inhibition of dopamine release may partially explain antidepressant activity.
▶ Serotonin syndrome (see Clinical Presentation below) is a result of overstimulation of serotonin receptors related to SSRIs, TCAs, MAOIs, or other serotonergic agents.

CLINICAL PRESENTATION

▶ Many SSRI overdoses are asymptomatic.
▶ SSRI overdose may cause vomiting, dizziness, blurred vision, drowsiness, hyponatremia, seizures, and QRS prolongation (rarely).
▶ Citalopram specifically has been linked to more frequent seizures and QT prolongation in overdose; bupropion and venlafaxine are also associated with seizure activity.
▶ Serotonin syndrome is a constellation of symptoms including behavioral (confusion, agitation, coma, insomnia), autonomic (fever, hyperhidrosis, tachycardia, hypotension or HTN, tachypnea), and neurologic (myoclonus, tremors, rigidity, hyperreflexia, ataxia, akathisia); diarrhea may be present.
▶ Serotonin syndrome is a diagnosis of exclusion, after infectious, metabolic, psychiatric, and other toxic causes have been eliminated; diagnosis can only be made with a recent addition (or increase in dose of) a serotonergic agent.

DIFFERENTIAL DIAGNOSIS

▶ Depends on presenting symptoms: overdose of SSRI agents can present as sedation similar to opiate or benzodiazepine intoxication; GI symptoms similar to a viral illness; seizures, if present, have a wide differential including metabolic, infectious, and traumatic causes; for ECG changes (QT prolongation or QRS widening), consider TCAs, antipsychotics, antiarrhythmics (class IA, IC, III), or electrolyte disorder (hypokalemia, hypomagnesemia).

▶ Neuroleptic malignant syndrome (NMS) is the diagnosis most often confused with serotonin syndrome—distinguish based on known exposure (neuroleptics vs. serotonergic agents) and symptoms. NMS develops gradually (days to weeks) and persists for days after exposure is removed; serotonin syndrome usually develops within hours of exposure to new agent (or increased dose) and resolves quickly when exposure is removed.

▶ NMS usually shows more pronounced hyperthermia, akinesia, and "lead pipe" rigidity vs. agitation, myoclonus, and hyperreflexia of serotonin syndrome; mortality is much higher with NMS (15–20%).

EMERGENCY DEPARTMENT MANAGEMENT

Diagnosis

▶ In intentional overdose, patients are typically brought in with empty pill bottles; attempt to quantify overdose.

▶ In patients without a clear overdose history, take a detailed history of psychotropic medications (which ones taken, compliance, dosages, recent adjustment in dosages or frequency).

▶ Serotonin syndrome is a diagnosis of exclusion and must consider other possibilities first: alternative ingestions, metabolic or infectious causes, NMS (make sure a neuroleptic agent has not recently been introduced nor dose increased).

▶ All patients should have a 12-lead ECG performed to rule out prolongation of the QT (most frequently with citalopram) and also as a screen for more serious co-ingestants (TCAs, etc.).

▶ See Chap. 88 for other appropriate lab testing.

Management

▶ Supportive care is the mainstay of treatment—IVF and observation.

▶ As most ingestions are not life-threatening, orogastric or NG lavage is generally not indicated.

▶ Activated charcoal (1 g/kg) is generally recommended for more than minimal ingestions.

▶ For patients with suspected serotonin syndrome, all potentially offending medications should be held; treatment depends on nature and severity of symptoms.

▶ Cyproheptadine (antihistamine and serotonin receptor antagonist) may play a beneficial role; consultation with a toxicologist or poison center is recommended.

Disposition

▶ Most patients with pure SSRI overdoses can be discharged home or transferred to a psychiatric facility if their ECG and mental status are normal after 2–4 hours of observation.

▶ Reasons for inpatient admission include co-ingestants, ongoing CNS depression, ECG changes, serotonin syndrome, and suicidality.

CHAPTER 95

MONOAMINE OXIDASE INHIBITORS (MAOIs)

Brian D. McBeth

▸ Most commonly used for treatment of atypical depression, Parkinson's disease, post-traumatic stress disorder, phobias, and other psychiatric disorders.
▸ Specific agents include phenelzine and tranylcypromine (antidepressants), selegiline (anti-Parkinson), and procarbazine (chemotherapeutic); St. John's wort also has MAOI-like properties.

PATHOPHYSIOLOGY

▸ Monoamine oxidase is a ubiquitous intracellular enzyme that degrades bioactive amines (epinephrine, serotonin, dopamine, tyramine, amphetamines).
▸ MAOIs selectively or non-selectively block components of this enzyme (MAO-A and MAO-B) by competitive antagonism.
▸ Result is elevation of level of bioactive amines (dopamine, epinephrine, serotonin), which leads to antidepressive effects.
▸ MAOIs can cause sympathomimetic effects from the acute release of neurotransmitters or sympatholytic effects from their depletion with long-term use; serotonin syndrome is also described, especially when used in combination with other serotonin reuptake inhibitors.
▸ Tyramine-related hypertensive crisis can result from blockage of MAO-A and consumption of excessive amounts of exogenous tyramine contained in certain foods (red wine, cheese, smoked/aged meats and fish, etc.).

CLINICAL PRESENTATION

▸ In overdose, MAOI ingestion typically causes tachycardia (less commonly bradycardia) and may present with either hypotension or HTN. CNS symptoms are also frequent and include increased activity (agitation, hallucinations, muscle rigidity, hyperreflexia, seizures) and decreased activity (somnolence, coma). Hyperpyrexia and rhabdomyolysis may be present. Late complications include MI, disseminated intravascular coagulation, and ARDS; death has resulted from significant overdoses (> 2 mg/kg).

▶ Symptoms are typically delayed: usually begin 6–12 hours after ingestion but may be delayed as long as 24–32 hours after acute overdose.

▶ Tyramine crisis presents more acutely (minutes to hours) with HTN, tachycardia, hyperpyrexia, disorientation, flushing, rigidity, seizures; intracranial hemorrhage and death have been reported.

▶ MAOIs have numerous drug–drug interactions, so addition of a new antidepressant, neuroleptic, sympathomimetic, opiate, or other medication may cause acute symptoms similar to a tyramine crisis; commonly implicated medications include SSRIs, methylxanthines, cocaine, amphetamines, lithium, opiates (especially meperidine), and antihistamines.

EMERGENCY DEPARTMENT MANAGEMENT

Diagnosis

▶ Primarily a clinical diagnosis based on history of exposure, symptoms, and physical exam findings.

▶ Although screening for MAOIs is not available on most urine toxicology screens, certain MAOIs (selegiline and tranylcypromine) will cross-react and give positive amphetamine results.

▶ See Chap. 88 for other appropriate lab testing.

Management

▶ Supportive care: cardiac and BP monitoring, IVF, external cooling for hyperthermia.

▶ A toxicology or regional poison center consultation should occur early with a suspected significant exposure.

▶ All significant acute overdoses should be treated with activated charcoal (1 g/kg) PO or NG; activated charcoal is not recommended for tyramine food exposure.

▶ Gastric lavage may be considered for large or symptomatic ingestions up to 4 hours post-ingestion (gastric motility may be delayed).

► HTN should be treated with nitroprusside (0.5 mcg/kg/minute infusion) or phentolamine (1–5 mg bolus in adults, followed by infusion, 5 mg/hour); these agents are easily titratable and can be discontinued if hypotension occurs; continuous arterial monitoring of BP is indicated in these patients.

► Bradycardia, if present, should be treated with atropine (up to 3 mg in an adult); if unsuccessful, isoproterenol or external/transvenous pacing may be required.

► Hypotension typically occurs later and should first be treated with fluid hydration; if unsuccessful, norepinephrine is the pressor of choice (start low: 0.1 mcg/kg/minute).

► CNS overstimulation may respond to benzodiazepines; these are also first-line treatment for seizures.

► Cyproheptadine, an antihistamine and serotonin antagonist, has theoretical benefit if serotonin syndrome or symptoms predominate; discussion with a toxicologist is warranted if considering treatment.

Disposition

► All patients with suspicion of significant MAOI overdose or exposure should be admitted with cardiac monitoring for 24–36 hours of observation, even if asymptomatic.

► Any patient with hemodynamic instability should be admitted to an ICU setting.

CHAPTER 96

LITHIUM

James C. Mitchiner

▶ Serum toxic levels are generally > 1.5 mEq/L; may be normal early in the course of acute intoxication and do not correlate with CNS lithium levels.

▶ Consider early hemodialysis (HD) for patients with significant acute or chronic toxicity.

PATHOPHYSIOLOGY

▶ May inhibit release of norepinephrine and serotonin and increase reuptake of norepinephrine; may also affect expression of serotonin and adrenergic receptors.

▶ Lithium can cause nephrogenic diabetes insipidus by decreasing cAMP in the kidney and blocking the action of antidiuretic hormone (ADH); the resulting hyperosmolar state can subsequently lead to increased lithium toxicity.

▶ Certain drugs decrease renal clearance of lithium and cause elevated levels: thiazide diuretics, NSAIDs, phenytoin, metronidazole, tetracycline, doxycycline.

▶ Neuroleptic agents and carbamazepine can cause increased toxicity at therapeutic levels.

CLINICAL PRESENTATION

▶ Acute toxicity.
- Neurologic: dysarthria, ataxia, tinnitus, nystagmus, hand tremor (up to 65%), weakness, extrapyramidal symptoms, seizures, coma
- GI: abdominal pain, nausea, vomiting, diarrhea
- Renal: polyuria, renal failure
- Cardiac: QT interval prolongation, non-specific ST-T wave changes, first-degree AV block, and sinus node dysfunction

▶ Chronic toxicity.
  • Neurologic: same as acute, and can also develop Parkinsonism, memory deficits, psychosis, and intracranial HTN
  • Renal: nephrogenic diabetes insipidus, interstitial nephritis, renal failure
  • Cardiac: same as acute, and can also develop myocarditis
  • Endocrine: hypothyroidism
  • Hematologic: aplastic anemia
▶ Chronic toxicity may occur in the setting of reduced salt or water intake, or conditions predisposing to dehydration (vomiting, diarrhea, diuretics, heat, exercise, polyuria, etc.).

DIFFERENTIAL DIAGNOSIS

▶ Depends on clinical signs and symptoms.
▶ Other drugs presenting with nystagmus: anticonvulsants, alcohols, phencyclidine, solvents, and sedative/hypnotics.
▶ Other drugs presenting with tremors: sympathomimetic agents, anticholinergics, antihistamines, cocaine, drug withdrawal syndromes.
▶ See Table 99-1 for differential diagnosis of altered mental status.

EMERGENCY DEPARTMENT MANAGEMENT

Diagnosis

▶ Diagnosis may be difficult due to varied and subtle clinical presentations.
▶ Serum lithium levels do not always correlate with neurologic symptoms and may be normal early in the course of acute intoxication.
▶ Therapeutic lithium levels are generally 0.6–1.2 mEq/L; in an acute ingestion, concentrations between 1.5 and 2.5 mEq/L indicate moderate intoxication; concentrations between 2.5 and 3.5 mEq/L suggest severe intoxication; levels > 4.0 mEq/L are potentially lethal.
▶ In chronic toxicity, the lithium level may not be as impressively elevated, though severe toxicity may result from levels > 1.5 mEq/L.
▶ Lab/ancillary evaluation in the ED should also include
  • Electrolytes, BUN, creatinine, glucose.

- ECG.
- Continuous monitoring of urinary output (UOP).
- See Chap. 88 for other appropriate lab testing.
- Serial lithium levels should be considered to follow distribution/response to treatment in a significant intoxication.

Treatment

▶ ED management is generally supportive, with aggressive infusion of IVF, continuous cardiac monitoring, and airway management as needed.

▶ Orogastric/NG lavage may be considered in an early presentation of an acute overdose of a sustained-release lithium formulation; absorption is rapid for non–sustained-release formulations, and thus gastric emptying is generally not helpful.

▶ Although activated charcoal does not bind lithium, this agent should be used if there is possibility of co-ingestants.

▶ Whole bowel irrigation using polyethylene glycol solution (GoLYTELY™) may be helpful, especially in the setting of acute sustained-release exposures; infusion rates per orogastric/NG tube are doses of 2 L/hour in adults, 500 ml/hour in children; endpoint is clear rectal effluent.

▶ Multiple doses of oral sodium polystyrene sulfonate (Kayexalate™) have been shown in basic science trials and case reports to increase GI excretion of lithium; consultation with a toxicologist or poison control center is recommended, and close monitoring for hypokalemia is mandatory.

▶ HD indications include
  - Serum lithium level of 2.0–4.0 mEq/L in the setting of severe symptoms
  - Serum lithium level > 4.0 mEq/L regardless of symptoms
  - ARF
  - Significant neurologic symptoms including altered mental status
  - Significant ingestion of sustained-release preparations with anticipated toxicity
  - Rapidly increasing or persistently elevated lithium levels (relative)

▶ Seizures should be treated with standard doses of IV benzodiazepines. Avoid phenytoin, as it decreases renal excretion of lithium.

Disposition

▶ Indications for admission:
  • Patients with acute overdose and toxic levels (> 1.5 mEq/L)
  • Patients with symptoms regardless of their lithium levels or acuity of ingestion
▶ If patient has altered mental status, seizures, or any cardiac toxicity, admission should be to an ICU setting.
▶ If dialysis is likely to be required, the on-call nephrologist should be consulted at the time of admission.

CHAPTER 97

BARBITURATES

Swagata Mandal

▶ Once a very popular recreational drug of abuse, causing physical dependence and a life-threatening withdrawal syndrome.
▶ Mainly used today for procedural sedation and anesthesia and as an adjunct to anticonvulsant therapy.
▶ Lethal dose is 3 g of short-acting agents or 5–10 g of long-acting agents.

PATHOPHYSIOLOGY

▶ Classified by onset and duration of action.
- Ultrashort (methohexital, thiopental)
  ○ Onset immediate after IV, duration minutes
- Short-acting (pentobarbital, secobarbital)
  ○ Onset 10–15 minutes after PO, duration 6–8 hours
- Long-acting (phenobarbital)
  ○ Onset 1 hour, duration 10–12 hours
▶ Barbiturates cause CNS depression by binding to GABA-sensitive ion channels in the CNS and potentiating the effects of GABA.
▶ Act on the medulla to cause respiratory depression in a dose-dependent fashion.
▶ In overdose, cause decreased transmission in autonomic ganglia and decrease myocardial and GI tract activity.

CLINICAL PRESENTATION

▶ Respiratory depression in a spectrum from sedation to stupor to coma and death; respiratory failure is the most common cause of death in early intoxication.
▶ Abdominal distention secondary to ileus and delayed gastric emptying.
▶ Mild-to-moderate intoxication presents with ataxia, slurred speech, drowsiness, and impaired memory and judgment.

▶ Severe intoxication.
- Significant hypotension, especially in patients with heart failure or hypovolemia.
- Hypothermia (31°–36.6° C) common in intoxication with short-acting agents.
- Cyanosis corresponding to level of hypoxemia.
- Non-cardiogenic pulmonary edema.
- Neurologic signs are variable and do not necessarily correlate with level of intoxication or CNS depression.
    ○ Pupils: normal or small; reactive; nystagmus and disconjugate gaze possible
    ○ Gag: diminished or absent
    ○ Flaccid muscle tone
    ○ Decerebrate or decorticate posturing
▶ Withdrawal presents similarly to ethanol withdrawal with tremors, hallucinations, and seizures.
▶ 50% of patients with lethal intoxications and 6% of all patients with barbiturate poisoning develop tense, clear, bullous skin lesions on the hand, knees, and buttocks within 24 hours.

EMERGENCY DEPARTMENT MANAGEMENT
Diagnosis
▶ Exclude other causes of respiratory/CNS depression; see Table 99-1 for differential diagnosis of altered mental status.
▶ CXR may show non-cardiogenic pulmonary edema.
▶ Urine and blood tests for barbiturates:
- Qualitative tests only establish presence of barbiturates, not presence of toxic level.
- Serum barbiturate levels do not reflect CNS concentrations and may not be available in a timely fashion.

Treatment
▶ Cardiovascular and respiratory support
- ABCs, IV, O_2, monitor
▶ Decontamination and elimination
- Activated charcoal for recent ingestion: 50–100 g PO or per NG tube.

- Multiple dose activated charcoal reduces enterohepatic recirculation: 25 g PO every 2 hours.
  - Increases clearance, decreases elimination half-life
  - May adsorb toxin from a gastric bezoar and interrupt enterohepatic circulation
- Alkalinization of urine with $NaHCO_3$ reduces the elimination half-life of phenobarbital and increases its renal clearance.
  - 1–2 mEq/kg bolus followed by 2–3 ampules of $NaHCO_3$ in 1 L of D5W titrated to maintain urine pH of 7.5–8.0
- Gastric lavage for drug removal is indicated only in the setting of acute life-threatening overdose that presents within 1 hour of ingestion.
- Hemodialysis (HD) is rarely indicated.
  - May consider for phenobarbital poisoning with anuric renal failure or with shock and ileus.

Disposition

▶ Patients with barbiturate ingestion should be observed and monitored in the ED for at least 6 hours. Asymptomatic patients may be discharged or transferred for psychiatric evaluation.

▶ Those who are symptomatic should be admitted for further observation and treatment.

CHAPTER 98

BENZODIAZEPINES

Elke G. Marksteiner

- ▶ Introduced in the 1950s, these are the most commonly prescribed sedative-hypnotics; also have anxiolytic, muscle relaxant, amnestic, and anticonvulsant properties.
- ▶ Fatalities due to pure benzodiazepine overdose are relatively rare; poor outcomes are commonly due to co-ingestion of other substances. Approximately 20 deaths were reported in 2003 that were attributed to benzodiazepine toxicity.

PATHOPHYSIOLOGY

- ▶ Main site of action is CNS, where they potentiate the effect of the inhibitory neurotransmitter GABA by opening receptor chloride channels.
- ▶ Cardiac toxicity can occur from vascular smooth muscle dilatation and direct depression of cardiac contractility.
- ▶ Tolerance can develop with chronic benzodiazepine exposure, and withdrawal is common (especially with short-acting agents).
- ▶ Flunitrazepam (Rohypnol) is an illegal benzodiazepine in the United States that is often used as a "date rape" drug; it is long-acting (8–12 hours) and can cause profound amnesia, which is enhanced by ethanol.

CLINICAL PRESENTATION

- ▶ Lethargy, drowsiness, and CNS depression (ranges from mild depression to coma).
- ▶ Ataxia, dysarthria, nystagmus, hallucinations.
- ▶ Respiratory depression, hypoventilation, hypercarbia, hypoxia, aspiration.
- ▶ Hypotension, tachycardia.
- ▶ Hypothermia.

TABLE 98-1.
HALF-LIVES OF THE BENZODIAZEPINES

Ultrashort-acting	Short-acting	Long-acting
Midazolam 2–5 hours Triazolam 2–3 hours	Alprazolam 11–16 hours Chlordiazepoxide 5–15 hours Lorazepam 10–20 hours Oxazepam 5–15 hours Temazepam 10–16 hours	Diazepam 20–50 hours Clonazepam 18–50 hours Clorazepate 30–200 hours

▶ Paradoxical excitation can occur (more common in pediatric or geriatric patients).

▶ Benzodiazepine withdrawal can resemble severe ethanol withdrawal—agitation, tachycardia, HTN, hyperthermia, and seizures.

▶ Approximate half-lives of parent compounds: Table 98-1.

DIFFERENTIAL DIAGNOSIS

▶ Other drugs that cause CNS and respiratory depression: ethanol, barbiturates, TCAs, opiates, GHB, chloral hydrate, meprobamate, neuroleptics, CO.

▶ Consider co-ingestion, especially if significant CNS depression is present—morbidity and mortality are correlated with other substances ingested.

▶ See Table 99-1 for differential diagnosis of altered mental status.

EMERGENCY DEPARTMENT MANAGEMENT
Diagnosis

▶ Urine drug screen for qualitative confirmation of benzodiazepine overdose has multiple limitations; not all benzodiazepines are present in large enough concentrations to be detected, and many active metabolites are also not detected. A negative urine screen does not exclude the possibility of benzodiazepine exposure or toxicity.

▶ Flunitrazepam is rapidly metabolized and therefore difficult to detect on standardized urine drug screens. An active metabolite

(7-amino-flunitrazepam) may be detectable in urine up to 72 hours after ingestion; consider freezing 30 ml of urine for later diagnostic testing.

▶ See Chap. 88 for other appropriate lab testing.

Treatment

▶ ABCs:
- Monitor carefully for airway problems and worsening respiratory depression; early intubation to protect airway for significant CNS depression and concern for aspiration.
- Significant hypotension is unusual in isolated benzodiazepine overdose; should be initially treated with IVF and consideration of other causes.

▶ Consider giving naloxone if co-ingestion with opioids is suspected.

▶ Gastric lavage is generally not necessary and may put patient at risk for aspiration; it may be considered for co-ingestants, but intubation should generally precede attempt if any significant CNS depression is present.

▶ Significant ingestions should generally receive decontamination with single dose activated charcoal (1 g/kg) PO or orogastric/NG tube; consider intubation prior to administration if significant CNS depression or concern for aspiration.

▶ Flumazenil:
- Competitive antagonist at the benzodiazepine receptor, which can reverse sedative effects of benzodiazepines.
- Main indications are accidental benzodiazepine overdose in non-habituated user or reversal of conscious sedation.
- Contraindications (may precipitate seizures):
  ○ Chronic benzodiazepine use
  ○ Concomitant or suspected ingestion of drugs that lower seizure threshold (TCAs, cocaine, lithium, theophylline, chloral hydrate)
  ○ History of prior seizures
  ○ ECG abnormality suggestive of TCA exposure (QRS or QT prolongation, prominent R wave in terminal 40 milliseconds of aVR)
  ○ Hemodynamic instability or hypoxia
- Dose: 0.1–0.2 mg IV slowly over 1 minute; this can be repeated every 2 minutes as needed. Total dose should not exceed 3 mg (some authorities suggest total dose should not

exceed 1 mg); initial pediatric dose is 0.01 mg/kg (total dose should not exceed 1 mg).

- Half-life is approximately 50 minutes, so expect re-sedation with most benzodiazepines.

▶ Benzodiazepine withdrawal may be treated with diazepam loading intravenously with titration to improvement in symptoms; phenobarbital is an appropriate alternative agent.

▶ Counseling, STD, and pregnancy prophylaxis in appropriate cases if suspicion of sexual assault and flunitrazepam exposure.

Disposition

▶ Any patient with continued altered mental status, respiratory depression, cardiovascular compromise, or exposure to toxic co-ingestions requires admission.

▶ Admission to an ICU setting is generally indicated for respiratory depression, obtundation, or cardiovascular compromise.

▶ All patients should be monitored for 4–6 hours; may consider discharge to home with family member if patient's mental status is normal, hemodynamically stable, and not suicidal.

CHAPTER 99

OPIOIDS

Joshua A. Small and Brian D. McBeth

▶ Opioids are a broad group of drugs including natural opium-derived alkaloids like morphine and codeine (opiates) and synthetic compounds like fentanyl and meperidine.

▶ Generally used as analgesics, but also as antitussives (codeine) and antidiarrheals (diphenoxylate).

▶ Oral opiates (hydrocodone, oxycodone) are being abused at increasing rates: 4.7% of young adults in the U.S. reported past-month, non-medicinal analgesic use in 2003.

PATHOPHYSIOLOGY

▶ Clinical effects are related to stimulation of three major groups of opioid receptors: μ (mu), κ (kappa), and σ (sigma); signaling occurs by a G protein mechanism, and receptor effects include analgesia, sedation, euphoria, dependence, GI dysmotility, respiratory depression, etc.

▶ Half-lives vary widely based on specific compound consumed (from short-acting fentanyl to long-acting methadone).

CLINICAL PRESENTATION

▶ Signs and symptoms of intoxication: depressed level of consciousness, decreased respiratory effort or apnea, bronchospasm, slurred speech, miosis, orthostatic hypotension, decreased gastric motility/bowel sounds, and pruritus (due to histamine release).

▶ Chronic IV users may have stigmata of chronic opiate abuse including track marks, multiple skin abscesses (from "skin popping"—injecting directly into the skin), or suspicious scarring of the extremities.

▶ Seizures can be seen with meperidine or propoxyphene.

▶ Non-cardiogenic pulmonary edema can be seen with almost any opioid overdose.

TABLE 99-1.
NON-TOXICOLOGIC CAUSES OF ALTERED MENTAL STATUS

Hypoglycemia
Hypoxia
Trauma or elevated ICP (mass lesion)
Infectious (meningitis, encephalitis)
Seizures
Stroke (pontine stroke typically has miotic pupils as well)
Hypertensive encephalopathy
Metabolic/electrolyte (hypo/hypernatremia, hypo/hypercalcemia, hyperkalemia, uremia)
Endocrine (DKA, hyperosmolar coma, hypothyroidism, adrenal insufficiency, etc.)
Psychiatric (severe depression, conversion disorder, malingering)

▶ IV drug users may present with other systemic complications of their use, including bacterial endocarditis, sepsis, CNS infections (meningitis, epidural abscesses, intracranial abscesses), infectious hepatitis, and HIV/AIDS.

DIFFERENTIAL DIAGNOSIS

▶ Other drugs that cause CNS and respiratory depression: ethanol, barbiturates, benzodiazepines, toxic alcohols, TCAs, GHB, chloral hydrate, meprobamate, neuroleptics, clonidine, CO.
▶ Consider non-toxicologic causes for altered mental status (Table 99-1).

EMERGENCY DEPARTMENT MANAGEMENT
Diagnosis

▶ Diagnosis is clinical, based on consistent history, physical exam, and response to naloxone (see below).
▶ Urine drugs of abuse screens have variable sensitivity and may commonly show false negatives for patients exposed to synthetic opioids (fentanyl, methadone are commonly missed).
▶ False positives can also result if patient has consumed large amount of poppy seeds; urine screening positives should generally be considered preliminary, pending definitive assays.
▶ Consider co-ingestants and combination products; patients taking Vicodin, Tylox, Darvon, etc. may have acetaminophen (APAP) or salicylate toxicity from products taken in large quantity.

Treatment

▶ The mainstay of opioid overdose treatment is respiratory support (bag-valve-mask ventilation, intubation) and naloxone (Narcan) administration.

▶ Naloxone is a non-specific opioid receptor antagonist with a half-life of 60–90 minutes in adults.

▶ **Dosing of naloxone is 0.05–2.0 mg IV** (can also be given via ETT or IM) titrated to effect of spontaneous respirations; this can be re-dosed every 3–5 minutes as necessary. Patients suspected to be opioid dependent should receive smaller doses (starting with 0.05 mg) because administration can precipitate withdrawal.

▶ In addition, because many of the opioids have longer half-lives than naloxone, repeated administration or a continuous infusion may be necessary; a starting estimate for naloxone drip infusion is to administer two-thirds of the reversal dose required continuously per hour, titrated to adequate respiration.

Disposition

▶ Patients on continuous naloxone infusions or requiring repeated dosing require admission to a monitored setting for neurologic checks and respiratory monitoring.

▶ Patients presenting with profound obtundation are at risk for development of pulmonary edema and warrant admission for 24 hours of observation.

▶ Patients who require only a single dose of naloxone and have taken a short-acting opioid without co-ingestants who have a normal mental status and no respiratory complaints after a 4-hour observation period may be discharged with a family member.

▶ Referral for drug abuse/dependence counseling and treatment may be appropriate.

OPIOID WITHDRAWAL

▶ Opioid withdrawal can occur in patients who are chronically using opioids and who either stop taking their medications or are given an antagonist such as naloxone.

▶ Clinical presentation includes mydriasis, lacrimation, diarrhea, nausea, vomiting, yawning, diaphoresis, rhinorrhea, piloerection, anxiety, and restlessness.

▶ Opioid withdrawal, though distressing and uncomfortable for the patient, is generally not life-threatening.

▶ Depending on the situation, signs and symptoms of opioid withdrawal may be treated by judicious administration of small amounts of opiate medication or clonidine, a centrally-acting alpha-agonist, which can ameliorate some of the catecholamine stimulation associated with withdrawal.

CHAPTER 100

COCAINE

Brian D. McBeth

- ▶ Most frequent drug-related cause of ED visits in the U.S.
- ▶ 1.5 million regular users of cocaine in the U.S. today
- ▶ Increasing incidence of cocaine use (934,000 new users in 1998) due to increased availability, low cost, and highly addictive forms of drug

PATHOPHYSIOLOGY

- ▶ Blocks fast sodium channels and stabilizes axonal membranes
- ▶ Blocks reuptake of dopamine, serotonin, epinephrine, and norepinephrine, which leads to CNS hyperstimulation
- ▶ Acutely, can induce vasoconstriction, vasospasm, MI, supraventricular and ventricular arrhythmia, aortic dissection, stroke, SAH and other intracranial bleeding, seizures, hyperthermia, rhabdomyolysis, bronchospasm, pulmonary edema, pulmonary infarcts, uteroplacental insufficiency, placental abruption, and acute psychosis
- ▶ Chronically, causes increased atherosclerosis, platelet aggregation, increased LV hypertrophy and dysfunction, cardiomyopathies, drug tolerance, and physical and psychological addiction

CLINICAL PRESENTATION

- ▶ Classically a sympathomimetic toxidrome: tachycardia, HTN, mydriasis, hyperthermia, diaphoresis (Table 100-1).
- ▶ Psychomotor agitation ranges from restlessness and mild increase in motor activity to agitation and disorientation to tonic-clonic seizure activity or frank psychosis.
- ▶ Cocaine chest pain can signify myocardial ischemia or an infarction, even in a young patient with no evidence of pre-existing cardiac disease; an ECG in this setting is less sensitive and less specific with recent cocaine use.
- ▶ Focal neurologic deficits in a cocaine-intoxicated individual suggest an ischemic or hemorrhagic stroke or SAH.

TABLE 100-1.
DIFFERENTIAL DIAGNOSIS OF SYMPATHOMIMETIC TOXIDROME

PCP
Amphetamines, including MDMA (ecstasy)
Ephedrine and related decongestants
Caffeine
Ethanol withdrawal
MAOI crisis
Thyrotoxicosis
Hypertensive encephalopathy
Neuroleptic malignant syndrome
Pheochromocytoma
Psychiatric (mania, psychosis)

▶ Tonic-clonic seizure activity is common and may include status epilepticus.

▶ Cardiac dysrhythmias are varied and may result from primary cocaine toxicity or as a result of a complication (e.g., hyperkalemia from rhabdomyolysis-induced renal failure).

▶ Dyspnea and respiratory failure can result from non-cardiogenic pulmonary edema, bronchospasm, PTX, pulmonary infarcts, and thermal burns.

▶ CHF can result from injury, ischemia, and dysrhythmia.

▶ Pregnant patients may present with abdominal pain (signaling placental abruption), spontaneous abortion, premature labor and delivery, and tocographic evidence of fetal distress.

EMERGENCY DEPARTMENT MANAGEMENT
Diagnosis

▶ Mild, uncomplicated intoxication requires no diagnostic testing.

▶ Patients with chest pain require ECG, CXR, and cardiac enzyme rule-out per protocol.

▶ Patients with focal neurologic deficits, status epilepticus, or persistent altered mental status should receive head CT evaluation.

▶ Dyspneic or hypoxic patients should have a CXR; if clinical suspicion warrants, a chest CT may be required to evaluate for pulmonary hemorrhage or infarct.

▶ Suspicion of rhabdomyolysis (oliguria, tea-colored urine, myalgia) should prompt checking of CPK, serum creatinine, and electrolytes (especially potassium).

▶ Pregnant women should receive fetal HR monitoring and obstetric consultation.

▶ Cocaine use can be confirmed by urine evaluation (gas chromatography or thin-layer chromatography) for cocaine metabolite benzoylecgonine; sensitivity depends on the assay, but most pick up metabolite up to 48–72 hours after last use.

Treatment

▶ Benzodiazepines are the most important treatment for most presentations of acute cocaine intoxication. Lorazepam (1–2 mg IV) or diazepam (5–10 mg IV) initially, titrated to improvement in BP, HR, and agitation.

▶ Cocaine chest pain should be treated primarily with benzodiazepines and NTG. Morphine sulfate can also be used. Beta-blockers should **not** be used, as beta-blockade may increase BP and worsen cardiac ischemia secondary to unopposed alpha stimulation. Persistent severe HTN may be treated with phentolamine (1 mg IV initially, may be repeated). Thrombolytics should only be used in consultation with a cardiologist, as an acute injury pattern on ECG in the setting of cocaine intoxication may be a false positive.

▶ Dysrhythmias should be treated with benzodiazepines and by ACLS guidelines, avoiding beta-blockers.

▶ Seizures should be treated primarily with benzodiazepines. Second-line agents are phenobarbital (10–20 mg/kg IV) or phenytoin (15–20 mg/kg IV).

▶ Hyperthermia should be treated with benzodiazepines and rapid external cooling measures; core temperature should be continuously monitored.

▶ Hemorrhagic stroke or subarachnoid bleeding demands immediate neurosurgical consultation. Ischemic stroke requires observation and neurology consultation.

▶ Rhabdomyolysis should be treated with fluid resuscitation, monitoring of urinary output (UOP), and alkalinization of the urine.

Disposition

▶ Uncomplicated cocaine intoxication may be discharged home with counseling on the risks of continued abuse. Referral for detoxification and substance abuse counseling should be offered.

▶ Complications such as stroke, MI, rhabdomyolysis/renal failure, status epilepticus or persistent seizures, prolonged psychosis, and hyperthermia requiring treatment should be admitted. A single brief tonic-clonic seizure with a quick return to baseline may not require admission.

CHAPTER 101

MARIJUANA

Brian D. McBeth

- Most commonly abused illicit drug in the U.S. (14.6 million past month users in 2002)
- Almost 120,000 marijuana-related ED visits in 2002 (up 164% from 1995)

PATHOPHYSIOLOGY

- Marijuana is the common name for the Indian hemp plant, *Cannabis sativa.*
- Delta-9-tetrahydrocannabinol (d-9-THC) is the main psychoactive ingredient in marijuana.
- d-9-THC stimulates specific cannabinoid receptors in the cerebral cortex, hippocampus, and cerebellum, as well as interacting with noradrenergic, dopaminergic, serotonergic, and cholinergic neurotransmitter systems.
- Tolerance develops rapidly with regular use; withdrawal syndrome is seen with chronic heavy use (irritability, anorexia, tremor, and cholinergic signs).
- Marijuana is typically smoked in cigarettes or pipe, although it can be eaten. Hashish is a brown, oily substance obtained from extraction of plant material with solvents and contains higher concentrations of d-9-THC.

CLINICAL PRESENTATION

- Acutely, CNS symptoms predominate: euphoria, dysphoria, alterations in cognition, sensory perception, depersonalization, loss of psychomotor ability and judgment, and impaired short-term memory.
- Cardiovascular effects can include vasodilatation, tachycardia, and hypotension (in large doses).

▶ Other effects include increased appetite, antiemetic effects, muscle tremors and weakness, and conjunctival injection.

▶ Psychiatric presentations may include panic, paranoia, hallucinations (rarely), and acute psychosis in patients without a psychiatric history.

▶ Pediatric ingestions have been associated with significant respiratory depression and coma.

▶ Dyspnea and chest pain due to PTX or pneumomediastinum from barotrauma are not infrequent.

▶ Chronic effects of marijuana abuse include amnesia (blackout spells), impaired short-term memory, attention deficits, obstructive and restrictive pulmonary disease, increased risk for pulmonary carcinoma, and infertility.

▶ Marijuana use in pregnancy has been associated with hyperactivity, inattention, and delinquency in school-aged children.

EMERGENCY DEPARTMENT MANAGEMENT
Diagnosis

▶ Mild, uncomplicated intoxication requires no diagnostic testing.

▶ Patients with chest pain or dyspnea require a CXR to exclude barotrauma.

▶ Marijuana-intoxicated patients often have impaired judgment and present with concomitant trauma.

▶ Marijuana use can be confirmed by urine evaluation if desired; tests include qualitative immunoassay screen for THC or metabolites included on most drugs of abuse panels. These have a significant number of false positives and negatives, depending on the assay, and can be affected by timing of last use, acute vs. chronic consumption, second-hand smoke inhalation, and urine concentration.

Treatment

▶ Most presentations require no intervention and respond to supportive care and observation.

▶ Benzodiazepines are appropriate treatment for acute psychosis or significant agitation; lorazepam (1–2 mg IV) or diazepam (5–10 mg IV) initially, titrated to clinical improvement.

▶ Patients presenting with significant oral ingestions, especially pediatric patients (ingestion of plant material or cigarettes, brownies, etc.), may be considered for treatment with activated charcoal (1 g/kg), though there are not clearly established clinical guidelines; consultation with a regional poison center or toxicologist is warranted.

Disposition

▶ Uncomplicated marijuana intoxication may be discharged home with counseling on the risks of continued abuse. Referral for detoxification and substance abuse counseling should be offered.

▶ Rarely, psychosis may be prolonged and require an inpatient admission for further observation and evaluation; significant co-ingestion may require inpatient admission and evaluation.

CHAPTER 102

AMPHETAMINES

Jonathan Shenk

- ▶ Long history of abuse dating back to the early 20th century.
- ▶ Low cost of production and wide availability have led to increasing rates of abuse, especially in the mid-western and western U.S.
- ▶ Current medical uses of amphetamines include treatment of obesity, narcolepsy, and attention deficit disorder.

PATHOPHYSIOLOGY

- ▶ Amphetamines stimulate release of catecholamines, especially dopamine and norepinephrine, and block their reuptake.
- ▶ Central and peripheral adrenergic receptors are stimulated by released catecholamines, resulting in alpha- and beta-effects (see below).
- ▶ Amphetamines are well absorbed, and common routes of administration include smoking, ingestion, snorting, or injection.

CLINICAL PRESENTATION

- ▶ Sympathomimetic toxidrome: tachycardia, HTN, hyperthermia, mydriasis, diaphoresis, agitation, tremor; similar to cocaine intoxication.
- ▶ Hallucinations (visual and tactile) and psychosis are common.
- ▶ Rhabdomyolysis and renal failure are seen, especially in the setting of severe hyperthermia.
- ▶ Myocardial ischemia and infarct can result from vasospasm and thrombosis.
- ▶ Death most commonly occurs from severe hyperthermia, dysrhythmias (VT, VF), and intracranial hemorrhage.
- ▶ Chronic effects include necrotizing vasculitis, pulmonary HTN, valvular heart disease (especially aortic and mitral regurgita-

tion), schizophrenia, permanent memory loss, and all complications of IV administration (endocarditis, HIV, etc.).

DIFFERENTIAL DIAGNOSIS OF SYMPATHOMIMETIC TOXIDROME

► See Chap. 100.

EMERGENCY DEPARTMENT MANAGEMENT

Diagnosis

► Diagnosis is clinical, based on history or suspicion of exposure and consistent clinical presentation.

► Consider co-ingestants and other causes of altered mental status.

► Qualitative urine immunoassay testing is frequently performed, but both false positives and false negatives are common (false positives are seen with pseudoephedrine, ephedrine, phenylpropanolamine, selegiline, etc.).

► Head CT (if seizure activity present or significant altered mental status) to rule out intracranial bleed.

► See Chap. 88 for other appropriate lab testing.

Treatment

► ABCs and supportive care (IVF, O_2, cardiac monitor)

► Agitation
   • Benzodiazepines are first-line; large doses may be required.
   • Antipsychotics (haloperidol, droperidol) are another option for sedation, though they have the disadvantage of decreased seizure threshold.

► Hyperthermia (> 40° C)
   • Aggressive external cooling with mist and fans.
   • Sedation with benzodiazepines.
   • Frequent core temperature monitoring: if unable to control temperature with above measures, neuromuscular blockade may be necessary.

► HTN
   • Repeated dosing of benzodiazepines generally effective at reducing BP.
   • Phentolamine: pre- and post-synaptic alpha-blocker, often used in hypertensive crisis due to sympathomimetic toxicity.

- Like in cocaine toxicity, beta-blockers have the theoretical risk of allowing unopposed alpha stimulation; however, several agents have been used with some success.
    ○ Labetalol has both alpha- and beta-blocking effects.
    ○ Esmolol has a very short duration of action and can be readily titrated.
    ○ Nitroprusside may be effective if other agents fail.
▶ Seizures
- Benzodiazepines are first line of therapy.
- Add phenobarbital if seizures are recurrent or difficult to control.
- Patients with seizures or mental status changes not responsive to medications require head CT to exclude hemorrhage.
▶ Rhabdomyolysis
- Aggressive sedation to prevent further muscle injury.
- IVF resuscitation with NS, bladder catheterization, and target urinary output (UOP) to 1–2 cc/kg/hour.
- Serial CPK, BUN, creatinine.
- Alkalinization of urine is generally not indicated.
    ○ No strong evidence that alkalinization reduces nephrotoxicity
    ○ Increases half-life of amphetamines
▶ Chest pain
- ECG and cardiac enzymes for a rule-out MI protocol.
- MI: thrombolytics and cardiac catheterization are indicated as they would be for other causes of MI.

Disposition

▶ Patients with mild symptoms may safely be discharged with a responsible adult when they are asymptomatic.
▶ Patients with complications (rhabdomyolysis, significant hyperthermia, psychosis, HTN requiring parenteral agents) require admission, monitoring, and directed care.

CHAPTER 103

ECSTASY

Amer Z. Aldeen

- ► One of the most commonly used designer drugs among the adolescent and young adult population due to ease of oral use, perception of lower toxicity, and low cost.
- ► 2.1 million adolescents and adults in the U.S. reported ecstasy use in the past year.
- ► Use is very highly correlated with attendance at rave dance parties (available at up to 70% of raves).

PATHOPHYSIOLOGY

- ► Chemical structure: 3,4-methylenedioxymethamphetamine, or MDMA.
- ► Structure is similar to both methamphetamine (stimulant) and mescaline (hallucinogen); effects of MDMA are both stimulatory and hallucinogenic.
- ► Acts primarily to increase serotonin and norepinephrine by increasing release and inhibiting reuptake; also has a minor similar function on dopamine.
- ► Other MDMA-like compounds (MDEA, MDA, etc.) have similar chemical structures and effects and may be sold as "ecstasy."

CLINICAL PRESENTATION

- ► Serotonergic symptoms include euphoria, sociability, extroversion, closeness to others, loss of sexual inhibition, and visual changes.
- ► Adrenergic symptoms include HTN, tachycardia, increased arousal, and diminished hunger.
- ► Characteristic adverse effects include
  - Hyponatremia: may be life-threatening and results from excessive sweating, concomitant increase in free water consumption, and an SIADH-like mechanism.

- Serotonin syndrome: hyperthermia, rigidity, altered mental status, and potential multi-system organ failure.
- Cardiovascular: severe HTN and tachycardia are common. VTs and MI can also occur.
- Cerebral: seizures and intracranial hemorrhage.
- Rhabdomyolysis and ARF, especially in the setting of hyperthermia.
- Acute hepatic failure: may be due to depletion of glutathione and other antioxidants necessary for adequate metabolism of drug (suspect MDMA in young patients with acute or recurrent hepatitis and negative viral serologies).

▶ Myalgias are very common during and after use, especially in the jaws (due to bruxism, the reason why users often suck on lollipops or pacifiers).

▶ Users can exhibit stimulant-like crash related to catecholamine depletion after discontinuing drug use.

▶ Long-term neurologic dysfunction (related to serotonergic neuronal destruction) and psychiatric effects (memory loss, schizophrenia-like psychosis) are seen and can be irreversible.

DIFFERENTIAL DIAGNOSIS

▶ See differential diagnosis of sympathomimetic toxidrome (Table 100-1).

EMERGENCY DEPARTMENT MANAGEMENT
Diagnosis

▶ Obtain a good history if possible. Rave party attendance is suggestive of exposure.

▶ No specific lab test available in the ED exists for MDMA; urine toxicology screens may show qualitative positive for amphetamines if MDMA consumed in sufficient quantity.

▶ Lab studies that may be useful: CBC, metabolic panel (including electrolytes and renal function tests), ethanol level, UA, urine toxicology screen, pregnancy test, and LFTs.

▶ Check CPK if rhabdomyolysis is suspected, cardiac troponin if the patient is having chest pain, and salicylate/acetaminophen (APAP) levels if an intentional overdose is suspected.

▶ ECG to assess for arrhythmias and myocardial damage.

▶ Focal neurologic deficits mandate head CT.

Treatment

▶ ABCs and stabilization of vital signs should be addressed first.
▶ Generally, supportive care is indicated: observe, monitor, and perform serial examinations until mental status returns to baseline.
▶ For acutely agitated states, persistent hallucinations, seizures, or sympathetic hyperstimulation, benzodiazepines are the drug of choice: **lorazepam (1–2 mg IV) or diazepam (5–10 mg IV)** titrated to effect.
▶ For specific conditions:
  • Seizures: benzodiazepines as above, phenobarbital (10–20 mg/kg IV), or propofol, if intubated (10 mg IV bolus, then drip at 10 mcg/kg/minute).
  • Hyponatremia: free water restriction and gentle hydration with NS; use hypertonic saline only for seizures refractory to benzodiazepines.
  • Rhabdomyolysis: IVF, consider urine alkalinization with urine pH > 6.5.
  • Serotonin syndrome: aggressive cooling measures (cooled IVF, spray mist cooling, icepacks), cyproheptadine (0.25 mg/kg divided tid per NGT), dantrolene (1 mg/kg IV push q6h), benzodiazepines as above.
▶ Consultation with a toxicologist or regional poison center is recommended for complicated ingestions, especially with multisystem involvement.

Disposition

▶ Uncomplicated MDMA intoxication may be discharged home with responsible adult when mental status has returned to normal.
▶ Patient education is essential with regards to permanent neurologic damage caused by chronic use of MDMA.

CHAPTER 104

HALLUCINOGENS

Brian D. McBeth

▶ Frequently abused drugs among young people, with increasing prevalence in the mid- to late 1990s.

▶ Mushroom exposures range from benign GI irritants to deadly hepatotoxins.

LYSERGIC ACID DIETHYLAMIDE (LSD)

▶ Significant resurgence in prevalence in 1990s associated with rave dance parties and culture; most commonly abused by suburban youth, aged 15–25.

Pathophysiology

▶ Ergot alkaloid that acts as a serotonin and dopamine receptor agonist and also stimulates release of excitatory glutamate

▶ May be taken sublingually, ingested, smoked, or injected

Clinical Presentation

▶ Physiologic effects include tachycardia, mydriasis, tachypnea, hyperthermia, GI distress, dizziness, generalized weakness, and ataxia.

▶ Psychological effects include loss of body image, altered perceptions, illusions, and depersonalization.

▶ Hallucinations range from visual to auditory, olfactory, and tactile.

▶ Psychiatric reactions include panic and frank psychosis; flashbacks or hallucinogen persisting perception disorder (HPPD) may present days to years after exposure.

▶ Rarely can present with significant hyperthermia and/or rhabdomyolysis.

Management

▶ Generally supportive: IVF, observation.

▶ Active cooling if significant hyperthermia is present.

▶ GI decontamination is usually unnecessary.

▶ Low-stimulation environment (quiet dark room) and benzodiazepines as needed.

▶ Disposition is usually discharge to home unless complications are present (prolonged psychosis, multiple ingestions, rhabdomyolysis, etc.).

PHENCYCLIDINE (PCP)

▶ Developed originally as an anesthetic, but its use was discontinued in the 1960s when severe dysphoria and post-operative psychosis were frequent.

Pathophysiology

▶ Primarily an NMDA receptor antagonist.

▶ Complex receptor activity also includes inhibition of reuptake of dopamine and norepinephrine, leading to increases of these neurotransmitters at a synapse level.

▶ May be smoked (most common), snorted, ingested, injected, or added to other drugs (marijuana cigarettes, most commonly).

Clinical Presentation

▶ Dissociative anesthesia (think ketamine: PCP has similar chemical structure); patients relate decreased sensory perception, feelings of depersonalization, alterations in body image/perception.

▶ Hallucinations are common; auditory more often than visual.

▶ Nystagmus, ataxia, delirium, and seizures; with larger doses, decreasing mental status and obtundation may be present.

▶ Psychosis is not unusual, accompanied by bizarre and violent behavior.

▶ Hyperthermia and rhabdomyolysis are more common than with LSD; physical restraints may put patients at increased risk for these complications.

Management

▶ Protect patients from self-induced injury (and caregivers from patient violence).

▶ Active cooling if significant hyperthermia is present.

► GI decontamination should be considered for significant intoxication; activated charcoal (1 g/kg) effectively absorbs PCP and increases clearance.

► Urinary acidification was recommended in the past (will increase urinary excretion) but increases risk of rhabdomyolysis and is **not** recommended today.

► Treat rhabdomyolysis aggressively (fluids, alkalinization of urine), and avoid restraints that may put patients at risk.

► Benzodiazepines are recommended for agitation, but watch mental status closely; additive effects of multiple CNS depressants can result in an obtunded patient.

► Haloperidol may be used for acute psychosis, but use caution as this can lower the seizure threshold in predisposed patients.

► Disposition is usually discharge to home unless complications are present (prolonged psychosis, multiple ingestions, rhabdomyolysis, etc.).

TOXIC MUSHROOMS

► Vast majority of mushroom ingestions are benign; lethal ingestions are very rare.

► There are many mushroom species that cause GI symptoms of diarrhea, nausea, vomiting, abdominal pain; most, but not all, of these patients present with self-limited symptoms and respond to supportive care.

► Most physicians have little or no training or ability to identify mushrooms accurately, making clinical decision-making difficult.

► In any questionable case or one with potential toxicity, involvement of a mycologist (through a regional poison control center) is recommended.

Cyclopeptides (*Amanita phalloides* and Other Species)

Pathophysiology

► Heat-stable amatoxin is taken up by hepatocytes and inhibits mRNA synthesis, leading to acute hepatitis and fulminant liver failure.

Clinical Presentation

► Stage 1 (6–24 hours): vomiting, diarrhea, abdominal pain, dehydration, tachycardia, hypotension, and hyperglycemia.

▶ Stage 2 (24–48 hours): symptoms improve, but worsening hepatitis and azotemia demonstrated by lab evaluation.

▶ Stage 3 (3–5 days): fulminant hepatic failure, hepatic encephalopathy, coma, and death.

Management

▶ Immediate consultation with regional poison center.

▶ Aggressive fluid resuscitation.

▶ Gastric lavage is recommended in most cases with early presentation; may interrupt enterohepatic circulation and diminish absorption.

▶ Multi-dose activated charcoal.

▶ Other adjunctive therapies are unproven and should be done only in consultation with a toxicologist: high-dose IV penicillin, cimetidine, silibinin, and N-acetylcysteine.

▶ Liver transplantation may be appropriate for candidates with fulminant liver failure.

▶ Disposition is hospital admission for any patient with suspected cyclopeptide ingestion even if asymptomatic.

Gyromitrins (*Gyromitra* Species)

Pathophysiology

▶ Monomethylhydrazine is released, which binds pyridoxine, which disrupts function of the inhibitory neurotransmitter GABA.

Clinical Presentation

▶ Vomiting, diarrhea, abdominal pain, diffuse muscle cramping (common)

▶ Delirium, seizures, coma, hepatorenal failure (rare)

Management

▶ Consultation with a regional poison center.

▶ Supportive care: IVF, antiemetics.

▶ Activated charcoal (1 g/kg) is generally recommended.

▶ Seizures may be treated with benzodiazepines or with pyridoxine (70 mg/kg IV); pyridoxine may limit toxicity especially in cases of status epilepticus and severe intoxication.

▶ Disposition is hospital admission for any ingestion with persistent symptoms.

Hallucinogenic Mushrooms (Psilocybin-, Ibotenic Acid–, and Muscimol-Containing Species)

Pathophysiology
► Psilocybin acts as a serotonin agonist, with a pathophysiology similar to LSD.
► Ibotenic acid acts as a glutamic acid analogue, with resulting CNS stimulation.
► Muscimol has a similar chemical structure to GABA, which may result in CNS depression.

Clinical Presentation
► GI symptoms may include vomiting, diarrhea, and abdominal pain.
► CNS manifestations range from depressive (somnolence, delirium) to excitatory (agitation, hallucinations, seizures, ataxia), depending on the species ingested.
► Rhabdomyolysis and renal failure have been reported with psilocybin-containing species, but are very rare.

Management
► Care is supportive: IVF, observation.
► Occasionally, benzodiazepines may be required for agitation or seizures.
► Disposition is discharge to home in most cases after observation if symptoms resolve.

CHAPTER 105

ANTICHOLINERGICS

John P. Erpelding

▶ The term *anticholinergic* is somewhat misleading, as these drugs generally affect only muscarinic and not nicotinic (skeletal muscle) receptors.

▶ In 2002, there were over 65,000 antihistamine and anticholinergic exposures reported to U.S. poison control centers resulting in 80 deaths.

PATHOPHYSIOLOGY

▶ Exert clinical effects by competitive inhibition of acetylcholine muscarinic receptors.

▶ Several classes of drugs exhibit anticholinergic toxic effects when taken in overdose, including

- Antihistamines (first generation, sedating; e.g., brompheniramine, chlorpheniramine, cyproheptadine, diphenhydramine, dimenhydrinate, doxylamine, hydroxyzine, meclizine)
- Anti-parkinsonian drugs (e.g., benztropine, procyclidine, trihexyphenidyl, etc.)
- Belladonna alkaloids and derivatives (e.g., atropine, homatropine, scopolamine)
- Carbamazepine
- GI antispasmodics (e.g., dicyclomine, glycopyrrolate, hyoscyamine)
- Ipratropium bromide
- Muscle relaxants (e.g., cyclobenzaprine, orphenadrine)
- Mydriatic/cycloplegic agents (e.g., atropine, cyclopentolate, homatropine, tropicamide)
- Some antiemetics (e.g., promethazine)
- Some antipsychotics (e.g., mesoridazine, thioridazine)
- TCAs (e.g., amitriptyline, clomipramine, desipramine, doxepin, imipramine, nortriptyline, protriptyline)

- • Urinary tract antispasmodics (e.g., flavoxate, oxybutynin, tolterodine)
► Several toxic plants containing belladonna alkaloids also cause anticholinergic toxidrome, including
  - • *Atropa belladonna* (deadly nightshade)
  - • *Brugmansia x candida* (angel's trumpet)
  - • *Datura stramonium* (Jimson weed)
  - • *Hyoscyamus niger* (black henbane)
  - • *Solandra* species (chalice vine, cup-of-gold)

CLINICAL PRESENTATION

► The classic toxidrome includes the following:
  - • Altered mental status: delirium, hallucinations, coma ("mad as a hatter")
  - • Dry mouth, dry axilla ("dry as a bone")
  - • Hyperthermia ("hotter than Hades")
  - • Mydriasis ("blind as a bat")
  - • Peripheral vasodilation: warm, red skin ("red as a beet")
► Other common findings include hypoactive bowel sounds, HTN (occasionally hypotension), seizures, tachycardia, and urinary retention.

DIFFERENTIAL DIAGNOSIS

► Adrenergic toxicity.
  - • Same: tachycardia, hyperthermia, HTN, altered mental status, mydriasis
  - • Differ: moist mucous membranes, diaphoresis, hyperreflexia, active bowel sounds, increased urination
► Hallucinogen toxicity (LSD, PCP, mescaline, hallucinogenic mushrooms, MDMA).
► Sedative-hypnotic withdrawal.
► Acute thyrotoxicosis.
► Meningitis, encephalitis, or other CNS infection.
► SAH.
► Neuroleptic malignant syndrome (NMS).
► Acute psychosis.
► See Table 99-1 for differential diagnosis of altered mental status.

EMERGENCY DEPARTMENT MANAGEMENT
Diagnosis

▶ Clinical diagnosis with appropriate history and physical exam: no specific tests to confirm most substances

▶ Lab/ancillary studies that may be helpful:
- Electrolytes with BUN and creatinine to evaluate metabolic cause of altered mental status.
- CPK to evaluate for rhabdomyolysis.
- TSH and free T_4 if concern for thyrotoxicosis.
- Urinary toxicologic screen may show qualitative results for TCAs, cocaine, PCP, etc.
- ECG to evaluate QRS and QTc intervals.
- See Chap. 88 for other appropriate lab testing.

Treatment

▶ External cooling indicated for hyperthermia; do **not** use phenothiazines.

▶ Intubation for coma, refractory seizures, or airway protection if gastric lavage needed in presence of altered mental status.

▶ Generous IV hydration with isotonic fluids for initial treatment of hypotension and maintenance of adequate urinary output (UOP) (2–3 ml/kg/hour) and to prevent/treat rhabdomyolysis.

▶ Gastric lavage should be considered in potentially life-threatening ingestions if performed within 1–2 hours of ingestion. Because of anticholinergic slowing of GI motility, it may be effective even when performed later; also consider for sustained-release preparations and those known to form concretions or bezoars.

▶ Activated charcoal (without cathartics) should be given to most patients.

▶ Agitation, seizures, HTN, and sinus tachycardia should be treated with IV benzodiazepines (typically lorazepam or diazepam).

▶ Hypotension refractory to crystalloid solution may respond to dopamine or norepinephrine infusions.

▶ Tachyarrhythmias refractory to fluids and benzodiazepines can be treated with esmolol for narrow-complex or lidocaine for ventricular arrhythmias; consider $NaHCO_3$ if evidence of QRS widening or magnesium sulfate for QTc prolongation.

▶ Severe HTN unresponsive to benzodiazepines may require nitroprusside (alternatives: NTG and phentolamine).

▶ Physostigmine can be used to reverse anticholinergic effects for both diagnosis and therapy, although it is not considered a first-line agent.

  • Dose is 1–2 mg IV in adults, or, in children, 0.02 mg/kg (maximum 0.5 mg/dose, 2 mg total), given over 5 minutes.

  • Physostigmine should not be given if there is any suspicion of TCA ingestion (including widened QRS and R wave in aVR on ECG). Physostigmine has been associated with seizures and refractory cardiac arrest in TCA-intoxicated patients; these effects have also been associated with too rapid IV administration.

  • May be used diagnostically to differentiate anticholinergic delirium from other causes of altered mental status; effects generally last from 20–60 minutes.

  • Although there have been impressive case reports demonstrating success with physostigmine, its practical use has been limited due to its potential complications, and consultation with regional poison control center or toxicologist is recommended before its use.

Disposition

▶ Admit all those who are persistently symptomatic; those with any ECG changes should be observed in an ICU setting.

▶ If completely asymptomatic 6 hours post-ingestion, can be discharged (8 hours for *Datura stramonium* or cyclobenzaprine) with close observation at home for 24 hours in the appropriate social setting.

CHAPTER 106

ORGANOPHOSPHATES

Victor S. Roth

- ▶ Pesticides account for approximately 4% of human exposures annually in the U.S. (> 97,000 cases in 2003).
- ▶ 41 deaths in the U.S. in 2003 related to pesticide exposure; organophosphate compounds make up the largest component of fatalities.
- ▶ High-risk exposures include children < 6 years (> 50% of all cases) and occupational exposures (pesticide applicators, farmers, families of these workers, health care workers during decontamination).

PATHOPHYSIOLOGY

- ▶ Organophosphates are direct and indirect AChE inhibitors, resulting in accumulation of acetylcholine at cholinergic muscarinic and nicotinic receptors.
- ▶ Unopposed stimulation of receptors causes both CNS and peripheral signs and symptoms.

CLINICAL PRESENTATION

- ▶ Muscarinic signs: bronchorrhea, SLUDGE syndrome (salivation, lacrimation, urination, diarrhea, GI distress, emesis), sweating, miosis, bradycardia, bronchospasm.
- ▶ Nicotinic signs: mydriasis, tachycardia, weakness, HTN, fasciculations, urinary retention, hyperglycemia.
- ▶ CNS signs: confusion, agitation, seizures, coma.
- ▶ Cardiovascular signs: hypotension or HTN, AV nodal blocks, prolonged QT, torsades de pointes (rare).
- ▶ Respiratory failure is the primary cause of death in acute toxicity, usually precipitated by profuse bronchorrhea and muscle weakness.

▶ Some organophosphates can result in a characteristic garlic-like odor that may be apparent on initial presentation.

DIFFERENTIAL DIAGNOSIS

▶ Other toxins that can cause similar signs and symptoms to organophosphate pesticides:
  - Carbamate insecticides
  - Paraquat and diquat
  - Phosphene
  - AChE-inhibiting nerve agents (sarin, tabun, etc.)
  - Muscarine-containing mushrooms
  - Medicinal AChE-inhibiting agents (physostigmine, pyridostigmine, etc.)
  - Medicinal cholinomimetics (pilocarpine, bethanechol, etc.)

EMERGENCY DEPARTMENT MANAGEMENT

Diagnosis

▶ Primarily a clinical diagnosis: careful history and physical exam are key; consider important historical clues.
  - High-risk occupations (chemical factory, farm worker, groundskeeper, pesticide applicator, veterinarian)
  - General: contaminated drinking water, recent pesticide application in neighborhood, home, or garden
▶ AChE levels:
  - RBC AChE (true cholinesterase) has activity very similar to nervous system AChE and more closely correlates with organophosphate clinical toxicity.
  - Plasma AChE (pseudocholinesterase) levels do not correlate with symptoms related to depression of nervous system or RBC AChE.
  - Depression of RBC AChE levels < 50% of standards is most commonly seen with symptoms of organophosphate toxicity.
  - Draw RBC and plasma AChE levels before initiating medical therapy if possible.
  - Do not delay treatment while awaiting results of cholinesterase levels.
▶ Please see Chap. 88 for other appropriate lab testing.

Treatment

▸ Protect safety of caregivers and other patients. Patient with an organophosphate poisoning should be disrobed and decontaminated prior to entry into the ED.

▸ Decontamination: removal of clothing, triple washing with soap and water, and removal of all contaminated body hair if necessary; caregivers should use rubber gloves (not vinyl or latex).

▸ ABCs including early intubation and suctioning if necessary for severe bronchorrhea and respiratory failure; succinylcholine should **not** be used for intubation, as prolonged paralysis can result (use a non-depolarizing agent instead).

▸ GI decontamination:
  • Induction of emesis is contraindicated.
  • Orogastric/NG lavage is indicated if patient is seen within 1 hour of ingestion.
  • Activated charcoal (with cathartic), single dose of 1 g/kg is usually indicated; multiple doses are generally not given, as ileus may develop with atropine therapy.

▸ Atropine:
  • Very large doses may be required with endpoint of control of bronchorrhea.
  • Reverses muscarinic symptoms but will not affect nicotinic symptoms.
  • Start with 2–5 mg IV q2–3min as needed (adults and children > 12 years).
  • Start with 0.05 mg/kg IV dose q2–3min as needed (children ≤ 12).
  • Infusions may be necessary: start with 0.5–1 mg/hour in adults and 0.025 mg/kg/hour in children and titrate to effect.
  • Every patient undergoing atropine therapy should receive bladder catheterization to prevent urinary retention.

▸ Pralidoxime:
  • Hydrolyzes and regenerates bound AChE, if enzyme has not undergone aging (most of which has occurred by 24–48 hours).
  • Initial dose is 1–2 g IV (adults) administered over 10 minutes, 20–50 mg/kg IV (children < 12 years) over 30 minutes.
  • Continuous infusion is usually required: 2–4 mg/kg/hour in adults, 10–20 mg/kg/hour in children.

▶ Diazepam:
  • Use for seizures and sedation after intubation; may help improve survival and decrease neuropathy.

Disposition

▶ Any symptomatic patient requires hospital admission, and most should be observed in an ICU setting even if not intubated.
▶ Large amounts of atropine often result in delayed confusion and agitation and require close monitoring.

CHAPTER 107

ETHANOL

Rebecca M. Cunningham

▶ Ethanol is the leading cause of death of persons age 15–45 years, in association with MVAs, homicides, suicides, and other trauma.

▶ Over 100,000 deaths per year related to ethanol in the U.S.

▶ 8% of all ED visits attributable to ethanol.

▶ A single alcohol-related ED visit predicts continued problem drinking.

PATHOPHYSIOLOGY

▶ Enhances GABA receptor activation and inhibits NMDA receptor activation.

▶ Antidiuretic hormone (ADH) metabolizes ethanol to acetaldehyde; acetaldehyde is then metabolized to acetate.

▶ Ethanol level falls 15–20 mg/dl/hour for occasional drinkers, 30–40 mg/dl/hour for chronic drinkers (though there is considerable individual variation).

CLINICAL PRESENTATION

▶ Degree of intoxication and symptoms depend on degree of habituation and tolerance.

▶ Mild intoxication:
  • Selective depression of the cerebral cortex
  • Euphoria, giddiness, loss of inhibition, impaired concentration and judgment, loss of restraint

▶ Severe intoxication:
  • Generalized CNS depression
  • Diaphoresis, flushing, nausea, vomiting, ataxia, coma, hypothermia, hypotension, loss of protective reflexes, respiratory depression/aspiration

- Generally seen with serum ethanol levels > 150 mg/dl in non-habituated drinker, > 250 mg/dl in habituated drinker

DIFFERENTIAL DIAGNOSIS

▶ Consider toxic alcohol (ethylene glycol, methanol) exposure in high-risk patients.
▶ See Table 99-1 for differential diagnosis of altered mental status.

EMERGENCY DEPARTMENT MANAGEMENT

Diagnosis

▶ Careful history should include the time of last drink, as well as preceding pattern of drinking (quantity, frequency, etc.).
▶ Focus on potential for trauma and history of seizures and falls.
▶ Screen for symptoms suggestive of infection (fevers, cough), presence of complications of alcoholism (encephalopathy, GI bleed, etc.).
▶ Check bedside glucose to rule out hypoglycemia (ethanol depletes hepatic glycogen and impairs gluconeogenesis).
▶ Mild, uncomplicated intoxication requires no additional diagnostic testing.
▶ Serum ethanol level is helpful in severe intoxication to correlate to severity of symptoms (a low level should prompt a search for alternative diagnoses).
▶ See Chap. 88 for other appropriate lab testing.

Treatment

▶ ABCs.
▶ If trauma by history, C-spine immobilization.
▶ Isotonic fluid for dehydration.
▶ Dextrose infusion for hypoglycemia.
▶ Restraints (physical or chemical) for the intoxicated, uncooperative patient may be necessary to assure safety of patient and ED staff.
▶ Observe, monitor, and serial examinations until mental status returns to baseline.
▶ Electrolyte and nutritional abnormalities are common in chronic alcoholics; low magnesium is very common. Additional vitamin/electrolyte therapy as needed:
  - Thiamine, 100 mg IV, for Wernicke's encephalopathy (see below)

- Magnesium, 2 g IV, for documented deficits
- Folate, 1 mg IV, and multivitamin in IVF
▶ Ethanol cessation counseling and referral.

Disposition

▶ Discharge with a sober adult when ambulatory; observe until clinically sober if no sober adult is available.
▶ Admission may be required for complicating medical or surgical issues, if airway management is required, or if major withdrawal symptoms (see below) occur.

ETHANOL WITHDRAWAL
Pathophysiology

▶ Syndrome of CNS excitability occurs 4–72 hours after decreasing ethanol intake; can occur in people with measurable ethanol level.
▶ Repeated bouts of milder ethanol withdrawal sensitize the brain to the development of a severe withdrawal syndrome.

Clinical Presentation

▶ Minor withdrawal (tremulousness)
  - 4–24 hours after the last drink
  - Tremor, anxiety, nausea, vomiting, and insomnia
▶ Major withdrawal (hallucinations)
  - 10–72 hours after the last drink
  - Visual and auditory hallucinations, whole body tremor, vomiting, diaphoresis, and HTN
▶ Withdrawal seizures
  - 6–48 hours after the last drink.
  - Generalized seizures in patients who do not have a seizure diagnosis and have a normal EEG.
  - 30–40% of patients with withdrawal seizures progress to DTs.
▶ DTs
  - 3–10 days following the last drink.
  - Agitation, global confusion, disorientation, hallucinations, fever, tachycardia, and HTN.
  - Mortality for patients with DTs ranges from 5–15%, usually due to respiratory failure and cardiac arrhythmias.

Emergency Department Management

Diagnosis

▶ Usually by history: heavy ethanol consumption, followed by abrupt decrease or halt in intake.

▶ Consider differential diagnosis of sympathomimetic or anticholinergic ingestion, TCA overdose, other sedative withdrawal, thyrotoxicosis, infection (meningitis, encephalitis), or acute psychosis.

▶ Labs are generally not helpful, except for eliminating alternative diagnoses.

Treatment

▶ Benzodiazepines: primary treatment (can require high doses)
   • Lorazepam, 2 mg IV q20–30min until symptoms and signs improve
   • Outpatient protocol: chlordiazepoxide, 50 mg q6h for 4 days, then taper for 3 more days

▶ Haloperidol, 5 mg IV (may be useful adjunct)

Disposition

▶ Major withdrawal, seizures, or DTs: admission is recommended.

▶ ICU level care is warranted for severe delirium or hemodynamic instability.

▶ Mild withdrawal (with normal vital signs and normal mental status) may be released after 4 hours of observation with planned close follow-up.

WERNICKE'S ENCEPHALOPATHY

▶ Triad of confusion, ataxia, and oculomotor disturbances (although only a minority of patients have all three).

▶ Mortality rate is 10–20%. Prognosis depends on prompt treatment.

Pathophysiology

▶ Due to thiamine deficiency, but exact pathophysiology is not well understood

Clinical Presentation

▶ Confusion (80%): encephalopathy characterized by profound disorientation

▶ Ataxia (23%), often with a wide, short-stepping gait due to a combination of polyneuropathy, cerebellar involvement, and vestibular paresis

▶ Oculomotor disturbances (11%): nystagmus and ocular palsies are most common

▶ Korsakoff's psychosis: severe memory loss and confabulation, chronic continuum of Wernicke's encephalopathy; generally irreversible

Emergency Department Management

Diagnosis

▶ Heavy ethanol consumption by history is most common; thiamine deficiency without ethanol consumption can also prompt Wernicke's encephalopathy.

▶ Consider broad differential diagnosis for altered mental status (see Table 99-1).

▶ Labs are generally not helpful, except for eliminating alternative diagnoses.

Treatment

▶ Thiamine hydrochloride, 100 mg IV; dose may need to be repeated if delirium or neurologic deficits persist. Patient should subsequently be started on daily thiamine therapy.

▶ Thiamine improves the reversible lesions of Wernicke's encephalopathy (ophthalmoplegia, ataxia).

Disposition

▶ Patients with newly diagnosed Wernicke's encephalopathy or deterioration in mental status or function should be admitted.

ADDENDUM: CAGE QUESTIONS

▶ Have you ever felt the need to **C**ut down on drinking?

▶ Have you ever felt **A**nnoyed by criticism of your drinking?

▶ Have you ever had **G**uilty feelings about your drinking?

▶ Have you ever taken a morning **E**ye-opener?

▶ One positive response suggests the need for closer assessment; two positive responses indicate high likelihood of alcohol abuse and/or dependence.

CHAPTER 108

TOXIC ALCOHOLS

Amit R. Trivedi

▶ **Ethylene glycol:** commonly found in antifreeze, de-icing solutions, hydraulic brake fluid, glycerin substitutes (paints, lacquers, detergents, cosmetics), and chemical solvents; high degree of toxicity

▶ **Methanol:** commonly found in windshield-washing solutions, paints, varnishes, antifreeze, fuel (picnic stoves and torches), solvents, and copier fluids; high degree of toxicity

▶ **Isopropanol:** found in rubbing alcohol, paints, inks, thinners, hair tonics, aftershaves, and industrial solvents

PATHOPHYSIOLOGY

▶ Toxic alcohols are all rapidly absorbed from the GI tract and are metabolized by antidiuretic hormone (ADH) into their respective metabolites.

▶ Ethylene glycol causes calcium chelation and resulting hypocalcemia, which can cause QT prolongation and cardiac dysrhythmias. Calcium oxalate can precipitate in the kidney and result in ATN. Neurologic toxicity is also common and may be related to ethylene glycol–induced pyridoxine deficiency.

▶ Methanol causes retinal toxicity and results in many of the visual symptoms associated with poisoning.

▶ Isopropanol does not generally cause major toxicity unless present in very large amounts.

CLINICAL PRESENTATION

▶ See Table 108-1.

▶ Methanol also causes specific damage to the ophthalmologic system, which can include blurred vision (described as "snowstorm"), photophobia, partial to complete blindness, papilledema, hyperemic optic discs, retinal edema, and retinal hemorrhages; early methanol intoxication may have normal vision.

▶ Isopropanol has been reported to cause hemolytic anemia.

TABLE 108-1.
CLINICAL PRESENTATION OF TOXIC ALCOHOL INGESTION

	Ethylene glycol	Methanol	Isopropanol
CNS	Inebriation, ataxia, stupor, coma, seizures, cerebral edema	Alert or inebriated, headache, dizziness, agitation, stupor, coma, cerebral edema	Inebriation, ataxia, headache, confusion, stupor, and coma
Cardiopulmonary	Hypotension/HTN, tachycardia, dysrhythmias, myocarditis, tachypnea, Kussmaul respirations, pneumonitis, pulmonary edema	Hypotension/HTN, tachycardia or bradycardia, tachypnea, Kussmaul respirations	Hypothermia and/or hypotension (may mimic sepsis), respiratory depression, tracheobronchitis
Renal	ARF, calcium oxalate crystalluria	ARF	ARF, rhabdomyolysis
GI	Nausea and vomiting	Nausea, vomiting, abdominal pain, pancreatitis	Nausea, vomiting, gastritis, hematemesis, abdominal pain
Metabolic	Anion-gap acidosis and hypocalcemia	Anion-gap acidosis	None

DIFFERENTIAL DIAGNOSIS

▶ The pneumonic MUDPILES is frequently used to evaluate potential causes of anion-gap acidosis:
- **M**ethanol
- **U**remia
- **D**KA
- **P**araldehyde
- **I**soniazid (INH)/iron/ibuprofen (propionic acid)
- **L**actic acidosis
- **E**thanol/ethylene glycol
- **S**alicylates

▶ Consider a co-ingestion if clinically warranted: barbiturates, TCAs, opiates, GHB, other CNS depressants.

▶ Consider non-toxicologic causes for altered mental status (see Table 99-1).

EMERGENCY DEPARTMENT MANAGEMENT

Diagnosis

▶ Most important factor is to consider the diagnosis and take a complete history, including access to "alternative" alcohol sources; obtain relevant information from family members, friends, paramedics, etc., regarding empty bottles found at scene.

▶ The first step in evaluating for possible toxic alcohol ingestion is to determine if an anion-gap acidosis is present.
- Anion gap = $Na - (HCO_3 + Cl)$
- A normal anion gap is 8–12 mEq/L.

▶ Next, calculate the osmol gap.
- Osmol gap = osmolarity (serum) – osmolarity (calculated)
- Osmolarity (calculated) = $2(Na) + BUN/2.8 + glucose/18 + ethanol/4.6$
- A normal osmol gap is generally about 10 mOsm/L, though there is enormous individual variability.
- An elevated osmol gap (> 50 mOsm/L) is very suggestive of a toxic alcohol exposure.
- A normal or negative osmol gap is non-diagnostic.

▶ There are four instances when anion and osmol gap may **not** be helpful:
- In a very acute ingestion, enough time may not have passed for the breakdown by ADH into toxic metabo-

lites; this could result in a normal anion gap and osmol gap.

- In a very delayed presentation, most of the parent compound has been metabolized to the toxic acids and the osmol gap is no longer elevated.
- When ethanol is a concomitant ingestion, it will competitively inhibit ADH and will delay the metabolism of a toxic alcohol to its acid byproducts; anion gap may be normal. The half-life of ethylene glycol can be ≤ 17 hours and the half-life of methanol ≤ 30–50 hours.
- The range for a patient's baseline osmol gap can be large (from −14 to +10 mOsm/L), and this can make interpretation of the osmol gap complex.

▶ Quantitative serum ethylene glycol and methanol levels (determined by gas chromatography and mass spectrophotometry) should be obtained and are diagnostic; however, these determinations are rarely helpful in acute diagnosis and management. Also, in a delayed presentation with extensive metabolism, serum levels may be low or normal.

▶ UA can show the presence of ketones (suggestive of isopropanol exposure, though non-specific) and calcium oxalate crystals (suggestive of ethylene glycol exposure); the absence of crystals does not rule out ethylene glycol exposure.

▶ Urinary fluorescence is not helpful; it is neither sensitive nor specific.

▶ Serum ethanol level should be sent on every patient.

▶ Baseline renal function (BUN, creatinine), a full set of electrolytes including calcium, and a serum glucose should be sent on every patient.

▶ See Chap. 88 for other appropriate lab testing.

Treatment

Supportive Care

▶ IVF boluses for hypotension.

▶ Dextrose for hypoglycemia.

▶ Activated charcoal is ineffective with alcohols but may be considered if there is a concern for co-ingestants.

▶ NaHCO$_3$ may be necessary for severe acidemia.

▶ Isopropanol intoxication generally responds to supportive care and observation alone.

▶ Early consultation with a toxicologist or poison center is recommended for significant intoxication.

ADH Inhibitor

▶ Two competitive inhibitors of ADH currently available: fomepizole (Antizol) and ethanol; ADH inhibition should be considered for any known ingestion or high degree of clinical suspicion.

▶ Fomepizole loading dose is 15 mg/kg, which is diluted in 250 cc of NS or D5W and given IV over 30 minutes; maintenance dose is 10 mg/kg q12h for 4 doses and then 15 mg/kg q12h as long as necessary.

▶ Ethanol has a loading dose of 0.8 g/kg (about 1 ml/kg) of 100% ethanol, which is diluted to a 10% concentration in D5W; loading dose is given over 20–60 minutes. Maintenance dose of 130 mg (0.16 ml)/kg/hour of 100% ethanol diluted as above should be given, with serum ethanol levels monitored with a goal of 100–150 mg/dl.

Cofactor Therapy

▶ For ethylene glycol ingestion, give 100 mg thiamine and 100 mg pyridoxine IV (repeat every 6 hours).

▶ For methanol, administer folinic acid (leucovorin) at 1 mg/kg/dose (maximum 50 mg) q4h.

Hemodialysis

▶ Most suggest hemodialysis (HD) if there is severe acidosis or evidence of end organ damage regardless of levels; decision is best based on clinical status of the patient.

▶ Another possible indication is confirmed exposure to large toxic dose of methanol or ethylene glycol prior to onset of severe symptoms.

▶ Methanol or ethylene glycol levels > 25 mg/dl have traditionally been used as indications for HD.

▶ ADH inhibitor therapy should be continued during dialysis, though dosing needs adjustment.

Disposition

▶ All patients should be admitted if there is a known or suspected ingestion of methanol or ethylene glycol, especially if alcohol is a co-ingestant, as the acidosis may appear later.

▶ All patients requiring antidotal therapy clearly need admission and monitoring. Patients on ethanol infusion drips generally require ICU care. A hemodynamically stable patient with a stable mental status receiving fomepizole may be appropriate for a hospital ward setting.

▶ With isopropanol, most can be observed as long as the CNS depression is mild; most patients are able to be discharged home after 4–6 hours of observation if repeat lab evaluation is normal and mental status is improved.

CHAPTER 109

NON-STEROIDAL ANTI-INFLAMMATORY DRUGS (NSAIDs)

Joshua A. Small and Brian D. McBeth

▶ NSAIDs are commonly used for control of pain and inflammation in many disease processes, ranging from minor muscle or ligamentous injuries to severe rheumatological disease (over 73 million prescriptions annually in the U.S.).

▶ Two main classes of drugs: non-selective (e.g., ibuprofen, naproxen, indomethacin), which inhibit both cyclooxygenase systems (COX-1 and COX-2), and COX-2 selective agents (celecoxib, rofecoxib).

▶ Over 70,000 ibuprofen exposures reported to U.S. poison centers in 2003, with 13 related deaths.

PATHOPHYSIOLOGY

▶ NSAIDs work by reversibly blocking the cyclooxygenase enzymes (COX-1 and COX-2), which block the production of prostacyclin, prostaglandins, and thromboxanes from arachidonic acid.

▶ However, inhibition of protective prostaglandins (PGI_2 and PGE_2) leads to irritation of GI mucosa and can cause GI bleeding and perforation.

▶ NSAIDs can have numerous renal effects including anion-gap acidosis, decreased GFR, and interstitial nephritis.

▶ Hematologic effects include platelet inhibition and severe idiosyncratic reactions (aplastic anemia, agranulocytosis, thrombocytopenia, hemolysis). Recently, there has been a reported association between certain NSAIDs (rofecoxib, celecoxib, valdecoxib) and increased risk of heart attack and stroke.

CLINICAL PRESENTATION

▶ Many acute NSAID exposures are asymptomatic.

▶ High-risk ingestions: phenylbutazone (veterinary NSAID), mefenamic acid, ibuprofen ingestions > 400 mg/kg.

▶ Following overdose, GI symptoms are most common and range from nausea and vomiting to GI hemorrhage (hematemesis, melena) to severe abdominal pain from perforation.

▶ ARF can occur by acute interstitial nephritis (AIN) (usually chronic toxicity) or by decreased GFR and renal hypoperfusion related to inhibition of prostaglandin synthesis.

▶ Severe GI and renal toxicity are seen more commonly in chronic exposure than in acute exposure.

▶ Neurologic symptoms can include dizziness, confusion, tinnitus, visual disturbances, psychosis, seizures, and coma.

▶ Hypersensitivity-type reactions can occur and include asthma exacerbations, anaphylaxis, and Stevens-Johnson syndrome.

DIFFERENTIAL DIAGNOSIS

▶ Symptoms are often non-specific. Consider co-ingestants and other disease processes.

▶ Salicylates can have similar presentation and poorer prognosis (see Chap. 90 for details).

▶ Other etiologies of GI bleeding: esophageal varices, liver disease, PUD, IBD, malignancies, hematologic disorders.

EMERGENCY DEPARTMENT MANAGEMENT
Diagnosis

▶ Diagnosis is made by history of exposure. There is no readily available lab test to confirm toxicity or exposure.

▶ Acetaminophen (APAP) and salicylate levels are recommended in most circumstances to rule out dangerous co-ingestions.

▶ Renal function studies and electrolytes should be ordered for all significant exposures.

▶ CBC and type and cross-match for significant GI hemorrhage.

▶ Please see Chap. 88 for details on additional lab/ancillary testing that may be appropriate.

Treatment

▶ ABCs including large-bore IV access, IVF, and blood administration for significant GI hemorrhage.

- ▶ Gastric lavage is unnecessary for most ingestions but may be considered for massive overdoses seen within 30 minutes or agents with high risk for toxicity (phenylbutazone, mefenamic acid).
- ▶ Single-dose activated charcoal is recommended for all significant ingestions.
- ▶ Proton-pump inhibitors and misoprostol (prostaglandin analogue) may be considered for severe GI bleeding.
- ▶ Most ingestions respond to supportive care without lasting sequelae.

Disposition

- ▶ Patients with significant GI bleeding (especially older patients with comorbidities), acidosis, renal failure, or persistent altered mental status require admission.
- ▶ An asymptomatic patient who has been observed for 4–6 hours after ingestion may be safely discharged with primary care follow-up.

CHAPTER 110

BETA-BLOCKERS

James Pribble

- ▶ Approximately 15,000 beta-blocker overdoses were reported in 2003 (most common cardiovascular drug class seen in overdose).
- ▶ Approximately 14 deaths in 2003 attributed primarily to beta-blocker ingestions (most were intentional or suicidal ingestions).

PATHOPHYSIOLOGY

- ▶ Beta-blockers inhibit the activation of G proteins needed for intracellular calcium release and cardiac contractility.
- ▶ Calcium release is modulated by adenylate cyclase, which increases production of cAMP; beta-blockers antagonize this pathway.

CLINICAL PRESENTATION

- ▶ Many beta-blocker overdoses are asymptomatic; patients with intrinsic cardiac disease, co-ingestions, or large overdoses are more likely to show signs of toxicity.
- ▶ Hypotension and bradycardia are predominant symptoms; CHF may develop or be exacerbated in predisposed patients.
- ▶ Onset is usually rapid but varies based on lipid solubility; most cases of beta-blocker toxicity become symptomatic within the first 6 hours (sotalol can have delayed presentation). Half-lives vary from 8 minutes (esmolol) to > 30 hours (nebivolol).
- ▶ ECG changes include sinus bradycardia, sinus pause, sinus arrest, prolonged PR or high-grade AV block (uncommon), widened QRS, prolonged QT, and asystole.
- ▶ Delirium, coma, and seizures can occur due to membrane-stabilizing effect/inhibition of fast sodium channels and high lipid solubility; propranolol is commonly associated with these symptoms.

TABLE 110-1.
TOXIN-INDUCED BRADYCARDIA

Beta-blockers
CCBs
Digoxin/cardiac glycosides
TCA toxicity
AChE drugs
Opioids
Clonidine
GHB
Phenylpropanolamine

▶ Sotalol has intrinsic potassium channel–blocking activity and can delay cardiac repolarization; it prolongs the QT interval and predisposes to torsades de pointes and ventricular dysrhythmias.

▶ Some beta-blockers also have intrinsic sympathomimetic activity (pindolol, acebutolol) so may paradoxically result in tachycardia and HTN.

▶ Hypoglycemia is common in pediatric ingestions.

DIFFERENTIAL DIAGNOSIS OF BRADYCARDIA

▶ Toxin induced (Table 110-1)
▶ Other causes (Table 110-2)

EMERGENCY DEPARTMENT MANAGEMENT
Diagnosis

▶ History and physical exam: hypotension and bradycardia should raise immediate suspicion for beta-blocker or other cardiotoxic drug ingestion.

TABLE 110-2.
OTHER CAUSES OF BRADYCARDIA

MI/structural heart disease
Hyperkalemia
Hypothyroidism
Hypothermia
Elevated ICP (due to hemorrhage, mass lesion, etc.)

▶ If evidence of prolonged QT, consider sotalol.
▶ If altered mental status or seizures, consider propranolol or other lipophilic agents.
▶ A 12-lead ECG should be obtained on every patient with suspected beta-blocker toxicity.
▶ Serum glucose should be checked.
  • See Chap. 88 for other appropriate lab testing.

Treatment

▶ ABCs, with early intubation if required for seizures, decreased mental status, or concern for airway stability.
▶ IV access, O_2, and continuous cardiac monitoring.
▶ Induction of emesis is contraindicated.
▶ Consider NG/orogastric lavage for massive overdoses or sustained-release drugs, ingestion of more toxic compounds (propranolol, acebutolol, metoprolol, oxprenolol, or sotalol), or if patient presents within 1 hour of ingestion.
  • Vagal stimulation can cause worsening bradycardia.
  • Pre-treat with atropine if lavage performed.
▶ Activated charcoal:
  • 1 g/kg for all patients (even asymptomatic patients).
  • Multiple doses may be considered in the setting of sustained-release compounds.
▶ Whole bowel irrigation recommended for sustained-release compounds.
▶ Treat seizures with benzodiazepines.
▶ Specific interventions:
  • IVF/atropine
    ○ Fluid boluses of 0.9% NS, 500 ml or 20 ml/kg for hypotension (monitor for pulmonary edema)
    ○ Atropine, 1 mg or 0.02 mg/kg IV (minimum dose 0.1 mg), may be repeated
  • Vasopressors
    ○ Epinephrine, norepinephrine, dopamine, isoproterenol, and dobutamine can all be used (epinephrine may be an appropriate initial choice due to its non-specific alpha- and beta-agonism).
    ○ Very high doses may be required in significant intoxication (invasive hemodynamic monitoring is usually necessary).

- Indicated for patients with hypotension and bradycardia unresponsive to initial supportive care and atropine.
- Initial doses:
  - Epinephrine, start at 0.02 mcg/kg/minute
  - Isoproterenol, start at 0.1 mcg/kg/minute
  - Norepinephrine, start at 0.1 mcg/kg/minute
  - Dobutamine, start at 2.5 mcg/kg/minute
- Glucagon
  - Improves contractility and bradycardia.
  - Initial bolus, 2–5 mg IV over 60 seconds (50 mcg/kg in children); may repeat up to 10 mg. Duration of effect is 15 minutes.
  - Infusion: use bolus dose/hour (i.e., if patient responds to 5 mg, start infusion at 5 mg/hour).
- Calcium
  - May help improve hypotension, though effect may be transient.
  - Initial dose is 1 g of calcium chloride or 10–20 ml of 10% calcium chloride (20 mg/kg in children); calcium gluconate may also be used, 30–60 ml of 10% solution.
  - Repeat boluses (maximum of three) q20min or infusion (0.2 ml/kg/hour calcium chloride or 0.6 ml/kg/hour calcium gluconate) may be required.
  - Calcium should be avoided in any patient taking a cardiac glycoside such as digoxin.
- Insulin and glucose
  - Experimentally has been shown to improve outcome in beta-blocker toxicity by improving myocardial glucose and calcium utilization.
- Phosphodiesterase inhibitors (milrinone)
  - May be considered for patients unresponsive to glucagons, calcium, and initial vasopressor therapy
- Other supportive measures
  - Transvenous or transcutaneous pacing; may not be effective secondary to failure to capture.
  - Intra-aortic balloon pump may be considered to increase cardiac output.
  - Cardiopulmonary bypass may be appropriate for severe toxicity.

Disposition

▶ Asymptomatic patients.
- Monitor for 6–8 hours for non–sustained-release beta-blocker, and if remains asymptomatic with normal vital signs, consider discharge.
- Sotalol overdose requires a minimum of 12 hours of observation.
- Sustained-release compounds require hospital admission and 24 hours of observation.

▶ Symptomatic patients: all should be admitted, and most to ICU setting for hypotension, bradycardia, ECG changes, or altered mental status.

CHAPTER 111

CALCIUM CHANNEL BLOCKERS

James Pribble

▶ CCBs widely used for the treatment of HTN and tachyarrhythmias.
▶ Number one cause of cardiovascular drug overdose deaths (> 50 deaths associated with CCB overdose in 2003).

PATHOPHYSIOLOGY

▶ CCBs act on the L-type calcium channels in cardiac, vascular smooth muscle, and pancreatic islet cells; influx of calcium is impaired, which leads to decreased myocardial contractility.
▶ CCBs also inhibit SA and AV nodal function, reducing HR and myocardial electrical conduction.

CLINICAL PRESENTATION

▶ Commonly asymptomatic at initial presentation, with onset of symptoms at 2–3 hours (6–10 hours for sustained-release compounds).
▶ Signs and symptoms include hypotension, bradycardia, dizziness, hyperglycemia, acidosis, pulmonary edema, and cardiogenic shock.
▶ ECG findings include sinus bradycardia, AV nodal blocks including complete heart block, and idioventricular and junctional escape rhythms.
▶ Decreased cerebral perfusion may lead to confusion, lethargy, seizures, and strokes.
▶ Decreased systemic perfusion may lead to renal failure and ischemic bowel.
▶ Degree of toxicity is likely to be increased with co-ingestions (especially beta-blockers) and pre-existing structural heart disease.

DIFFERENTIAL DIAGNOSIS

▶ See Chap. 110 for differential diagnosis of bradycardia.
▶ See Table 99-1 for differential diagnosis of altered mental status.

EMERGENCY DEPARTMENT MANAGEMENT
Diagnosis

▶ History and physical exam: hypotension and bradycardia should raise immediate suspicion for CCB or other cardiotoxic drug ingestion.

▶ A 12-lead ECG should be obtained on every patient with suspected CCB toxicity.

▶ Serum glucose should be checked.

▶ Serum levels of most CCBs are generally not available at most hospital labs and are not helpful acutely.

▶ See Chap. 88 for other appropriate lab testing.

Treatment

▶ ABCs, with early intubation if required for seizures, decreased mental status, or concern for airway stability.

▶ IV access, O_2, and continuous cardiac monitoring.

▶ Induction of emesis is contraindicated.

▶ Consider orogastric/NG lavage in large overdose, exposure to sustained-release compounds, or presentation within 1 hour of ingestion.
   • Vagal stimulation can worsen bradycardia.
   • Pre-treat with atropine if lavage performed.

▶ Activated charcoal:
   • 1 g/kg for all patients (even asymptomatic patients).
   • Multiple doses may be considered in the setting of sustained-release compounds.

▶ Whole bowel irrigation recommended for sustained-release CCBs.

▶ Treat seizures with benzodiazepines.

▶ Specific interventions:
   • Atropine/IVF
      ○ Fluid boluses of 0.9% NS, 500 ml or 20 ml/kg, for hypotension (monitor for pulmonary edema)
      ○ Atropine, 1 mg or 0.02 mg/kg IV (minimum dose, 0.1 mg); may be repeated
   • Vasopressors
      ○ Epinephrine, norepinephrine, dopamine, isoproterenol, and dobutamine can all be used (epinephrine may be an appropriate initial choice due to its non-specific alpha- and beta-agonism).

- ○ Very high doses may be required in significant intoxication (invasive hemodynamic monitoring is usually necessary).
- ○ Indicated for patients with hypotension and bradycardia unresponsive to initial supportive care and atropine.
- ○ Initial doses: see Chap. 110.
- Calcium
  - ○ Initial dose is 1 g of calcium chloride or 10–20 ml of 10% calcium chloride (20 mg/kg in children); calcium gluconate may also be used: 30–60 ml of 10% solution.
  - ○ Repeat bolus q20min may be required (maximum of three total doses).
  - ○ Infusion: 0.2 ml/kg/hour calcium chloride or 0.6 ml/kg/hour calcium gluconate.
  - ○ Serum calcium, phosphorus, and potassium need to be closely monitored in patients receiving ongoing calcium therapy.
  - ○ Calcium administration should be avoided in any patient taking a cardiac glycoside such as digoxin.
- Glucagon
  - ○ Consider in patients with significant CCB overdose who do not respond to fluids, calcium, and vasopressor therapy.
  - ○ Initial bolus 2–5 mg IV over 60 seconds (50 mcg/kg in children); may repeat up to 10 mg. Duration of effect is 15 minutes.
  - ○ Infusion: use bolus dose/hour (i.e., if patient responds to 5 mg, start infusion at 5 mg/hour).
- Insulin and glucose
  - ○ Basic science evidence that therapy may improve outcomes when used to treat significant CCB toxicity
- Phosphodiesterase inhibitors (milrinone)
  - ○ May be considered for patients unresponsive to glucagon, calcium, and initial vasopressor therapy
- Other supportive measures
  - ○ Transvenous or transcutaneous pacing: may not be effective secondary to failure to capture.
  - ○ Intra-aortic balloon pump may be considered to increase cardiac output.
  - ○ Cardiopulmonary bypass may be appropriate for severe toxicity.

Disposition

► Asymptomatic patients
  - Monitor for at least 6–8 hours for non–sustained-release CCB.
  - Sustained-release compounds require hospital admission and at least 24 hours of observation.
  - An asymptomatic patient with serial normal ECGs and normal vital signs without co-ingestion or exposure to a sustained-release compound may be discharged after observation period.
► All symptomatic patients should be admitted, and most to ICU setting for hypotension, bradycardia, ECG changes, or altered mental status.

CHAPTER 112

CLONIDINE

John P. Erpelding

▶ Clonidine is most commonly used to treat HTN but is also used for nicotine, alcohol, and opiate addiction; migraine headaches; Tourette's syndrome; attention-deficit hyperactivity disorder; panic attacks; obsessive-compulsive disorder; and post-traumatic stress disorder.

▶ Increasingly problematic poisoning in children: over 5400 exposures reported to poison centers in 2003 (majority in children and teens), with seven deaths.

▶ Consider clonidine overdose in the patient with an opioid toxidrome that fails to improve with naloxone administration.

PATHOPHYSIOLOGY

▶ A centrally acting alpha-2 adrenergic agonist, which reduces sympathetic outflow from the vasomotor center in the medulla oblongata, causing decreased vascular tone and HR.

▶ When taken in large doses, clonidine can transiently activate peripheral post-synaptic alpha-2 receptors, giving rise to HTN and tachycardia before exerting its primary central effects.

▶ Toxic dose can be as little as 0.1 mg in children, yet patients have survived acute ingestions ≤ 100 mg in adults and 50 mg in a child.

▶ Even after 7 days of use, transdermal patches may retain up to 75% of initial drug concentration and can cause severe toxicity if ingested.

CLINICAL PRESENTATION

▶ Altered mental status (ranging from somnolence and lethargy to coma) is most common; other CNS manifestations include hypotonia, hyporeflexia, miosis, and seizures (rare).

► Cardiovascular toxicity includes bradycardia, hypotension, HTN (usually transient), tachycardia (usually transient), and AV nodal blocks (including complete heart block).

► Respiratory depression is associated with CNS depression and is more common in children.

► Hypothermia is common, especially in children.

► In chronic use, severe rebound HTN can result with abrupt cessation of use; other symptoms of clonidine withdrawal include agitation, tremor, palpitations, vomiting, and insomnia.

► Clonidine patches can be mistaken for Band-Aids by children and can cause significant toxicity with dermal application or ingestion; complete exposure and careful examination of all skin and visible mucus membrane surfaces (e.g., roof of mouth) are key in identifying this problem and to remove the patch(es) to prevent further absorption.

DIFFERENTIAL DIAGNOSIS

► Depends on clinical signs and symptoms but may include
  • Barbiturate or benzodiazepine intoxication
  • Beta-blocker, CCB, or digoxin toxicity
  • Opioid intoxication
  • Phenothiazine intoxication
  • Severe alcohol intoxication (ethanol, methanol, isopropanol, ethylene glycol)
  • Intracranial hemorrhage (especially pontine and thalamic hemorrhages, which can also have miosis)

► See Table 99-1 for differential diagnosis of altered mental status.

► See Chap. 110 for differential diagnosis of bradycardia.

EMERGENCY DEPARTMENT MANAGEMENT

Diagnosis

► Must be diagnosed clinically: no specific tests to confirm.

► A 12-lead ECG should be obtained on every patient with suspected clonidine toxicity.

► Serum glucose should be checked.

► See Chap. 88 for other appropriate lab testing.

Treatment

► ABCs: intubation is indicated for severe respiratory depression and/or CNS depression.

► IV access, O_2, and continuous cardiac monitoring.

► Induction of emesis is contraindicated.

► Orogastric/NG lavage can be considered in large ingestions if performed within 1 hour after ingestion.

► Activated charcoal, 1 g/kg by mouth or NG, is generally recommended.

► Whole bowel irrigation has been used for transdermal patch ingestion.

► Hypotension typically responds to crystalloid fluid boluses, though occasionally vasopressors such as dopamine or norepinephrine are necessary.

► Atropine can be used for significant bradycardia.

► Occasionally, patients with severe HTN require antihypertensive therapy such as sodium nitroprusside (caution with use of beta-blockers as risk of unopposed alpha stimulation exists); this is rare. Only if HTN is threatening end-organ damage should antihypertensives be started.

► Paradoxical HTN is usually transient, and patients can rapidly become hypotensive if HTN is being aggressively treated; continuous BP monitoring and titration of BP-lowering agents are advised.

► Naloxone may be tried, although its use and efficacy as an antidote remain inconsistent and controversial; generally reserved for severe intoxications where intubation or vasopressors might be required. Severe HTN can also result.

Disposition

► Symptomatic patients all require admission, typically to an ICU setting.

► Asymptomatic patients 6 hours post-ingestion of oral clonidine with serial normal ECGs and vital signs may be discharged if no suspicion for co-ingestions.

CHAPTER 113

CAUSTIC INGESTIONS

Dominic A. Borgialli

► Most caustic ingestions are unintentional and occur in children < 6 years of age, though adult intentional ingestions are more likely to result in serious injury.

► Injury severity depends on the form (solid or liquid), concentration, and volume of the agent.

ALKALI

► Alkali caustics include industrial compounds like sodium hydroxide and potassium hydroxide (cleaning fluids), household compounds (sodium hydroxide in drain and oven cleaners), household bleach (sodium hypochlorite), and button batteries.

Pathophysiology

► Alkali corrosives saponify fat in cell membranes causing liquefaction necrosis and deep tissue injury.

► Severe ingestions may cause multi-system organ injuries, including gastric perforation, necrosis of abdominal viscera, and eventual esophageal strictures.

► Household liquid bleach (3–6% sodium hypochlorite, pH ~11) is not corrosive to the esophagus, but gastric and pulmonary irritation occurs.

► Solid or granular alkali ingestions have greater potential for proximal esophageal injury; liquid alkali ingestions are characterized by generalized esophageal injury.

Clinical Presentation

► Drooling, odynophagia, vomiting, dyspnea, hoarseness, oropharyngeal burns, and stridor are common symptoms following significant ingestions.

▶ Inhalation exposure can cause wheezing, upper-airway edema, or pulmonary edema; rapid airway compromise can result with significant burns.

▶ Esophageal burns are more common than gastric burns.

▶ Children with two or more of the following symptoms (vomiting, drooling, or stridor) have been found to have a significant esophageal injury.

▶ Shock, metabolic acidosis (severe GI bleeding or massive tissue necrosis), and renal failure are rare complications found with severe exposures.

▶ Peritoneal signs and mental status changes are ominous findings; tachycardia and hypotension are frequently associated with esophageal perforation.

▶ Pneumomediastinum, pleural effusion, and pneumoperitoneum on an upright chest radiograph suggest viscus perforation requiring surgical management.

▶ Immediate injury is followed in 2–3 days by tissue sloughing with increased risk of perforation in 5–14 days.

Emergency Department Management

Diagnosis

▶ Inspection of the oropharynx and assessment of the airway, vital signs, and mental status, followed by a thorough history of the exposure, are required.

▶ Direct visualization of the vocal cords with a fiberoptic nasopharyngoscope can provide additional information for the need for intubation.

▶ Lab studies of value include type and cross-match, HCT, coagulation parameters, electrolytes, and serum pH.

▶ CXR can demonstrate evidence of pneumomediastinum, pleural effusion, or pneumoperitoneum, though a normal film does not rule out significant injury.

Treatment

▶ Any signs of airway edema or depressed mental status should prompt consideration of airway protection as edema may rapidly evolve; paralytics should be used with caution and preparation for a prompt surgical airway should be made.

▶ Hypotension often indicates perforation and significant blood loss; large-bore IV access and aggressive resuscitation for anticipated operative intervention.

▶ Dilution with a small amount of water or milk within minutes of ingestion in the stable, awake, asymptomatic patient may be considered.

▶ Activated charcoal, induction of emesis, neutralization, NGT placement, and NG lavage are all contraindicated.

▶ Button battery ingestions need chest and abdomen radiographs to determine location (endoscopy indicated if it has not passed the gastroesophageal junction); otherwise, follow with stool straining and serial X-rays in the asymptomatic patient.

▶ Endoscopy indications: stridor (after airway stabilization), children with vomiting and drooling, any intentional ingestion; consider in every symptomatic exposure.

▶ Patients who require endoscopy should have it performed within 12–24 hours.

▶ Surgical intervention is indicated for patients with evidence of perforation on physical exam or X-rays, persistent hypotension, or evidence of deep ulcers or necrosis on endoscopy.

▶ Steroids (prednisolone, 2 mg/kg/day) and antibiotics should be considered for patients with significant injury on endoscopy.

Disposition

▶ Children with unintentional caustic ingestions who remain asymptomatic and tolerate liquids after a few hours of observation can be discharged.

▶ Any symptomatic patient or individual with an intentional ingestion requires admission and observation.

ACIDS

▶ Common acids include industrial agents like hydrochloric and sulfuric acids (cleaning agents), hydrofluoric acid (HF) (etching and metal cleaning), and household products containing sulfuric acid (drain cleaners) and HF (rust removers).

Pathophysiology

▶ Injuries by strong acids produce coagulation necrosis with severe injury to superficial tissues; tissue destruction results in eschar formation.

▶ Ingested acids settle in the stomach, where gastric necrosis, perforation, and hemorrhage may result; esophageal injury is common as well.

▶ Due to the systemic penetration of acids, there is more commonly damage to the spleen, liver, biliary tract, and pancreas, as well as systemic acidosis.

Clinical Presentation

▶ Similar initial presentation to alkali ingestions, consisting of chest and abdominal pain, respiratory distress, and vomiting (see above).
▶ Metabolic acidosis, shock, hemolysis, and renal failure may occur.
▶ Hematemesis, melena, and GI hemorrhage with gastric perforation and peritonitis can occur; gastric outlet obstruction is a late complication.
▶ HF can cause extensive tissue penetration; classically, patients have benign wounds with pain out of proportion. Hypocalcemia, hypomagnesemia, hyperkalemia, acidosis, ventricular dysrhythmias, and death may occur.

Emergency Department Management

Diagnosis
▶ Same as alkali agents (see above)

Treatment
▶ Initial stabilization, supportive care, and dilution are the same as for alkali exposures (see above).
▶ Activated charcoal, cathartics, and neutralizing agents are contraindicated.
▶ $NaHCO_3$ may be required with a serum pH < 7.1.
▶ Steroid and antibiotic use is the same as in alkali ingestions.
▶ Patients with a depressed mental status, unstable vital signs, acidemia, or peritoneal signs should be considered for acute surgical intervention.
▶ Indications for endoscopy are the same as for alkali ingestions.
▶ HF exposure is potentially rapidly fatal and requires specific treatment with calcium and magnesium. Consultation with a poison center is recommended.

Disposition
▶ Same as alkali agents (see above)

CHAPTER 114

HYDROCARBONS

Constance J. Doyle

- ▶ Hydrocarbons are a group of chemical compounds that contain carbon and hydrogen derived from plant and animal material, as well as petroleum and natural gases.
- ▶ Most common exposures are gasoline and fuels, mineral spirits, oil, lighter fluid (naphtha), kerosene, and turpentine.
- ▶ Off-gassing from contaminated patients and clothing can occur in the absence of decontamination and presents a risk to emergency staff.

PATHOPHYSIOLOGY

- ▶ Hydrocarbons can be aliphatic (straight chained and branched) or aromatic (cyclic: include a benzene ring); halogenated or substituted hydrocarbons contain hydroxyl or halide groups.
- ▶ Aspiration: severe pneumonitis can occur with ingestion; vomiting does not necessarily have to occur.
  - Common exposures: adults siphoning gasoline; children consuming poorly-stored, fragrant lamp oils.
  - Potential for aspiration is increased for substances with lower viscosity, greater volatility, and lower surface tension.
- ▶ Cutaneous: irritation of skin and mucosal surfaces and transcutaneous absorption depend on number of carbons and additives; dermatitis and chemical burns occur and are proportional to length of exposure.

CLINICAL PRESENTATION

- ▶ Pulmonary symptoms are common with any aspiration: cough, tachypnea, hemoptysis, hypoxemia, pulmonary edema, respiratory distress, hemorrhagic pneumonitis, and barotraumas can all occur.

► Cardiovascular symptoms include ventricular irritability and arrhythmias, sensitization of myocardium, myocardial depression, and sudden death.

► CNS symptoms consist of lethargy, CNS depression, headaches, lightheadedness, dizziness, confusion, seizures, and coma; chronic exposure can lead to leukoencephalopathy (especially toluene) and generalized neuronal destruction.

► Peripheral neuropathy occurs with many occupational exposures.

► Hepatic failure is common with chlorinated hydrocarbons (especially carbon tetrachloride, vinyl chloride) and benzene; renal failure is more common with halogenated hydrocarbons and usually occurs by ATN.

► Nausea and vomiting are common and increase the risk of aspiration; cutaneous and mucosal burns occur as well (see above).

► Bone marrow suppression and hematologic malignancies are associated with chronic exposure.

DIFFERENTIAL DIAGNOSIS

► See Table 99-1 for differential diagnosis of altered mental status.

► Patients with predominantly respiratory symptoms may have other pulmonary pathology: asthma, FB aspiration, PTX, PE, and anaphylaxis.

► Consider possibility of impurity in hydrocarbon; adulteration with insecticides, heavy metals, etc., is not uncommon.

EMERGENCY DEPARTMENT MANAGEMENT
Diagnosis

► Typically made by history of exposure and consistent symptoms.

► Exact product identification and specifics regarding the amount, concentration, and time of exposure are helpful in directing subsequent care.

► Consultation with a regional poison center early in care is recommended to assist in directing treatment.

► Other lab and ancillary testing should be directed by clinical symptoms and specific substance exposure:

• Pulse oximetry, ABG, and CXR (for patients with pulmonary symptoms)

- ECG and cardiac monitoring (especially for halogenated hydrocarbons and benzene)
- Electrolytes, BUN, creatinine, CPK (especially for halogenated hydrocarbons and toluene)
- Transaminases and coagulation studies (especially for carbon tetrachloride and other halogenated hydrocarbons)
- CBC (especially for benzene, which can cause hemolysis, aplastic anemia, and hematologic malignancies)

Treatment

▶ Remove from exposure and decontaminate the skin and wounds with soap and water; irrigate eyes with NS if splash or exposure.

▶ Remove and bag clothing and place in an area that will not further contaminate treatment area; vomitus should be placed in a closed container and isolated away from treatment areas.

▶ Supportive care should be initiated, including supplemental O_2, IVF, ventilatory support, or intubation as needed.

▶ Gastric emptying is controversial but may be considered in intentional or large-volume ingestions (> 30 ml), or in compounds with a high degree of toxicity (camphor, halogenated hydrocarbons, and compounds with metals or pesticides).

▶ Activated charcoal is generally not helpful.

▶ Prophylactic antibiotics are controversial but may be justified with severe pulmonary toxicity.

▶ Hyperbaric O_2 (HBO) therapy may be considered for carbon tetrachloride exposures (consultation with poison and hyperbaric centers is recommended).

Disposition

▶ Any patient with evidence of toxicity or persistent symptoms should be hospitalized.

▶ Asymptomatic patients without expected delayed effects and a normal repeat CXR after 6 hours may be discharged with primary care follow-up.

CHAPTER 115

HEAVY METALS

Troy Christian Sims

LEAD

▶ Lead is the most common cause of chronic metal poisoning encountered due in great part to its abundance in the industrialized world.

▶ It exists in two forms, inorganic and organic, which differ in their route of absorption.
  - Inorganic: batteries, soldering, automobile radiators, paint, pipes, cable sheathing, fishing weights, ammunition
  - Organic: gasoline (especially in developing countries)

▶ Inhalation of lead fumes or fine particulates is the major route of exposure in industrial settings, while ingestion is seen more commonly in non-industrial settings, particularly in young children with pica.

▶ Percutaneous absorption is significant with organic lead, but negligible with inorganic forms.

Pathophysiology

▶ Following absorption, lead is extensively bound to RBCs, which redistribute it to the bone, where over 90% of it is stored.

▶ It interferes with many cellular processes, mainly by interfering with cellular calcium handling and heme production; it also binds sulfhydryl groups, affecting many different cellular proteins and enzymes.

Clinical Presentation

▶ See Table 115-1.

Differential Diagnosis

▶ May include other peripheral neuropathies, infectious encephalitis or meningitis, Guillain-Barré, renal colic, acute appendicitis

TABLE 115-1.
CLINICAL PRESENTATION OF LEAD INGESTION

System	Acute	Chronic
CNS	Fatigue, irritability, headache, memory loss, ataxia, seizures, encephalopathy	Same + depressed mood, decreased libido
Peripheral nervous system	—	Weakness and atrophy, foot drop, wrist drop
GI	Anorexia, nausea, and abdominal pain (lead colic)	Same + weight loss, chronic constipation
Hematopoietic	Anemia (basophilic stippling is non-specific)	Anemia (usually microcytic/hypochromic)
Renal	Fanconi syndrome (glycosuria, hyperphosphaturia, aminoaciduria), renal tubular acidosis	Renal insufficiency, saturnine gout (secondary to hypouricuria)
Cardiovascular	—	HTN

or other surgical causes of abdominal pain, infectious gastroenteritis, behavioral or psychiatric problems

Emergency Department Management

Diagnosis
▶ Complete history, including potential exposures (industrial, occupational, pica behavior, past GSWs), is key to diagnosis.
▶ Should be considered in anyone presenting with the combination of abdominal symptoms, neurologic dysfunction, and anemia, as well as in all children with encephalopathy or irritability.
▶ Lab studies:
  • Serum lead level is the most useful test, with levels ≥ 10 mcg/dl in children and ≥ 40 mcg/dl in adults raising concern (see below).
  • CBC may reveal anemia and basophilic stippling on peripheral smear.
  • Electrolytes, BUN, and creatinine may reveal evidence of renal impairment.
  • UA may reveal proteinuria or Fanconi syndrome in children.
  • Liver enzymes may show elevated transaminases.

- Plain film radiographs may reveal *lead lines* in children, which are transverse, linear opacities at the metaphyses.
- Head CT may reveal cerebral edema in severe cases.
- Radiographs may reveal bullet or ingested lead material.

Treatment

▶ Removal from environmental lead exposure.

▶ If signs of acute ingestion, then activated charcoal with whole bowel irrigation.

▶ Chelation therapy usually recommended for symptomatic adults and/or those with serum lead levels ≥ 70 mcg/dl.

▶ Chelation therapy usually recommended for symptomatic children and/or those with serum lead levels ≥ 45 mcg/dl; controversial for asymptomatic children with levels 20–44 mcg/dl (studies under way).

▶ Chelators include British antilewisite (BAL), CaNa$_2$-EDTA, and succimer [dimercaptosuccinic acid (DMSA)]; dosing is complex, and consultation with a poison control center is recommended when initiating therapy.

ARSENIC

▶ Arsenic is the most common cause of acute metal poisoning, with soil, water, and food being the most common sources of contamination.

▶ Most common industrial use of arsenic is as a wood preservative, so wood burning may cause poisonings.

▶ It is a tasteless and odorless metal that is readily absorbed after ingestion and inhalation but has insignificant dermal absorption.

Pathophysiology

▶ On entering the blood, arsenic is rapidly re-distributed to various organs; as a result, blood and urine levels are unreliable in detecting exposure.

▶ Arsenic crosses the placenta and blood-brain barrier and interferes with ATP production and citric acid cycle; it can impair gluconeogenesis and cause hypoglycemia.

▶ It can also uncouple oxidative phosphorylation and induce mutagenesis.

TABLE 115-2.
CLINICAL PRESENTATION OF ARSENIC INGESTION

System	Acute/subacute (< 1 month)	Chronic (> 1 month)
CNS	Headache, irritability, seizures, encephalopathy	Headache, confusion, encephalopathy
Peripheral nervous system	Dysphagia with metallic taste, stocking-glove sensory neuropathy	Stocking-glove sensory neuropathy, ascending motor paralysis in severe cases
GI	Nausea, vomiting, abdominal pain, cholera-like diarrhea	Nausea, vomiting, diarrhea, or constipation
Cardiovascular	Hypotension, prolonged QTc, brady- and tachydysrhythmia	Prolonged QTc
Respiratory	Pulmonary edema, ARDS, respiratory failure	Restrictive and obstructive lung disease
Hematopoietic	Anemia (normocytic, normochromic)	Anemia (may show basophilic stippling)
Renal	ARF, rhabdomyolysis	Renal failure
Dermatologic	—	Hyperkeratosis, Mees' lines (transverse white line just above lunula of fingernail), alopecia

Clinical Presentation

▶ See Table 115-2.

Differential Diagnosis

▶ See Differential Diagnosis under Lead.

Emergency Department Management

Diagnosis

▶ Complete history, including potential exposures (seafood, well water, metallurgy, mining, wood preservatives, etc.), is key to diagnosis.
▶ Lab studies:
   • CBC may show anemia and basophilic stippling on peripheral smear.
   • Electrolytes, BUN, creatinine can reveal renal impairment; AST, ALT, and bilirubin may be elevated.

- ECG for dysrhythmias, T-wave changes, and prolonged QTc.
- Abdominal radiographs may reveal evidence of acute ingestion.
- Note blood levels will not be reliable except in acute exposure because arsenic remains in blood stream for only 2–4 hours.
- Urine spot tests, 24-hour collection, and hair/fingernail analysis for arsenic are helpful if positive, but rarely are immediately available.

Treatment

▶ Activated charcoal does not bind arsenic well, but it generally should be given for acute ingestions; consider whole bowel irrigation if metal seen on X-rays.

▶ If symptomatic and elevated blood (or other source) arsenic levels, start BAL chelation therapy; also start if strong suspicion for acute exposure, without lab results.

▶ Succimer is used for subacute or chronic toxicity.

MERCURY

▶ See Table 115-3.

Pathophysiology

▶ Toxicity is directly related to its ability to interrupt cellular metabolism; it binds sulfhydryl groups and disrupts cellular enzymes and structural proteins.

TABLE 115-3.
FORMS, SOURCES, AND PRIMARY ROUTES OF MERCURY EXPOSURE

Form	Source	Primary route of exposure
Elemental	Batteries, barometers, thermometers, electro-plating, fluorescent lights	Inhalation (no significant GI absorption)
Organic	Embalming processes, farming, seafood, paper manufacturing	Ingestion (more than 90% absorbed via GI tract)
Inorganic	Explosives, fur processing, dyes, cosmetics, taxidermy	GI and dermal

TABLE 115-4.
CLINICAL PRESENTATION OF MERCURY INGESTION

System	Elemental	Organic	Inorganic
CNS	Tremors, erethism (emotional lability, insomnia, anxiety), peripheral neuropathy	Same—neurologic symptoms predominate	Same
GI	Nausea, vomiting, diarrhea	Nausea, vomiting, diarrhea	Nausea, vomiting, hemorrhagic gastroenteritis
Renal	Proteinuria	Rare	ARF
CV/pulmonary	Pneumonitis, pulmonary fibrosis	Rare	Shock
Dermal	Acrodynia (swollen hands/feet with desquamation), stomatitis	Same	Same

Clinical Presentation

▶ The form of the mercury is important in determining the extent of absorption.
  • For example, ingestion of the elemental mercury in a thermometer will not be expected to cause toxicity as it is minimally absorbed by the GI tract (Table 115-4).

Differential Diagnosis

▶ See Differential Diagnosis under Lead.

Emergency Department Management

Diagnosis

▶ Complete history about potential exposures is key to diagnosis.
▶ Combination of unexplained neuropsychiatric symptoms and renal abnormalities is a typical presentation in a patient with potential exposure.
▶ Lab studies:
  • CBC, electrolytes, and UA for renal failure.

- Radiographs of abdomen if acute ingestion suspected.
- Spot urine and blood mercury levels may be helpful if elevated (< 10 mcg/L and < 20 mcg/L are considered normal in blood and urine respectively).
- However, mercury levels do not always correlate well with toxicity.

Treatment
- ▶ Decision to initiate chelation therapy should be made on basis of likely exposure and symptoms consistent with toxicity.
- ▶ If inorganic mercury salts were ingested, then activated charcoal, followed by whole bowel irrigation, and initiation of BAL chelation therapy.
- ▶ Succimer (DMSA) should be used in chronic poisoning with mild symptoms or in organic mercury poisoning, such as methyl mercury (BAL may potentially redistribute mercury to the CNS).
- ▶ In elemental mercury poisoning, either succimer or BAL can be used (d-penicillamine is an alternative as well).

DISPOSITION OF HEAVY METAL TOXICITY

- ▶ All patients requiring chelation therapy or with ongoing symptoms should be admitted to a monitored bed.
- ▶ Children with significantly elevated lead levels (> 45 mcg/L), regardless of symptoms, should be admitted.
- ▶ Admit any patient whose discharge environment is suspected to be contaminated.

CHAPTER 116

CYANIDE

Troy Christian Sims

▶ Extremely potent toxin, with a colorful history of use in suicides, murders, chemical warfare, and occupational exposures.

▶ 275 exposures to cyanide reported in the U.S. in 2003—most were unintentional; nine deaths reported.

PATHOPHYSIOLOGY

▶ Potential sources of cyanide poisoning include
  • Fires and inhalational injuries (released from nylon, wool, acrylic, polyurethane, silk, plastics, melamine, and polyacrylonitrile)
  • Sodium nitroprusside infusions
  • Ingestion of fruit seeds (pits of apricots, peaches, cherries, apples, pears, and bitter almonds) or cassava
  • Industrial exposure (chemists, metal refiners, photographers, and jewelers)
  • PCP manufacturers (by-product of PCP synthesis)
  • Ingestion of nail-polish removers containing acetonitrile

▶ Cyanide binds to cytochrome oxidase and blocks the final step in oxidative phosphorylation, rendering the cells incapable of utilizing oxygen.

▶ This binding blocks ATP production and forces anaerobic metabolism; there is increased production of lactic acid, which results in severe metabolic acidosis.

▶ CNS injury occurs by inducing cellular oxidative damage, enhanced release of excitatory neurotransmitters, and impaired oxygen utilization.

CLINICAL PRESENTATION

▶ Tachypnea from inability to utilize O_2.

▶ CNS symptoms include headache, agitation, confusion, convulsions, and coma.

▶ Cardiovascular effects may include HTN (early) and hypotension (later), typically from severe metabolic acidosis; tachycardia may be present early, but bradycardia predominates later. Cardiogenic pulmonary edema occurs with significant intoxication.

▶ GI symptoms include abdominal pain, vomiting, and hemorrhagic gastritis.

▶ Cyanosis is typically absent, but occasionally a cherry-red skin color has been seen due to increased venous O_2 saturation.

▶ Characteristic "bitter almonds" odor of cyanide (detectable by only 60–75% of people).

DIFFERENTIAL DIAGNOSIS

▶ CO.
▶ Hydrogen sulfide.
▶ Strychnine.
▶ Other simple asphyxiants.
▶ Salicylates, toxic alcohols, iron, isoniazid (INH), and sodium azide can all induce severe metabolic acidosis.
▶ Other causes of lactate-induced anion-gap metabolic acidosis are seizures and sepsis.

EMERGENCY DEPARTMENT MANAGEMENT

Diagnosis

▶ Consider in every patient with a metabolic acidosis, especially in the presence of a normal PaO_2 and tachypnea.

▶ Greatest barrier to diagnosis is not considering it. Remember to think about house fires, high-risk industrial settings, etc.

▶ Lab/ancillary studies that may be helpful:
  • Serum electrolytes and glucose: look for anion-gap acidosis.
  • Lactate level typically elevated.
  • CBC: assess for anemia.
  • ABG: normal PaO_2 (O_2 saturation is often 100%).
  • Serum cyanide level typically will not be available in time to aid decision to treat but can eventually confirm exposure; > 0.5 mg/L generally indicates toxicity.
  • COHb level to assess for CO exposure.

- Methemoglobin to assess for methemoglobinemia.
- Methanol, ethylene glycol, salicylate levels as indicated for alternative diagnoses.
- CXR may indicate pulmonary edema.

Treatment

▶ ABCs, including 100% O_2, establishment of IV access, and crystalloid boluses for hypotension.
▶ Decontamination:
  - Removal of any ongoing cutaneous exposure (removal of clothing, skin flushing, etc.).
  - Activated charcoal may be helpful in large oral exposures, even though absorption is somewhat limited.
▶ $NaHCO_3$ may be necessary for severe acidemia.

Antidote Kit

▶ Amyl nitrite pearls
  - Initiate methemoglobin formation; inhaled
  - Necessary only for patients with delayed IV access
▶ Sodium nitrite
  - Induces methemoglobinemia, which binds cyanide to yield cyanomethemoglobin.
  - Adult dose is 10 ml of 3% solution (300 mg) IV.
  - Goal is methemoglobin level of 20–30%.
  - Pediatric dosing is based on Hgb levels; consultation with a poison center or toxicologist is recommended prior to treatment.
  - Induction of methemoglobinemia in smoke inhalation patients can dangerously lower O_2 carrying capacity due to additive effects with COHb.
  - Side effect is hypotension, though this is not a contraindication in severe toxicity.
▶ Sodium thiosulfate
  - Sulfation of cyanide from cyanomethemoglobin induces thiocyanate formation; thiocyanate is safely excreted if renal function is normal.
  - Dose is 50 ml of 25% solution (12.5 g) IV.
  - May be used as single agent in smoke inhalation patients.

Disposition

▶ All symptomatic patients with high suspicion of cyanide exposure should be admitted, generally to an ICU setting.

▶ Asymptomatic patients with a possible inhalational exposure or cyanide salt ingestion should be monitored for at least 4 hours; if no evidence of acidosis or symptoms at 4 hours, may be discharged home with close primary care follow-up.

▶ All patients with an acetonitrile or cyanogenic glycoside (fruit pit) exposure should be admitted, as symptoms may be delayed up to 24 hours.

CHAPTER 117

HYPOGLYCEMIA

Scott Ferguson and Christopher R. H. Newton

▶ Defined as low serum glucose (usually < 50–60 mg/dl) associated with symptoms that resolve upon administration of carbohydrate.

▶ Hypoglycemia should be considered in any patient presenting to the ED with altered mental status or focal neurologic deficits.

▶ Seen most commonly in young diabetics either having missed meals, increased exercise, or increased dose of insulin. Also related to the increased emphasis on tight glycemic control.

PATHOPHYSIOLOGY

▶ Glucose homeostasis involves the intake of food as well as the complex interactions between insulin, glucagon, and the other counter-regulatory hormones.

▶ The brain requires a continuous supply of glucose for normal function. When glucose levels fall, patients develop symptoms as a direct effect of the lack of glucose on the brain, or adrenergic symptoms, caused by the increased levels of the counter-regulatory hormones.

▶ Insulin administration in diabetics is probably the most common cause of hypoglycemia. Most of these patients, however, self-treat at home and never present to the ED.

▶ Oral sulfonylurea hypoglycemic agents also cause hypoglycemia, particularly in the elderly, who may have decreased awareness of symptoms. Metformin is most commonly implicated.

▶ Alpha-glucosidase inhibitors (decreased glucose absorption) and thiazolidinediones (increased peripheral glucose use) rarely cause hypoglycemia.

CLINICAL PRESENTATION

▶ Hyperadrenergic symptoms: anxiety, nervousness, irritability, combativeness, tremor, nausea/vomiting, sweating, and palpitations. Caused by epinephrine/norepinephrine release. Often referred to as *warning symptoms* to which diabetics are able to respond by ingesting carbohydrate, preventing more serious sequelae. May be diminished with beta-blocker use, age, and autonomic neuropathy.

▶ Neuroglycopenic: altered mental status, lethargy, confusion, seizure, or focal neurologic deficit. Glucose transport from plasma to CSF to brain ECF requires active transport and, therefore, time to equilibrate. Therefore, once serum glucose is corrected, it may take several hours for the patient's mental status to normalize.

▶ Always ask about diabetic medications, last dose, and recent medication changes.

EMERGENCY DEPARTMENT MANAGEMENT
Diagnosis

▶ Diagnosis of hypoglycemia can be made at the patient's bedside with a capillary glucose level, which can be confirmed by a lab serum glucose testing.

▶ Rapid diagnosis is imperative so that treatment can be instituted in a timely fashion. Early diagnosis can also minimize costly work-ups for patients with altered mental status or focal neurologic deficits.

▶ Further work-up depends on the clinical improvement of the patient and possible precipitants. The response to IV dextrose is usually rapid. However, hypoglycemia and altered mental status can be an initial presentation of sepsis, and, if the clinical picture fits, the patient will require further work-up, including blood cultures, an LP, antibiotics, and admission.

Treatment

▶ Adults: 1 ampule 50% dextrose IV (D50 has only 100 calories per 50 cc, so while D50 is important in acutely correcting glucose, this effect is short lived).

▶ Children < 8 years old: 1 cc/kg of 25% dextrose IV, neonates use 10% dextrose.

▶ These doses may be repeated, and, if patient remains hypoglycemic, an infusion of dextrose should be initiated with a goal to maintain glucose above 100 mg/dl.

▶ As soon as mental status allows, attempt to feed patient a meal.

▶ Consider thiamine, 100 mg IV, prior to administering glucose in alcoholics or those malnourished to prevent Wernicke's encephalopathy.

▶ Octreotide is emerging as an effective agent to prevent rebound hypoglycemia with oral hypoglycemic agents. Octreotide is an analogue of somatostatin and inhibits insulin release. Optimal dose is yet to be defined, but 50–100 mcg SC q12h in adults seems to be effective.

▶ Glucagon may be used if patient has adequate glycogen stores, but normalization of serum glucose is slower than if IV dextrose is used. An advantage is that it may be given IM and SC as well as IV. The effect may be transient.

Disposition

▶ Although studies have shown that hypoglycemic diabetics refusing transport to the ED once the hypoglycemia is corrected in the field seem to do well, make sure that patients are able to eat and are not at risk of rebound/delayed hypoglycemia before discharging them from the ED. This usually requires a short 2- to 3-hour period of observation.

▶ Depending on the circumstances, insulin-dependent diabetics may be advised to cut back insulin pending follow-up to reduce risk of reoccurrence.

▶ Homeless and alcoholics require more prolonged observation and may benefit by seeing a social worker prior to discharge in an attempt to provide referrals and a plan for discharge.

▶ All patients with sulfonylurea-induced hypoglycemia should be admitted, as these drugs have long biological half-lives and a propensity for causing prolonged, severe hypoglycemia.

CHAPTER 118

DIABETIC KETOACIDOSIS

George M. Elliott and Christopher R. H. Newton

▶ 18.2 million people—6.3% of the U.S. population—have diabetes.
▶ 4.6–8 episodes of DKA per 1000 patients with diabetes.
▶ Most commonly observed in young type I diabetics related to either non-compliance or infection.

PATHOPHYSIOLOGY

▶ The primary abnormality in DKA is an absolute or relative insulin deficiency. This leads to a rise in the counter-regulatory hormones (catecholamines, glucagon, growth hormone, and cortisol). These changes in hormone levels produce three major effects:
  • Hyperglycemia resulting from decreased glucose utilization and increased hepatic gluconeogenesis
  • Increased lipolysis leading to ketone body formation
  • Increased metabolism of protein and reduction in protein synthesis
▶ Hyperglycemia causes a profound osmotic diuresis resulting in progressive dehydration. Ketonemia and acidosis may lead to nausea and vomiting, which may exacerbate both fluid and electrolyte losses.
▶ Precipitating causes include
  • Insulin omission (33%), infection (pneumonia and UTI), new-onset diabetes, pregnancy
  • Other acute illness: MI, CVA, pancreatitis, PE, surgery
▶ 25% of DKA patients have no clear precipitant.

CLINICAL PRESENTATION
History

▶ Classic presentation is the gradual onset of polyuria and polydipsia. Nausea, vomiting, and abdominal pain are common. This can lead to a misdiagnosis of gastroenteritis in early DKA.

▶ In known diabetics, inquire about insulin regime and compliance with it.

▶ Always ask about recent illness or symptoms of intercurrent infection.

▶ In older diabetics, consider MI, stroke, GI bleed as potential precipitants and always inquire about these in the history.

Exam

▶ The vital signs are often abnormal in DKA. Tachycardia is most frequently observed. As fluid deficits increase, orthostatic hypotension is common.

▶ Kussmaul respirations: increased rate and depth of respiration.

▶ Systemic ketosis is often associated with an unusual fruity odor that may be detected on the breath of patients.

▶ Progressive dehydration may also lead to mental status changes and coma.

▶ Evidence of infection should always be sought on examination of diabetics, with particular attention to elderly diabetics' feet and GU/rectal areas.

EMERGENCY DEPARTMENT MANAGEMENT
Diagnosis

▶ Guidelines published by the American Diabetic Association outline a triad of biochemical requirements for a diagnosis of DKA:
  • Glucose > 250 mg/dl
  • Arterial pH < 7.35, venous pH < 7.30, or bicarbonate < 15 mEq/L
  • Ketonemia or ketonuria

▶ Bedside capillary blood glucose test should be performed. This is usually accurate to around 500 mg/dl. If the bedside capillary glucose is above 300–400 mg/dl, fluid resuscitation should be initiated prior to obtaining the formal lab results.

▶ Other lab tests include serum electrolytes, BUN, creatinine, glucose, calcium, magnesium, phosphate, and a CBC. Serum ketones should also be ordered, as the urine dipstick for ketones can be falsely negative. A blood gas should be obtained to document the pH (venous pH is as good).

▶ Pseudohyponatremia is commonly seen and is caused by hyperglycemia. The sodium level can be corrected by adding 1.6 mEq for every 100 mg of glucose above 100 mg/dl.

▶ An ECG is essential to look for evidence of hyperkalemia and to search for a possible precipitant such as MI.

▶ Performance of a septic work-up, including blood and urine cultures and CXR, depends on the patient's presentation but should be considered, especially in febrile patients.

Treatment

▶ Fluids
  - 1 L/hour NS over the first 2 hours and then approximately 500 cc/hour (if no history of CHF or dialysis).
  - After that, fluid can be titrated to the patient's clinical improvement and perceived state of hydration.
  - Switch to 0.45 NS after initial 2 L with a goal of replacing one-half of deficit in the first 12 hours.
  - Switch fluids to 5% dextrose when glucose ≤ 250 mg/dl. Continue until insulin drip is stopped.

▶ Insulin
  - Bolus regular insulin at 0.1–0.15 units/kg IV (after initial potassium level to prevent potential complications if hypokalemic)—primes IV tubing.
  - Continuous insulin infusion at 0.1 unit/kg/hour.
  - Goal of decreasing glucose 10% in first hour, then 50–75 mg/dl per hour. If decreasing less than this, double the hourly rate.
  - Continue insulin infusion until serum ketones are cleared and anion gap has normalized.

▶ Potassium
  - Patients are usually severely potassium depleted but serum potassium (K^+) may initially be high, low, or normal.
  - Level will decrease as treatment progresses due to continued renal losses and intracellular shifts secondary to insulin administration.
  - Initially, start with IV replacement, switch to PO once patient can tolerate. Replace cautiously in the face of renal insufficiency.
  - Goal to maintain serum K^+ 4–5 mEq/L (Table 118-1).

▶ Bicarbonate
  - Bicarbonate replacement is controversial and is not routinely administered to patients in DKA. Despite a number of

TABLE 118-1.
RATE OF REPLACING K⁺ BASED ON INITIAL SERUM K⁺

Initial serum K^+ (mEq/L)	Replacement K^+ (mEq/hour)
< 4	20
4–6	10
> 6	0

clinical trials on the efficacy of bicarbonate, none has shown improvement in clinical outcomes.

- Bicarbonate can be considered for patients with an initial pH of < 7.0.

Disposition

▶ Most patients are admitted to the ICU setting as they require close monitoring, frequent vital sign checks, and blood draws.

▶ Serum electrolytes and glucose should be checked at 0, 2, and 4 hours from presentation and then every 4 hours during insulin infusion and potassium replacement. Capillary glucose should be checked at 0, 1, and 2 hours after presentation and then every 1–2 hours while on the insulin drip.

▶ Many hospitals now use DKA flow sheets that keep track of vital signs and lab results, making both documentation and patient management more efficient.

▶ Cerebral edema is a rare but life-threatening complication. It occurs primarily in young patients. It is manifest by progressive deterioration in mental status 6–10 hours after the initiation of therapy.

CHAPTER 119

HYPERGLYCEMIC HYPEROSMOLAR SYNDROME

Nima Afshar

▶ A decompensated diabetic state of severe hyperglycemia (glucose > 600), hyperosmolarity (serum osmolarity > 320), and lack of significant acidosis (bicarbonate > 15 and pH > 7.3) or ketosis (small urine/serum ketones).

▶ The name *hyperglycemic hyperosmolar syndrome* (HHS) is replacing hyperosmolar hyperglycemic non-ketotic coma as patients often have mild ketosis/acidosis, and although altered mental status is common, coma is not.

▶ On a continuum with DKA, and a significant minority of cases have overlapping features of both, but the fundamental difference is a *relative* insulin deficiency in HHS versus an *absolute* or *severe* insulin deficiency in DKA.

▶ HHS develops insidiously over days to weeks, causing volume and electrolyte deficits more profound than those seen in DKA.

▶ Mortality of at least 15%, partly due to age and co-morbidities.

▶ Degree of altered mental status is proportional to severity and rate of development of hyperosmolarity.

▶ Precipitating factors: infection (30–60%), acute illness (MI, CVA, PE, pancreatitis, mesenteric ischemia, thyrotoxicosis, etc.), new diabetes (25%), and non-compliance with hypoglycemic therapy.

CLINICAL PRESENTATION

▶ Typical patient is elderly, usually with mild or previously unknown diabetes mellitus, has limited fluid intake and several days to weeks of polyuria, and often finally presents with altered mental status.

▶ Severe dehydration usually with orthostatic hypotension, invariably with acute and/or chronic renal failure.

▶ Focal neurologic deficits may occur due to hypoperfusion with underlying cerebrovascular disease or due to a precipitating stroke.

- ▶ Seizures in up to 20%: usually partial and sometimes continuous (epilepsia partialis continua).
- ▶ Rhabdomyolysis: CK > 1000 in 25%, but pigment nephropathy is rare as osmotic diuresis dilutes myoglobin in renal tubules.
- ▶ Hemorrhagic gastritis in 25%, resolves with treatment of HHS.
- ▶ Symptoms/signs of precipitating illness.
- ▶ Differential diagnosis includes all causes of altered mental status; consider possibility that another cause of altered mental status resulted in poor fluid intake and consequent HHS; consider DKA as there is significant overlap.

EMERGENCY DEPARTMENT MANAGEMENT
Diagnosis

- ▶ Fingerstick glucose, blood gas immediately; consider obtaining electrolytes, especially potassium, from initial blood gas for rapid results.
- ▶ CBC, chemistry panel, calcium/magnesium/serum phosphate, serum osmolarity, serum ketones, CK, UA.
- ▶ Infection work-up performed in most patients, including blood cultures, CXR, UA.
- ▶ ECG and, in an elderly patient with severe altered mental status, strongly consider sending cardiac markers regardless of ECG findings.
- ▶ If necessary, further search for underlying precipitant of HHS.
- ▶ Average lab values on presentation: glucose 1000, serum osmolarity 365, BUN 65, creatinine 3.0, anion gap 23 (often partially a lactic acidosis).
- ▶ Typical sodium deficit is ~9 mEq/kg (the total sodium in 4 L NS for a 70-kg person), water deficit is ~150 ml/kg (or 10 L), and potassium deficit is ~5 mEq/kg (or 350 mEq).

Treatment

- ▶ IVF first
  - • Bolus 1–2 L of NS.
  - • Switch to hypotonic fluid (half-NS) if BP stable and corrected sodium is > 140.
  - • Give post-bolus fluid at 250–1000 cc/hour depending on age and cardiac function, hemodynamics, urinary output (UOP), and rapidity of glucose/electrolyte reduction.

- When glucose < 300 mg/dl, add 5% dextrose to IVF.
▶ Insulin
  - Regular insulin 0.15 U/kg bolus (~10 U), then 0.1 U/kg/hour infusion (~6 U/hour).
    ○ Do not start insulin until patient has received some IVF as there is a risk of rapid fluid shifts out of the extravascular space, which may cause hypotension and acute thrombosis.
    ○ Do not start insulin if patient is hypokalemic on presentation.
▶ Potassium
  - When potassium < 5.0 and patient has adequate UOP, add 20–40 mEq potassium to each liter of IVF (may give some as potassium phosphate for phosphate repletion).
  - Keep potassium at 4–5 mEq/L.
  - If potassium < 3.5, need to stop insulin and replete aggressively as there is high risk of arrhythmia and death from hypokalemia in this setting.
▶ Treat the precipitant
  - Unless another precipitant is identified, strongly consider early, empiric, broad-spectrum antibiotics to cover occult infection.

Monitoring

▶ Glucose every hour.
▶ Basic electrolytes (especially potassium) every 2 hours.
▶ Calcium, magnesium, serum phosphate, osmolarity every 4 hours.
▶ Cardiac monitor and continuous pulse oximetry.
▶ Foley catheter: follow UOP very closely.
▶ Consider CVP monitoring in patients with heart failure or chronic kidney disease.
▶ Consider using a flow sheet to follow vitals, fluid intake/output, glucose/electrolytes, etc.

Disposition

▶ Admit to step-down or ICU in most cases, as mortality is high, and patients usually have complicating co-morbidities.

CHAPTER 120

THYROID STORM

Jacques W. Kobersy

▶ Accelerated form of hyperthyroidism most commonly caused by Grave's disease
▶ Rare but life-threatening emergency (10–70% mortality)—untreated is usually fatal

PATHOPHYSIOLOGY

▶ Background:
  - Normal control: hypothalamus → anterior pituitary → thyroid → T_4/T_3.
  - T_4 is predominant (> 95%) form, and peripherally de-iodinated to T_3.
  - Free T_3 is more biologically active than T_4 but has a shorter half-life (day vs. week).
  - Unbound hormone is active, or "free." The rest is bound to plasma proteins, e.g., TBG and albumin.
  - Thyroid hormone has many diffuse metabolic functions.
  - Likely mechanism of thyroid storm: untreated or under-treated hyperthyroidism + stressful event → adrenergic hyperactivity.
  - Triggers include infection, MI, CVA, trauma, PE, DKA, parturition, dietary supplements/kelp, surgery (thyroid or other), iodine or thyroid hormone ingestion, medications (amiodarone/iodine contrast agents), withdrawal of thyroid medications, idiopathic.

CLINICAL PRESENTATION

▶ See Table 120-1.

DIFFERENTIAL DIAGNOSIS

▶ See Table 120-2.

TABLE 120-1.
CLINICAL PRESENTATION OF THYROID STORM

Tachycardia	Weakness/exhaustion
Dysrhythmia	GI (nausea/vomiting/diarrhea)
Fever (> 38.5° C)	CHF
Mental status changes (agitation/ delirium/psychosis/stupor/ seizures/coma)	

EMERGENCY DEPARTMENT MANAGEMENT

Diagnosis

▶ Elevated free T_4 and free T_3, low or undetectable TSH.

▶ Leukocytosis.

▶ Hyperglycemia.

▶ Calcium may be elevated due to increased osteoclast resorption.

▶ Possible increased LFTs/bilirubin.

Treatment

▶ Control the thyroid.

  • Decrease *de novo* hormone synthesis.

    ○ **Thionamides** work within 1–2 hours. Side effects: allergic reactions, hepatotoxicity, leukopenia, rare agranulocytopenia.

    ○ **Propylthiouracil (PTU),** 600–1000 mg PO, then 200–250 mg PO q4h.

      ■ **Preferred,** as it also decreases T_4 to T_3 conversion.
      or

    ○ **Methimazole,** 30–40 mg PO, then 25 mg PO q6h.

TABLE 120-2.
DIFFERENTIAL DIAGNOSIS OF THYROID STORM

Sepsis	Heat stroke
Medication withdrawal	DTs
Sympathomimetic ingestion	Neuroleptic malignant syndrome
Malignant hyperthermia	Pheochromocytoma

- Prevent release of hormone by giving **iodine** (at *least* 2–3 hours after blocking synthesis as above, or you will make *more* hormone).
    - ○ **Potassium iodide,** 5 drops PO q6h.
    - ○ **Lugol's solution,** 8–10 drops PO/per rectum q6h.
▶ Decrease effects of thyroid hormone on peripheral tissues.
  - Beta-blockade
    - ○ **Propanolol,** 0.5–1.0 mg IV q10–15min until HR is < 100 or until several mg given
               plus
    - ○ PO/NG **propanolol,** 60–120 mg q4h
               or
    - ○ **Esmolol,** 500 mcg/kg IV bolus, then 50–200 mcg/kg/minute maintenance
  - **Corticosteroids** (stress response; also decrease T_4 to T_3 peripheral conversion)
    - ○ **Hydrocortisone,** 100 mg IV q8h
               or
    - ○ **Dexamethasone,** 2 mg IV q6h
▶ Treatment of underlying disorder.
  - CXR, UA, pan-culture, ECG, CHF treatment.
  - Consider empiric antibiotics.
▶ Supportive measures.
  - ABCs, IVF, O_2, monitor.
  - Treat fever with cooling blankets, acetaminophen (APAP) (**do not** use salicylates, as they may increase T_4/T_3 by interfering with protein binding).
  - Admit to ICU setting. Definitive care is usually radioactive iodine.

CHAPTER 121

MYXEDEMA COMA

Jacques W. Kobersy

- ► Rare manifestation of extreme hypothyroidism characterized by decreased mental status and hypothermia
- ► Most commonly seen in winter months in elderly females with under- or untreated hypothyroidism
- ► High mortality (30–60%), therefore, must have high suspicion

PATHOPHYSIOLOGY

- ► See Chap. 120 for description of normal thyroid state.
- ► Can be due to any of the usual causes of hypothyroidism and precipitated by stressors such as cold exposure, infection, stroke, CHF, MI, trauma, burns, and some medications (lithium, amiodarone, analgesics/sedatives) (Table 121-1).

CLINICAL PRESENTATION

- ► See Table 121-2.

EMERGENCY DEPARTMENT MANAGEMENT

Diagnosis

- ► Mainly based on clinical suspicion, history, and physical exam. Lab results are usually unavailable to help with emergent management decisions.
- ► Electrolytes, TSH, free T_4/T_3, cortisol, as well as other labs/studies to evaluate for precipitants (CXR, ECG, cultures, etc.).
- ► Most patients with myxedema coma have primary hypothyroidism (high TSH and low free T_3/T_4).
- ► Normal or low TSH along with low free T_4 suggests pituitary or hypothalamic problems.

TABLE 121-1.
PATHOPHYSIOLOGY OF MYXEDEMA COMA

Prior thyroidectomy	Chronic autoimmune (Hashimoto's) thyroiditis
Radioactive iodine ablation	Iodine deficiency
External neck radiation	Medications (propylthiouracil, methimazole, lithium, amiodarone)
Hypopituitarism (tumors in hypothalamus or pituitary, trauma, Sheehan's)	Infiltrative disease [amyloidosis, hemochromatosis, scleroderma, leukemia, fibrous thyroiditis (Reidel's thyroiditis)]

Treatment

▶ Thyroid hormone and stress dose steroids:
- Levothyroxine (T_4) (200–500 mcg slow IV load initially, then 50–100 mcg IV/PO daily)

  plus
- Glucocorticoid (hydrocortisone, 100 mg IV q8h)

  and consider
- Liothyronine (T_3) (5–20 mcg IV, then 2.5–10 mcg PO q8h)

▶ Supportive measures:
- Hypothermia: usually passive rewarming is preferred to avoid vasodilation and further hypotension.
- Consider ventilator support.
- Electrolyte correction (glucose and sodium).

▶ Treat underlying causes and consider empiric antibiotics.

Disposition

▶ ICU admission

TABLE 121-2.
CLINICAL PRESENTATION OF MYXEDEMA COMA

All organ systems tend to be slowed.
- Hypothermia (~80%)
- Bradycardia
- Possible pericardial effusion
- Hypotension
- Hypoventilation with respiratory acidosis
- Decreased mental status
- Delayed deep tendon reflexes
- Electrolyte disturbance (hyponatremia, hypoglycemia)
- Periorbital edema
- Myxedema—generalized soft tissue swelling
- Macroglossia
- Normocytic anemia

CHAPTER 122

ADRENAL INSUFFICIENCY

Jacques W. Kobersy

▶ A rare disease that, if it goes unrecognized, has 100% mortality.
▶ Consider in any sick patient on chronic steroids.
▶ Adrenal **cortex** produces
   • Glucocorticoids—mainly cortisol, which helps regulate serum glucose and the distribution of intracellular and extracellular water and suppresses ACTH
   • Mineralocorticoids—mainly aldosterone, which increases sodium retention and potassium excretion in the renal distal tubules
   • Androgenic hormones (most important in women, but a trivial amount in men in comparison with the gonads)
▶ Adrenal **medulla** produces epinephrine and norepinephrine.

PATHOPHYSIOLOGY

▶ Adrenal insufficiency can be caused by either destruction of gland or decreased ACTH (Table 122-1).
▶ **Acute adrenal crisis** occurs when adrenal reserve is exhausted. It is usually seen when a patient with chronic insufficiency has replacement steroids abruptly discontinued and/or is stressed

TABLE 122-1.
PATHOPHYSIOLOGY OF ADRENAL INSUFFICIENCY

Primary—adrenal failure (Addison's)	Secondary—pituitary failure
Idiopathic atrophy Infiltrative/infectious (e.g., AIDS and TB) Hemorrhage or infarction [e.g., anticoagulant therapy, meningococcemia (Waterhouse-Friderichsen syndrome)] Medications	Most common cause is chronic steroid use Sheehan's syndrome Trauma Post-radiotherapy or surgery

TABLE 122-2.
CLINICAL PRESENTATION OF ADRENAL INSUFFICIENCY

History	Physical exam
Weakness, fatigue	Hypotension (especially postural)
Anorexia and weight loss	Confusion/coma
Nausea/vomiting	Decreased pulse and heart sounds
Abdominal pain	Fever (usually only if infection present)

(infections, trauma, burns, etc.) and diminishes endogenous supply.

CLINICAL PRESENTATION

▶ Symptoms are very non-specific and may be masked by those of concurrent illness (Table 122-2).

LAB VALUES

▶ Sodium may be slightly decreased or normal.
▶ Potassium may be slightly increased or normal.
▶ Hypoglycemia is usually marked.

EMERGENCY MANAGEMENT
Diagnosis

▶ Made clinically based on high index of suspicion in patients on long-term steroids.
▶ ACTH stimulation test can be performed in ED, but the more prolonged test is necessary to confirm adrenal insufficiency and differentiate primary from secondary failure.

Treatment

▶ Fluid replacement.
  • The fluid deficit is usually 20% of body weight, or ~2–3 L.
  • D5NS, 1 L over 1 hour, and additional 2 L over next 8 hours.
▶ Electrolyte correction and steroid replacement.
  • Dexamethasone, 4 mg IV, or hydrocortisone, 100 mg IV bolus, plus 100–200 mg PO/IV q6–8h for initial 24 hours.

- Mineralocorticoids are usually not required, but if necessary, desoxycorticosteroid acetate (Percorten), 2.5–5.0 mg IM qd–bid.
- Correct any hyperkalemia.
► Identify and treat precipitating cause.
    - Consider CXR, UA, cultures, CT as indicated.
► Admission for stabilization and further investigation.
    - The acute crisis should improve in 12–24 hours, but patients generally need ICU care for 24–48 hours.
    - Chronic glucocorticoid therapy is usually hydrocortisone, 20–30 mg daily, or prednisone, 5–7.5 mg daily.
    - If needed, chronic mineralocorticoid replacement can be provided with PO fludrocortisone, 50–200 mcg daily.

CHAPTER 123

HYPOTHERMIA

Steven Schmidt

▶ Defined as a decrease in body temperature that renders the body unable to adequately generate sufficient heat to continue its normal functions

▶ Can occur in any situation in which the ambient temperature is below the core body temperature

▶ More common in colder climates, though an aging population in conjunction with poverty and poor socioeconomic conditions increase chances even in warm climates

PATHOPHYSIOLOGY

▶ Heat regulation on exposure to cold
  • Shivering can increase basal metabolism up to five times the baseline.

▶ Mechanisms of heat loss
  • Radiation: approximately 60% of heat lost under normal conditions.
  • Conduction: proportion increases in cold, wet environments, especially in immersion incidents.
  • Convection: proportion increases in cold, wet environments.
  • Evaporation (including respiration): 25–30% of heat loss normally; proportion increases in cool, dry, windy environments.

▶ Cellular effects of hypothermia
  • Intracellular water crystallization, temperature-induced protein changes, membrane damage.
  • Vasoconstriction, endothelial injury, and thromboembolism contribute to vascular insufficiency and ischemia.
  • May have bleeding due to cold-induced inhibition of coagulation-cascade enzymes and platelet dysfunction.

TABLE 123-1.
CLINICAL PRESENTATION OF HYPOTHERMIA

	Mild hypothermia (core temperature > 32° C)	Moderate hypothermia (core temperature 28–32° C)	Severe hypothermia (core temperature < 28° C)
Thermoregulation	Shivering	Shivering lost, rapid cooling	Shivering lost, rapid cooling
Respiratory	Tachypnea	Hypoventilation, respiratory acidosis, hypoxemia, aspiration	Apnea, ARDS
Cardiovascular	Tachycardia, HTN	Hypotension, bradycardia, prolonged QT interval, J waves (Osborn wave)	AF, heart block, cardiac arrest
GU/fluids/electrolytes	Bladder atony, cold diuresis	Hyperkalemia, hyperglycemia, lactic acidosis	Hyperkalemia, hyperglycemia, lactic acidosis
Neurologic	Hyperreflexia, disorientation, ataxia	Hyporeflexia, delirium, decreased level of consciousness, dilated pupils	Areflexia, coma, absent pupillary response
Muscular	Hypertonia	Rigidity	Rhabdomyolysis

CLINICAL PRESENTATION

▶ See Table 123-1.

EMERGENCY DEPARTMENT MANAGEMENT
Diagnosis

▶ Establish core temperature—need low-reading thermometer as standard only measures accurately to 34° C.
  • Rectal, esophageal, or bladder catheter probe
▶ Lab.
  • Bedside glucose determination.

- CBC (HCT will increase 2% for 1° C decrease in body temperature, thrombocytopenia common), electrolytes, glucose, creatinine, CK, coags, UA, ethanol levels, LFTs, amylase/lipase.
- Consider ABG (assess ventilation, acid-base balance).
- Urine, blood cultures if infection is a consideration.
▶ Radiology.
  - CXR may reveal signs of aspiration pneumonia.
  - Other X-rays as needed to exclude trauma.

Treatment

▶ General
  - Remove all wet clothing.
  - Cardiac monitoring.
  - Careful transferring/movement of the patient (may precipitate arrhythmias).
▶ Venous access
▶ Intubation, mechanical ventilation as needed
▶ Cardiac life support (specific to hypothermia)
  - Monitor carotid pulse carefully.
    ○ Bradycardia common (palpate 30–45 seconds before beginning CPR).
    ○ Shivering may simulate VF on monitor.
  - Chest compressions more difficult due to rigid thorax.
  - VF may not respond to cardioversion or drugs until patient is rewarmed.
  - Drug of choice for VF is bretylium.
  - Hypothermic patients should not be pronounced dead until core temp > 34° C.
▶ Mild hypothermia
  - Passive rewarming (rewarms 0.5–2° C per hour, depending on amount of shivering)—remove all wet clothes and cover with warm blankets.
  - Active external rewarming (if unable to adequately shiver).
    ○ Heating blankets (0.8° C per hour)
    ○ Heated forced-air system (i.e., Bair Hugger)
▶ Moderate hypothermia
  - Active external: be sure to apply to trunk primarily, as applying to extremities may cause drop in temperature if cold blood is recirculated from periphery.

- Non-invasive internal (1–2° C per hour)
  - Warmed IV fluids
  - Warmed O_2
► Severe hypothermia
  - Active external
  - Non-invasive internal
  - Invasive internal
    - Heated irrigation techniques (1–4° C per hour)
      - Gastric and bladder lavage
      - Peritoneal exchange
      - Thoracostomy lavage
      - Esophageal warming tubes
    - Extracorporeal blood rewarming (1–2° C per 5 minutes)
      - Continuous venovenous or arteriovenous rewarming
      - Heated hemodialysis (HD)
      - Cardiopulmonary bypass

Disposition

► Mild hypothermia
  - May discharge home if hypothermia resolves, depending on cause.
  - Admit for all those with significant comorbidities/ongoing medical issues.
► Moderate hypothermia
  - Admission to monitored bed if temperature improves
► Severe hypothermia
  - ICU admission

CHAPTER 124

LOCAL COLD INJURY

Candice A. Sobanski

► Frostbite is caused by tissue freezing and includes a spectrum of tissue damage and loss.

► Immersion foot (trench foot): prolonged exposure to non-freezing, wet environment.

► Chilblains (pernio): exposure to non-freezing, dry environment.

► Risk factors for local cold injury include inappropriate clothing, homelessness, psychiatric disease, alcoholism, poor circulation, and tobacco use.

PATHOPHYSIOLOGY

► Cold leads to vasoconstriction of the periphery, which, if below freezing, eventually leads to direct cellular toxicity.

► Maximum vasoconstriction is at 15° C, significantly decreasing cutaneous flow.

► "Hunting response" occurs between 10 and 15° C and is a paradoxical vasodilation of the peripheral vessels in an attempt to prevent ischemic and freezing injuries.

► Below 10° C, the water in the extra-cellular space forms ice crystals, further decreasing blood flow and exposing the sensitive vascular endothelial membrane.

► Further temperature drop leads to plasma leakage, increased viscosity, RBC stasis, and vessel thrombosis.

► Permanent tissue damage occurs during re-warming, with the junction between normal and injured tissue susceptible to vasoconstriction and shunting, further propagating thrombosis and leading to irreversible injury.

► Repetitive freeze-thaw cycles promote worse injury and more severe thrombosis.

CLINICAL PRESENTATION

▶ **Immersion foot**
  • Numbness, painful paresthesia, and cramps
▶ **Chilblains**
  • Pruritus, erythema, and burning paresthesia
▶ **Frostnip**
  • Characterized by pain, then sudden loss of discomfort and cold sensation. Skin is pale and numb. Reversible.
▶ **Frostbite**
  • Loss of sensation, and color changes in the affected area. Develop pain as thawing takes place.
  • Skin is frozen. Once thawed, blisters develop (clear: superficial, hemorrhagic: deep).
  • Delayed presentation of a deep frostbite may have black eschar formation.
  • Initial presentation does not predict morbidity/tissue loss. Takes weeks to months to demarcate non-viable tissues.

EMERGENCY DEPARTMENT MANAGEMENT

Diagnosis

▶ Evaluate for signs or symptoms of hypothermia and treat appropriately.
▶ Diagnosis of local cold injury is made clinically, and tests are usually unnecessary.

Treatment

▶ Goal is rapid re-warming.
▶ Should be initiated pre-hospital only if there is no chance of re-freezing.
▶ Remove wet and constrictive clothing immediately.
▶ Soak affected areas in a circulating water bath at 40–42° C.
▶ Avoid dry heat and rubbing the affected area.
▶ Systemic analgesia often required during re-warming because of intense pain.
▶ Residual numbness can persist for weeks.
▶ Blister drainage is controversial, but most authors suggest debridement of clear blisters and leaving hemorrhagic blisters intact.

▶ Topical antibiotics and sterile dressing should be applied. Tetanus prophylaxis as indicated.

▶ Therapies such as NSAIDs, steroids, LMWH, and aloe vera have been studied in animals, but no benefit has been proven in humans.

▶ Phenoxybenzamine is a long-acting alpha-blocking agent that has theoretical benefit, but, again, no conclusive evidence exists.

▶ Decision regarding surgical intervention should be delayed until clear demarcation of injury.

Disposition

▶ If reliable and not homeless, a patient may be discharged with follow-up in a burn or wound care clinic.

▶ More often, a patient does not have adequate shelter or means to follow-up and needs admission to monitor progression and provide dressing changes, analgesia, hydrotherapy, and physical therapy.

CHAPTER 125

HEAT STROKE

Michael Baker

▶ 371 deaths annually in the U.S. between 1979 and 1997
▶ Mortality of up to 14%

PATHOPHYSIOLOGY

▶ Heat stroke is caused by loss of control of heat production and regulation, leading to cellular damage and death.
▶ Heat stroke differs from other forms of heat illness (e.g., heat edema, prickly heat, heat syncope, and heat cramps) in that it involves cell death and organ damage.
▶ Intrinsic heat production produced by exothermal reactions in the body can raise the body temperature by $2°$ F per hour at rest. This may be increased significantly by strenuous exertion.
▶ Risk of heat stroke increases with heat index (air temperature combined with humidity).

CLINICAL PRESENTATION

▶ Usually presents with severe neurologic dysfunction in face of elevated core body temperature.
▶ Neurologic damage can be profound, leading to hallucinations, cerebellar dysfunction, cerebral edema, seizures, and coma.
▶ Cardiovascular findings may include tachycardia with increased cardiac output, low peripheral resistance, and elevated CVP.
▶ Hepatic damage is almost always present, with AST and ALT usually elevated. Survivors typically have no permanent liver impairment.
▶ Hypoglycemia is common with exertional heat stroke.
▶ Coagulation abnormalities are a poor prognostic sign.
▶ Renal complications, such as proteinuria or ARF, may occur due to hypotension, decreased renal perfusion, and myoglobinuria.

▶ Usually divided into *classic* and *exertional*.
  • **Classic:** elderly, debilitated, or infants. Passive exposure to heat, which they are unable to avoid. Tends to occur over days. Very dehydrated.
  • **Exertional:** typically young men in good health with normal thermoregulatory system. Heat loss mechanism is overwhelmed by massive heat production secondary to strenuous activity in a hot environment. May be associated with lactic acidosis, rhabdomyolysis, and renal failure. Can also develop disseminated intravascular coagulation.

DIFFERENTIAL DIAGNOSIS
▶ Meningitis/encephalitis.
▶ Malaria, typhoid fever, typhus.
▶ Thyroid storm.
▶ Anticholinergic poisoning: presentation may be very similar other than mydriasis.
▶ DTs: search for history of ETOH abuse.
▶ Neuroleptic malignant syndrom (NMS): muscle rigidity, hyperthermia in patient on antipsychotic medications (commonly haloperidol).
▶ Malignant hyperthermia: muscle rigidity, hyperthermia, and acidosis in patients undergoing general anesthetic.

EMERGENCY DEPARTMENT MANAGEMENT
Diagnosis
▶ A heat stress exposure must exist.
▶ Elevated core temperature above 104° F (40° C).
▶ CNS dysfunction (e.g., coma, seizure, or delirium).
▶ Heat stroke patients classically have dry, hot skin due to failure of sweating mechanisms; however, sweating may persist in up to one-half of patients.
▶ Lab tests should include
  • CBC, coagulation profile, and fibrin split products (disseminated intravascular coagulation)
  • Chemistries (renal failure)
  • Blood glucose (hypoglycemia)
  • Liver panel (elevated transaminases)
  • UA (proteinuria, myoglobinuria)

- BUN/creatinine (renal failure)
- CPK (rhabdomyolysis)
- Lactic acid (lactic acidosis)
- Calcium (hypocalcemia)
- ABG (acidosis)

Treatment

▶ Airway/breathing management.
▶ Circulatory support.
  - Modest IVF required (< 1200 cc in first 4 hours).
  - Excessive fluids may increase the risk of pulmonary edema.
▶ Cooling is the mainstay of therapy.
  - Remove all clothes.
  - Evaporative cooling: regarded as best method for cooling in ED. Warm water mist is sprayed on patient while fans are directed at them.
  - Immersion therapy: ice water bath. Effective but controversial in ED setting. Causes shivering and also is impractical in ED.
  - Cooling adjuncts:
    ○ Ice packs: must watch for cold damage to skin
    ○ Cooling blanket
    ○ Peritoneal, rectal, or gastric lavage with hypothermic fluid: used only when no response to external cooling methods
    ○ Cardiopulmonary bypass
  - Cooling therapy treatment goals:
    ○ Lower core body temperature to < 102° F as quickly as possible, ideally within 20 minutes.
    ○ Hold aggressive cooling when temperature < 102° F to avoid over-cooling.
    ○ Constant body temperature monitoring required to keep temperature 98.6–100.4° F.
  - Dantrolene:
    ○ Conflicting evidence that dantrolene may decrease time required to cool core temperature and improve heat stroke outcome

Disposition

▶ ICU admission usually required due to thermodysregulation, hemodynamic instability, and neurologic and renal complications.

OTHER HEAT-RELATED ILLNESSES
Heat Edema

▶ Diagnosis: swollen feet/ankles in non-acclimatized individual without underlying disease. Often in first few days in hot climate

▶ Pathophysiology: caused by changes in hydrostatic pressure, vasodilation, and orthostatic pooling, leading to vascular leakage and interstitial fluid

▶ Treatment: leg elevation, support hose, and/or acclimatization/returning home

Prickly Heat (Miliaria, Rubra, Lichen Tropicus)

▶ Diagnosis: pruritic vesicles on an erythematous base usually confined to clothed areas

▶ Pathophysiology: caused by blocked sweat glands, leading to a macerated stratum corneum and secondary staphylococcal infection

▶ Treatment: chlorhexidine cream/lotion, salicylic acid (small areas), or oral erythromycin (large areas)

Heat Cramps

▶ Diagnosis: painful contraction of major muscle groups after exertion in hot environment (commonly calf and thigh).

▶ Pathophysiology: caused by copious sweating with exertion and hypotonic fluid replacement, resulting in salt deficiency in non-acclimatized workers/athletes.

▶ Treatment: rest and hydration. Can usually be done orally with commercially available electrolyte drinks or 0.1–0.2% salt solution. If severe, may need IV hydration with 0.9% NaCl. Avoid salt tablets, as they may cause gastric irritation.

Heat Exhaustion

▶ Diagnosis: malaise, nausea/vomiting, headache with core temperature normal to 104° F, and normal mental function. Differentiated from heat stroke by absence of major CNS dysfunction and temperature < 104° F.

▶ Pathophysiology: occurs by water depletion and/or salt depletion leading to hypovolemia and/or hyponatremia.

▶ Treatment: rest, cool environment, fluid replacement; consider admission for elderly or in case of severe electrolyte replacement.

CHAPTER 126

HYMENOPTERA ENVENOMATION

Edward Walton

- The order Hymenoptera includes bees, wasps, and ants.
  - Apidae (bees) leave venom apparatus behind.
  - Vespids (wasps, hornets, and yellow jackets) retain venom apparatus.
  - Formicidae (biting ants) introduce venom from mouth parts.
- The vast majority of those living in the U.S. have reported being stung by a wasp or bee at some point in their lives. Stings are most common from April to September.
- Approximately 40 deaths per year are attributed to insect stings.
- The red fire ant (*Solenopsis invicta*) was imported to the U.S. from Brazil in the 1940s. It is now endemic to the entire southern continental U.S. and continues to advance northward.

PATHOPHYSIOLOGY

- Venoms may include phospholipase A_2, hyaluronidase, acid phosphatase, and other antigenic proteins.
- Stings may cause local venom toxicity or allergic sensitivity with systemic reactions to later stings.

CLINICAL PRESENTATION

- Stings are most common on the head and neck, followed by the foot, leg, and hand.
- Fire ants: multiple stings in a small area.
- Usual reaction—due to local toxicity:
  - History of sting.
  - Immediate local pain, swelling, and erythema.
  - Usually resolves in 24 hours.
  - Fire ant stings have associated pustule formation (lasts 7–10 days).

► Large local reaction:
  • Cell-mediated (type IV) response
  • Pain, erythema, and swelling > 15 cm from sting site
  • Lasts > 24 hours post-sting
► Allergic reaction:
  • IgE mediated—0.4% of U.S. population at risk
  • Usually occurs within 20 minutes of sting
  • Urticaria and angioedema
  • Anaphylaxis
    ○ Airway obstruction: upper or lower airway edema with wheezing and/or respiratory distress
    ○ Hypotension/shock
► Multiple stings:
  • Toxic reaction
  • Generalized edema, vomiting, diarrhea, dyspnea, and hypotension/shock
► Other reported complications:
  • Serum sickness, Henoch-Schönlein purpura, MI, Guillain-Barré syndrome, encephalitis, myasthenia gravis, neuritis

EMERGENCY DEPARTMENT MANAGEMENT

► Retained stingers should be removed by scraping.
► Remove rings on affected extremity.
► Usual reaction:
  • Ice pack.
  • Non-steroid pain medications.
  • Oral antihistamine: H_1 blocker.
  • Leave pustule from fire ant sting intact.
► Large local reaction:
  • Ice pack.
  • Non-steroid pain medications.
  • Oral antihistamine: H_1 blocker.
  • Prescription for EpiPen (small risk of anaphylaxis with next sting).
  • Desensitization therapy has not been found to be effective.
  • Oral antibiotics if cannot distinguish from local cellulitis.
► Allergic reactions:
  • Urticaria and angioedema
    ○ Oral or IV/IM antihistamines: H_1 and consider H_2 blockers
    ○ Oral or IV/IM steroids

- ○ Discharge on antihistamines (H_1 blocker) and steroids
- ○ Disposition
    - ■ Discharge with epinephrine auto-injector
    - ■ Referral for desensitization therapy
- Anaphylaxis
    - ○ SC or IV epinephrine
    - ○ IV antihistamines: H_1 and H_2 blockers
    - ○ IV steroids
    - ○ Beta agonists via nebulizer for wheezing
    - ○ Observation/admission until symptoms resolve
    - ○ Disposition
        - ■ Discharge on antihistamines (H_1 blocker) and steroids.
        - ■ Discharge with epinephrine auto-injector.
        - ■ Referral for desensitization therapy.
- ► Multiple stings (500–1500 stings):
    - As per anaphylaxis
    - Supportive care if progress to rhabdomyolysis, renal failure, or diffuse intravascular coagulation
- ► Prevention of future stings:
    - Insect repellants not effective.
    - Avoid brightly colored clothes and perfumes.
    - Cover up with long sleeves and pants.

Commonly Used Medications for Envenomations

- ► Antihistamines: H_1 blockers
    - Diphenhydramine (Benadryl)
        - ○ Pediatric: 1.25 mg/kg dose PO/IV every 6 hours
        - ○ Adult: 25–50 mg/dose PO/IV every 6 hours
- ► Antihistamines: H_2 blockers
    - Cimetidine (Tagamet)
        - ○ Pediatric: 5 mg/kg IV every 6 hours
        - ○ Adult: 300 mg IV every 6 hours
- ► Steroids
    - Methylprednisolone (Solu-Medrol)
        - ○ Pediatric: 2 mg/kg IV loading dose, then 1 mg/kg every 6 hours
        - ○ Adult: 125 mg IV every 6 hours
    - Prednisone
        - ○ Adult: 60 mg PO day 1 then 40 mg PO daily × 5 days

- Prednisolone (Orapred)
  - Pediatric: 2 mg/kg PO day 1 then 1 mg/kg PO daily × 5 days
▶ Epinephrine
  - 1/1000 injectable
    - Pediatric: 0.01 mg/kg/dose SC/IM every 20 minutes up to maximum 0.5 mg
    - Adult: 0.3 mg SC every 20 minutes up to maximum of 1 mg
    - EpiPen auto injectors
      - < 30 kg: 0.15 mg IM (EpiPen Jr.)
      - > 30 kg: 0.3 mg IM (EpiPen)
  - 1/10,000 injectable
    - Pediatric: 0.1 ml/kg (0.01 mg/kg) IO/IV every 3–5 minutes for cardiovascular collapse
    - Adult: 1 mg IV every 3–5 minutes for cardiovascular collapse

CHAPTER 127

VENOMOUS ARACHNIDS/ SPIDER AND SCORPION BITES

Stuart A. Bradin

- ► Arachnids include spiders, scorpions, mites, and ticks. Almost all are predators.
- ► Venom delivered through fangs (chelicerae).
- ► Most do not cause clinically significant bites or envenomation because toxin is too weak to be harmful to humans and/or fangs are not large or strong enough to pierce human skin.
- ► Few poisonous spiders native to U.S. Two of the most clinically important in U.S. are the black widow and brown recluse.

BLACK WIDOW SPIDER

- ► *Latrodectus* species are ubiquitous in U.S. Found throughout temperate and tropical zones.
- ► Small black spider (approximately 1.5 in.) with characteristic red hourglass shape on ventral surface of abdomen.
- ► Only female has mouthparts large enough to envenomate a human.
- ► Venom is a potent neurotoxin with primary action at the neuromuscular junction. Results in overstimulation of motor endplate due to release/inhibition of acetylcholine and norepinephrine.
- ► Potentially deadly, although no recent reported deaths in U.S. Most significant morbidity seen in children and elderly.

Clinical Presentation

- ► Initial bite often missed. May produce brief pinprick sensation.
- ► At 1–2 hours, local erythema, cyanosis, urticaria, or "target lesion" at bite site with tender regional lymph nodes.
- ► Proximal muscle cramping in back, chest, or abdomen. Abdominal rigidity may mimic surgical abdomen.

► Pain may descend into lower extremities with "burning" soles of feet. Muscle fasciculations and flexor spasm of limbs.

► Autonomic symptoms: nausea, emesis, diaphoresis, salivation, seizures, weakness, fever, HTN, tachycardia, and priapism.

► Can progress to respiratory arrest or hypertensive crisis within 4–6 hours in very young or elderly.

► Symptoms can persist 36–72 hours.

Emergency Department Management

► Attempt to identify spider by history and description.

► Local wound care: cleansing, ice, and tetanus prophylaxis.

► If asymptomatic, may not require any further care. Usually observe in ED for 4–6 hours. Consider admitting children and elderly for 24-hour observation.

► If symptoms develop, treat symptomatically with analgesia, including IV opioids and benzodiazepines (smooth muscle relaxation and anxiolysis).

► No proven efficacy for calcium gluconate.

► Antivenin should be considered if < 12 years old, elderly, pregnant with definite exposure, or in patients with severe symptoms—rapidly effective but carries risk of anaphylaxis and serum sickness (horse serum product). Dose is 1 vial in 50 cc NS given over 15 minutes. Patients should be tested for horse serum sensitivity as described in product literature prior to getting antivenin.

BROWN RECLUSE SPIDER

► *Loxosceles reclusa*—typically non-aggressive. Bites when threatened, typically April through October.

► Worldwide distribution—in U.S., mainly central and southeast.

► Small brown spider with dark fiddle-shaped marking on dorsal cephalothorax.

► Venom contains sphingomyelinase D.

Clinical Presentation

► Victim often unaware of bite, seeking medical attention only when necrotic skin lesion develops.

► Clinical response ranges from cutaneous irritation (necrotic arachnidism) to systemic reaction (loxoscelism).

► Most commonly: pruritus, edema, erythema, and pain over bite site within hours. Erythematous halo surrounding violaceous center develops. At 3–4 days, wound progresses to necrotic base with central black eschar. At 2–5 weeks, eschar sloughs; poorly healing necrotic ulceration remains.

► Systemic reaction is much less common, higher morbidity. At 24–72 hours post-bite, develops fever, chills, emesis, myalgias, and arthralgias. May progress to disseminated intravascular coagulation with hemolytic anemia. Fatality most common in children and related to severe hemolysis.

Emergency Department Management

► Local wound care/supportive care recommended. Elevation, ice, analgesics, and tetanus prophylaxis.

► No proven benefit of steroids, antibiotics, hyperbaric O_2 (HBO), or early excision of bite. Surgical intervention should be delayed until demarcation of non-viable tissue.

► Dapsone may be helpful in preventing local effects of venom. However, it can induce methemoglobinemia and hemolysis in patients with G6PD deficiency and should, therefore, be given with caution.

► No antivenin available at present in U.S.

► Asymptomatic patients may be observed in ED for 4–6 hours and then discharged with close follow-up.

► All patients with systemic symptoms should be admitted for observation. Studies include a CBC, serum chemistry, coagulation profile, and UA. Treatment is mainly supportive with fluids to maintain urinary output (UOP) and observe for evidence of renal failure or hemolysis. Surgical consult should be obtained for consideration of wound debridement.

TARANTULAS

► Widely feared, largest of all spiders.

► Found in the deserts of western U.S., but also popular pets.

► Non-aggressive, rarely bite, relatively harmless. Bite in human rarely causes toxicity—local histamine reaction only.

▶ When agitated, they throw needle-like barbed hairs that can easily pierce skin or cornea. Medical attention is then sought as a result of allergic reaction to spider's body hairs.

▶ Reaction ranges from mild irritation/allergic reaction to severe conjunctivitis. Rarely can cause anaphylaxis.

Emergency Department Management

▶ Local wound care, tetanus prophylaxis

▶ Can use sticky tape to assist removal of hairs

▶ Analgesia, antihistamines, and consider steroids

SCORPIONS

▶ Only dangerous species in U.S. is the southwestern desert scorpion (*Centruroides exilicauda*). Known also as bark scorpion, it resides under bark of trees. Found mainly in arid southwestern U.S.—Arizona, Texas, California.

▶ Have paired venom glands in telson, just anterior to a stinger on end of tail. Most envenomations occur at night when scorpions are most active.

▶ Venom contains multiple digestive enzymes and several neurotoxins. Excessive stimulation of neuromuscular junctions and autonomic nervous system.

▶ Most serious stings in children younger than age 10.

Clinical Presentation

▶ Most stings result in local, immediate burning pain that peaks in 5 hours.

▶ Children often have more severe symptoms than adults. No reported deaths in 30 years, but significant sequelae can occur.

▶ Systemic symptoms include weakness, restlessness, roving eye movements, agitation, HTN, dysrhythmias, increased body temperature, increased secretions, slurred speech, muscle fasciculations of the tongue/face, diplopia , respiratory arrest, and paralysis.

▶ Movements may mimic seizure, but child remains awake and alert.

▶ Other complications include pancreatitis, rhabdomyolysis, renal failure, disseminated intravascular coagulation, and pulmonary edema.

▶ Recovery in 12–36 hours in most non-fatal cases.
▶ Tap test: tapping on wound elicits pain and withdrawal of affected part.

Emergency Department Management

▶ Most stings treated with symptomatic care/analgesia only: ice pack, local cleansing, and tetanus prophylaxis.
▶ Benzodiazepines for agitation.
▶ IV beta-blocker (propanolol) for severe tachycardia and HTN.
▶ Corticosteroids have shown no benefit.
▶ Antivenin is available in Arizona—rapidly effective but should only be given for significant systemic symptoms because of risk of anaphylaxis and serum sickness.

CHAPTER 128

SNAKE BITES

Troy Christian Sims

- ▶ Viperidae comprise the rattlesnakes and copperheads and are known as pit vipers. They may be identified by a heat-sensing pit antero-inferior to each eye, elliptical pupils, a triangular head, and undivided sub-caudal scales.
- ▶ Elapidae comprise the coral snakes and cobras.
- ▶ Coral snakes are the only Elapidae native to the U.S. known to cause serious envenomations and can be identified by a red, yellow, and black pattern, resulting in the caveat "red on yellow will kill a fellow; red on black, venom lack."
- ▶ Cobra envenomations have occurred at zoos and carnivals.

PATHOPHYSIOLOGY

- ▶ About half of all snake bites are "dry," or do not result in envenomation.
- ▶ Viperidae bites incur the highest occurrence of local necrosis, rhabdomyolysis, and coagulopathy due to the presence of phospholipase A_2.
- ▶ Elapidae bites possess a higher incidence of neurotoxicity caused by potent pre- and post-synaptic neurotoxins that block acetylcholine-binding sites.

CLINICAL PRESENTATION

- ▶ See Table 128-1.

DIAGNOSIS

- ▶ The bite marks are variable and should not be used to determine extent of envenomation or the type of snake.
- ▶ Care should be based on clinical presentation and history.

TABLE 128-1.
CLINICAL PRESENTATION OF SNAKE BITES

Findings	Viperidae	Elapidae of U.S.
Local	Severe burning, ecchymosis, swelling, and hemorrhagic blebs	Swelling is minimal, pain may be mild and transient, fang marks may be difficult to see.
Hematologic	Coagulopathy, thrombocytopenia, and, possibly, disseminated intravascular coagulation in rare instances	—
Neurologic	Weakness, odd taste in mouth, fasciculations, and paresthesias (especially in Mojave rattlesnakes)	Often delayed 12 hours, then progresses rapidly; paresthesias or numbness; altered mental status; peripheral muscle weakness; cranial nerve dysfunction, especially ptosis and impaired swallowing.
Musculoskeletal	Rhabdomyolysis, compartment syndrome	—
Cardiovascular	Pulmonary edema, hypotension in severe cases, but usually HTN due to pain	Respiratory depression due to neurologic involvement and risk of aspiration.
GI	Nausea and vomiting	Nausea, vomiting, abdominal pain.

► Lab studies are useful for Viperidae envenomations but not for Elapidae.
  • CBC with platelets, fibrinogen level, D dimer, and PT/PTT, all of which may be abnormal in Viperidae envenomations
  • UA, electrolyte panel, and CK looking for evidence of rhabdomyolysis in Viperidae envenomations
  • ECG
  • X-ray for retained FB
  • CXR for pulmonary edema in severe cases

PRE-HOSPITAL TREATMENT

► Always assume that envenomation has occurred.
► Wash with water to remove any residual venom.

TABLE 128-2.
TREATMENT OF SNAKE BITES

Severity of bite	Local/systemic	Labs	Anti-venom
Dry bite	Puncture wounds with no systemic effects	Normal	No
Minimal envenomation	Swelling locally, ecchymosis, and pain	Normal	Consider, but only start with 5 vials
Moderate envenomation	Swelling involves entire extremity ± abnormal vital signs	Abnormal	Seriously consider, and start with 10 vials
Severe envenomation	Hypotension, respiratory distress, bleeding	Abnormal	Yes, start with 15 vials

▶ Remove any jewelry in the anticipation of swelling.
▶ Immobilize the affected extremity and keep it below the level of the heart.

TREATMENT

▶ Definitive treatment for any poisonous snake bite is the administration of anti-venom.
▶ There is a significant potential for an anaphylactic reaction or serum sickness with conventional anti-venom, so administer anti-venom judiciously.
▶ For Viperidae, a grading scale based on clinical severity exists to help guide the decision to administer anti-venom (Table 128-2).
▶ If using anti-venom (Crotalidae) polyvalent (ACP), a skin test is recommended.
▶ If using CroFab®, no skin test is required.
▶ The skin test is not very reliable and takes 30 minutes to confirm a negative result; therefore, it is reasonable to forego in obvious dry bites and severe cases.
▶ Obtaining informed consent is imperative, as 20% of patients who receive the ACP by Wyeth-Ayerst Laboratories can be expected to have a type I, IgE-mediated hypersensitivity reaction, and 50–75% of patients can be expected to have a type III, IgG- and IgM-mediated hypersensitivity reaction, known as serum sickness, which can occur 3 days to 3 weeks after administration.

▶ Pre-medicate with a histamine blocker and have epinephrine available.

▶ The infusion should be started at a slow rate for 10–20 minutes and increased to a rate that allows the completion of the infusion over the next 1–2 hours.

▶ If findings progress, then repeat the infusion using 1–5 vials every 30 minutes to 2 hours, as needed.

▶ Avoid ASA and NSAIDs because they could potentiate a coagulopathy.

▶ Tetanus toxoid recommended.

▶ Consider measuring compartment pressures in moderate to severe cases.

▶ For the Elapidae, the approach to treatment is different.
  • Because the systemic effects may be delayed 12 hours, no grading scale is available to assess severity, and management should proceed as if significant envenomation had occurred.
  • Neurologic and respiratory status should be followed closely.
  • Preparation and administration of the anti-venom are similar to ACP; however, rarely are more than 10 vials required.
  • In the case of cobra envenomations, cardiovascular status should be monitored closely, and anti-venom should be given prophylactically, even though often not required.

▶ Antibiotics usually not required as wound infections are uncommon.

DISPOSITION

▶ Any Viperidae bites that require anti-venom should be admitted to an ICU, while those that are diagnosed as dry bites can be discharged with appropriate follow-up after a minimum of 8 hours monitoring.

▶ All Elapidae bites, regardless of symptom severity or whether diagnosed as being a dry bite, should be admitted to an ICU for 24-hour observation due to the delayed action and rapidly progressive effects of the venom's neurotoxin.

▶ Assistance with managing snake bites can be obtained from the University of Arizona Poison and Drug Information Center at 520-626-6016, Rocky Mountain Poison Control at 303-739-1123, or San Diego Regional Poison Control at 800-411-8080.

CHAPTER 129

MARINE ENVENOMATIONS

Troy Christian Sims

▶ The waters containing the most dangerous organisms are in tropical and sub-tropical areas of the world, especially the Indo-Pacific region.
▶ Both invertebrate and vertebrate marine organisms are capable of causing an envenomation injury, but invertebrate envenomations are more dangerous and occur with greater frequency.
▶ Jellyfish envenomations are among the most common of all.
▶ Sea snakes, however, are the most poisonous species in North American waters.

PATHOPHYSIOLOGY

▶ Marine venoms can induce any of the following:
  • Hypersensitivity reactions, including anaphylaxis
  • Neurologic impairment by impeding neuronal transmission
  • Muscle injury, including myonecrosis and cardiotoxicity, by interfering with cellular transport mechanisms and cellular metabolism
▶ Marine injuries themselves commonly cause significant bacterial infections, mainly by gram-negative organisms, such as *Vibrio* species.
▶ **Only** three species of poisonous sea creatures have an anti-venom available:
  • Box jellyfish, *Chironex fleckeri*
  • Stonefish, *Synanceja* species
  • Sea snakes, Hydrophiinae subfamily
▶ Because anti-venom administration is dependent upon identification of the offending organism, the history is vital and requires the following:
  • Locale in which the injury occurred
  • Site of injury on the body

- Venom delivery apparatus
- Clinical presentation of the victim

CLINICAL PRESENTATION

▶ Marine envenomations can present as shock, neurologic compromise, myalgias from myonecrosis, GI pain, or severe local pain.

▶ Venoms have variable time to onset of symptom, with the box jellyfish being the most rapid, which contributes to its deadliness.

▶ The type of wound is also a tell-tale sign of the type of envenomation.

TREATMENT

▶ See Table 129-1.

▶ In general, the approach to marine envenomation injuries has been three-fold:
- Inactivation of the venom and removal of the venom delivery apparatus
- Supportive care, including anaphylaxis treatment, antibiotic prophylaxis, pain control, and cardiopulmonary support
- Anti-venom, which is the definitive treatment in any serious envenomation

▶ The initial treatment of any marine injury is to remove the victim from the water.

▶ Attempt to identify organism and inactivate the venom.

▶ Remove the source of venom remaining on the victim.

▶ Consider a pressure immobilization dressing, which is a bandage wrapped around a piece of gauze covering the injury site to prevent lymphatic spread of the venom.

▶ Note that all marine envenomations carry a high potential for infection.
- The main offenders are gram-negative rods, especially the *Vibrio* species.
- Ciprofloxacin covers the broadest number of marine bacteria, but Bactrim and tetracycline are good alternatives.
- Tetanus prophylaxis should be updated accordingly.

◗ **PEARLS**
- Survival of a box jellyfish envenomation is dependent on how quickly the anti-venom can be administered, so all other measures of care should defer to acquiring it.

TABLE 129-1.
TREATMENT OF MARINE ENVENOMATIONS

Organism	Location	Clinical presentation	Treatment
Bluebottle jellyfish (*Physalia utriculus*) and Portuguese man-o'-war jellyfish (*Physalia physalis*)	Florida and Gulf of Mexico coasts and Indo-Pacific region	"String of beads" lesion with discrete wheals and surrounding erythema; pain is significant; systemic symptoms uncommon.	Remove victim from water; remove tentacles with forceps; analgesia; supportive care (vinegar **not** recommended as may cause discharge of nematocysts).
Box jellyfish (*Chironex fleckeri*)	Northern Queensland, Australia	Severe pain (worsened by moving victim as nematocysts are discharging); wide erythematous lines with blistering occurring within 6 hours and necrosis in 12–18 hours; pathognomonic for envenomation, but not always seen, is the "frosted" appearance of the lesions; hypotension; muscular and respiratory paralysis; resulting in cardiac arrest.	Remove victim from water; flood the skin with 5% acetic acid (vinegar) or use seawater, but do **not** use freshwater; remove tentacles with forceps; pressure immobilization dressing to limit absorption of venom; analgesia; *Chironex* antivenom preferably via IV route, but may be given IM (initial dose: 1 ampoule if IV and 3 if IM) and no skin testing necessary as it consists of purified sheep immunoglobulin; supportive care.
Irukandji jellyfish (*Carukia barnesi*)	Northern Queensland, Australia coastal and open waters	Irukandji syndrome: acute muscular chest pain; catecholamine surge resulting in sweating, vomiting, tachycardia, emergent HTN (diastolic in the 140s); possible SVT, and pulmonary edema; cardiopulmonary decompensation from a hypokinetic heart.	Remove from water; flood the skin with 5% acetic acid (vinegar) or use seawater, but do **not** use freshwater; remove tentacles with forceps; analgesia; supportive care, including phentolamine for HTN, positive pressure ventilation for pulmonary edema, and inotropic support.

(continued)

TABLE 129-1.
TREATMENT OF MARINE ENVENOMATIONS (CONTINUED)

Organism	Location	Clinical presentation	Treatment
Blue-ringed octopus (*Octopus maculosus*)	Indo-Pacific region (mainly shallow waters)	Pain is notably absent; venom contains tetrodotoxin (same as that of puffer fish) that causes blockade of sodium channels leading to numbness surrounding bitten appendage, face, and neck; severe injuries can progress to varying levels of paralysis and shock.	Remove from water; support cardiopulmonary functions until ET intubation is possible; pressure immobilization dressing; supportive care; effects of venom typically last 24–48 hours.
Cone shell (*Conus* sp.)	Indo-Pacific shallow waters and Florida coast	Pain is significant; numerous neurotoxic peptides that act pre- and post-synaptically leading to numbness surrounding bitten appendage, face, and neck; severe injuries can progress to varying levels of paralysis and shock.	Remove from water; support cardiopulmonary functions until ET intubation is possible; pressure immobilization dressing; supportive care (note that edrophonium may help paralysis).
Sea urchin (many species)	Ubiquitous	Intense pain; swelling; erythema; severe injuries may cause neurologic compromise, including weakness, paralysis, and shock.	Immerse injured appendage in non-scalding hot water for 30–90 minutes to alleviate pain and inactivate toxins; attempt extraction of spines as soon as possible; X-rays for broken spines; analgesia; supportive care.

Organism	Distribution	Presentation	Treatment
Stonefish (*Synanceja* sp.)	Tropical and temperate waters	Intense pain; swelling; severe injuries can cause neurologic compromise, including weakness, paralysis, and shock.	Immerse injured appendage in non-scalding hot water for 30–90 minutes to alleviate pain and inactivate toxins; vigorous irrigation with warmed saline to remove any remaining venom (slime); analgesia; stonefish anti-venom given IM, which consists of hyperimmune horse serum, so skin testing required (dose: 1 ampoule for 1–2 spines, 2 for 3–4 spines, and 3 for > 4 spines); X-rays for broken spines; supportive care.
Sea snake (*Hydrophiinae* sp.)	Indo-Pacific (including Hawaii); Central and South American Pacific waters (none exists in Atlantic Ocean)	Absence of pain; fang marks; myalgias and myonecrosis predominate; neurologic symptoms vary, including bulbar and lower-extremity paralysis.	Remove victim from water; pressure immobilization dressing; follow guidelines for terrestrial snake bite; sea snake anti-venom given IV from horse serum, so skin testing required (Australian tiger snake anti-venom can be substituted); treat for potential rhabdomyolysis; analgesia; supportive care. Note: If no symptoms manifest in 6–8 hours, then envenomation has not occurred.
Stingray (*Urolophus* sp. and *Dasyatis* sp.)	Ubiquitous in tropical, subtropical, and temperate waters	Trauma and envenomation injury; intense pain; swelling; severe injuries can cause neurologic compromise, including weakness, paralysis, and shock.	Immerse injured appendage in non-scalding hot water for 30–90 minutes to alleviate pain and inactivate toxins; attempt extraction of spines as soon as possible; analgesia; X-rays for broken spine; supportive care; incision and draining of wound are required, especially if abdomen or thorax penetrated.

- Do not flush jellyfish nematocysts with freshwater, as this will cause discharge.
- All three anti-venoms are available through CSL Ltd. in Melbourne, Australia.
- Pain can be excruciating, so analgesia is very important.
- Antibiotics are indicated in any serious marine injury.

CHAPTER 130

HIGH-ALTITUDE ILLNESS

Christopher R. Schmelzer and Christopher R. H. Newton

▶ Manifestations of high-altitude illness are often insidious in onset, occurring as low as 5000 feet.
▶ Represents an overlapping continuum of disease, from mild to quite severe.
▶ Rate of ascent, altitude, activity, and individual susceptibility are all contributing factors.

ACUTE MOUNTAIN SICKNESS

▶ Generally occurs in unacclimated persons rapidly ascending above 8200 ft
▶ Self-limiting disease

Clinical Presentation

▶ Presents with headache, nausea, vomiting, anorexia, and fatigue within a few hours and lasting for 3–6 days
▶ Often reports of sleeping difficulties

Treatment

▶ Mildest of symptoms may be treated with acclimatization at altitude, halting ascent. Symptomatic treatments for headache and vomiting.
▶ Advanced symptoms necessitate descent of 500 m (1500 ft) or more for 1–2 days.
▶ Acetazolamide at doses of 125–250 mg bid can improve subjective mild symptoms and speed acclimation.
▶ Progressive symptoms or inability to descend can be stabilized with low-flow O_2 and dexamethasone, 4 mg PO or IM q6h, until conditions allow descent.

HIGH-ALTITUDE PULMONARY EDEMA
Clinical Presentation

▶ Presents with classic pulmonary edema findings 1–4 days after ascent made
- Progressive exertional dyspnea, cough symptoms often worse at night
- Hypoxia, cyanosis, and rales on exam
- CXR: normal heart size (non-cardiogenic pulmonary edema)

Treatment

▶ Immediate and aggressive descent of 500–1000 m (1500–3000 ft) is curative.
▶ Temporary stabilization may be undertaken if immediate descent is not possible, including
- Supplemental O_2.
- Nifedipine at 10 mg PO, then extended release at 30 mg q12h may be beneficial in patients without evidence of high-altitude cerebral edema (HACE).
- Beta-agonists may also be helpful.
- Dexamethasone only helpful if evidence of cerebral edema.
- Portable low-pressure hyperbaric chamber is potentially life-saving if descent is difficult or delayed.

HIGH-ALTITUDE CEREBRAL EDEMA
Clinical Presentation

▶ Usually develops at altitudes of > 8000 ft
▶ Potentially fatal if not aggressively treated
▶ Often can present with insidious onset of CNS symptoms progressing from headache and vomiting to include confusion, ataxia, and progressive altered mental status leading to coma

Treatment

▶ Immediate and urgent descent of ≥ 1000 m below current altitude
▶ Portable hyperbaric therapy if available
▶ Dexamethasone, 8 mg PO/IM stat, followed by 4 mg PO/IM q6h
▶ Supplemental O_2

CHAPTER 131

DIVING EMERGENCIES

Christopher R. Schmelzer and Christopher R. H. Newton

▶ Medical complications of SCUBA diving affect approximately 1000 divers in the U.S. per year with approximately 10% mortality.

▶ Maintain a high index of suspicion for delayed presentations that may occur up to 48 hours after the last dive.

▶ Early consultation with a hyperbaric expert or the Divers Alert Network (DAN) Alert Line (919-684-8111) for all suspected cases.

DECOMPRESSION SICKNESS

▶ Multisystem disorder resulting from liberation of inert gas from solution with the formation of gas bubbles in blood and tissues when ambient pressure is decreased rapidly.

▶ Formation of the gas bubbles may result in either embolic phenomena or direct cellular damage.

Clinical Presentation

▶ Symptoms usually develop within 12 hours of diving (80% within an hour), but delayed presentations can occur up to 24 hours after last dive.

▶ Type 1 decompression sickness (DCS) is the mild form affecting skin, lymphatic, and musculoskeletal systems.

  • Common skin complaints are pruritus, SC emphysema, and mottled rashes.

  • Peri-articular pain in single or multiple joints that is classically worse with movement and relieved by direct pressure (also called "the bends").

  • Upper extremities most commonly involved.

▶ Type 2 DCS may present with a vast array of neurologic symptoms and signs. Classically involves the spine, can produce paresthesias, hypesthesias, or bowel or bladder symptoms. May also present with stroke-like symptoms.

- Neurologic findings in type 2 DCS may be dynamic and do not follow typical peripheral nerve distributions.
- The "chokes" from DCS consist of pleuritic chest pain, dyspnea, tachypnea, and cough.
- The "staggers" involve inner ear and cause nausea, vomiting, vertigo, tinnitus, and nystagmus.

▶ Patent foramen ovale in DCS allows right to left shunting of bubbles and more serious complications.

▶ May be difficult to differentiate DCS from air-gas embolism (AGE). Usually, AGE has rapid onset, but they can have very similar presentations. Treatment for both is fortunately the same.

Treatment

▶ 100% O_2.

▶ IVF hydration to prevent hemoconcentration and vascular occlusion.

▶ ASA, 325 mg PO.

▶ Avoid Trendelenburg position—previously thought to be beneficial.

▶ Rapid transport to hyperbaric chamber. Over 85% get complete resolution with hyperbaric therapy.

▶ Type 1 symptoms that resolve with high-flow O_2 may not require hyperbaric O_2 (HBO) but do need period of observation and consultation with hyperbaric expert. May develop more serious symptoms up to 24 hours after dive.

▶ Type 2 DCS requires HBO therapy.

AIR-GAS EMBOLISM

▶ Entry of gas bubbles into systemic circulation through ruptured pulmonary veins. From left heart can enter coronary or cerebral circulation, causing MI or stroke.

▶ Second most common cause of death in divers (first is drowning).

▶ Occurs on ascent; time from alveolar rupture to symptoms is usually < 10 minutes.

Clinical Presentation

▶ Abrupt onset of focal neurologic deficit after rapid ascent. May result in altered level of consciousness, headaches, and sensory or visual changes.

▶ May also cause apnea, dysrhythmias, and cardiac arrest.

Treatment

▶ High-flow O_2.

▶ Secure airway if indicated.

▶ IVF.

▶ Transport to facility with hyperbaric chamber; definitive care is recompression therapy.

▶ Early consultation with DAN may facilitate rapid transport to most appropriate facility.

▶ All patients are admitted.

MIDDLE EAR SQUEEZE

▶ Barotrauma of descent "squeeze": compression of gas in enclosed space as pressure increases with descent.

▶ Most commonly affects the ear. Diver experiences ear fullness or pain, which worsens until the TM ruptures or dive is aborted.

▶ No diving until healed. Decongestants may help symptoms.

NITROGEN NARCOSIS

▶ Nitrogen and other lipid-soluble, inert gases have an anesthetic effect at elevated partial pressures. Similar to the effects of alcohol, they increase with depth.

▶ Effects usually become evident at 90–100 feet of sea water (fsw). May impair diver's memory, concentration, and reaction times. At > 300 fsw, diver will lose consciousness.

CHAPTER 132

RADIATION INJURY

William E Lew

▶ Unstable isotopes release radioactivity as particles (alpha and beta) or waves (X- or gamma-rays).

▶ Alpha particles (helium nucleus) have poor penetration and can be blocked by paper or clothing. Toxicity develops when incorporated.

▶ Beta particles (electrons) can penetrate through skin approximately 1 cm. Toxicity develops from external contamination or incorporation.

▶ X-rays and gamma-rays induce ionization (resulting in highly reactive free radicals). Penetrate without difficulty, resulting in major external radiation hazard.

▶ Rad is the unit that describes absorbed radiation. Gy is equivalent to 100 rad.

▶ Radiation injury occurs via three mechanisms:
  • Irradiation (exposure to ionizing radiation)
  • Contamination (radioactive substance covers an object)
  • Incorporation (inhalation, ingestion, or wound contamination)

▶ Irradiation causes direct injury (DNA damage or mutation) or indirect injury (creates reactive species that induce molecular damage).

▶ Radiosensitivity is directly related to rate of cellular reproduction and inversely related to degree of differentiation.

CLINICAL PRESENTATION

▶ Acute radiation syndrome (ARS) develops from large whole body irradiation (> 2 Gy)
  • Stage 1 (early/prodromal): characterized by nausea and vomiting. Begins minutes to hours post-exposure (inversely proportional to dose received). Duration of a few hours to a few days (proportional to dose).
  • Stage 2 (latent): characterized by no clinical complaints. Duration of several days to weeks (proportional to dose).

- Stage 3 (symptomatic): characterized by nausea, vomiting, diarrhea, abdominal pain, sepsis, bleeding. Begins in third to fifth week after exposure.
- Stage 4 (recovery): lasts weeks to months.

▶ Sub-syndromes of ARS include
  - CNS syndrome: rapid development of cerebellar/motor/sensory dysfunction and mental status changes (due to neuronal cell death and cerebral edema). > 15 Gy exposure.
  - Cardiovascular syndrome: hypotension and dysrhythmias.
  - GI syndrome: nausea, vomiting, diarrhea, anorexia, hematochezia, sepsis, dehydration (due to mucosa cell death, colonization by enteric organisms). > 5 Gy exposure.
  - Hematopoietic syndrome: leukopenia, thrombocytopenia, anemia (due to consumption of platelets, hemorrhages, and direct effect on lymphocytes). 1–5 Gy exposure.
  - Pulmonary syndrome: pneumonitis leading to respiratory failure, pulmonary fibrosis, or cor pulmonale. 6–10 Gy exposure.

EMERGENCY DEPARTMENT MANAGEMENT
Diagnosis

▶ History of radiation exposure paramount in diagnosis.
▶ Send baseline CBC, T&S.
▶ Radiation exposure:
  - < 1.5 Gy: asymptomatic
  - 1.5–4 Gy: mild ARS (minimal mortality)
  - 4–6 Gy: moderate-severe ARS (> 50% mortality)
  - 6–15 Gy: severe ARS (mortality may approach 100%)
  - > 50 Gy: fulminating ARS (death < 48 hours)
▶ Median lethal dose of radiation is 4.5 Gy.
▶ Absolute lymphocyte count (ALC) at 48 hours post-exposure may aid in prognosis. > $1200/mm^3$, unlikely fatal dose. 300–$1200/mm^3$, possible fatal dose. < $300/mm^3$, critical dose received.

Treatment

▶ Irradiated patients pose no threat to health care workers once source is removed.
▶ Decontaminate patient. Remove all clothing. Wash patient with soap and water. Place clothing in radioactive waste containers.
▶ Radiation safety officer must be notified.

- ► Evaluate conventional injuries (burn, smoke inhalation, traumatic).
- ► Manage symptoms of ARS, including fluid replacement, antiemetics, pain control (avoid NSAIDs).
- ► If blood transfusion indicated, use irradiated blood products to avoid graft vs. host disease.
- ► Leukopenia may be treated with granulocyte colony-stimulating factor (G-CSF). Bone marrow transplantation may be an option for severe irradiation.

Disposition

- ► Symptoms of mild nausea/vomiting with resolution within hours of exposure, initial CBC unremarkable, estimated exposure < 2 Gy: may discharge home with mandatory outpatient follow-up.
- ► Symptoms of nausea and vomiting lasting < 48 hours with leukopenia: may need admission for dehydration, persistent emesis. If ALC at 48 hours < 1200/mm^3, admission is required for monitoring and potential bone marrow transplantation, G-CSF administration.
- ► Rapid onset of nausea, vomiting, diarrhea, pancytopenia: survival unlikely. Usually treated with comfort measures.

CHAPTER 133

TICK-BORNE DISEASES

Clifford W. Robins

- ▶ Ticks belong to the class Arachnida.
- ▶ Most common agents of vector-borne disease in the U.S.
- ▶ Transmit viruses, bacteria, spirochetes, parasites, and rickettsia.
- ▶ Nymphs and adults can be infectious.
  - Most diseases (90%) are transmitted by nymphs because they are small, can feed for long periods of time without being detected, and are present in larger numbers in the spring and summer when most humans are in the woods.

LYME DISEASE

- ▶ Vector: *Ixodes scapularis* (*I. dammini*) and *Ixodes pacificus.*
- ▶ Organism: *Borrelia burgdorferi.*
- ▶ Most common vector-borne disease in the U.S.
- ▶ Mainly in the northeastern, midwest, and north central regions (CT, RI, PN, DE, NJ, MD, MA, WI).
- ▶ Diagnosis is by history of a tick bite and characteristic clinical findings in an endemic area.

Clinical Presentation

- ▶ Early acute phase
  - Erythema migrans is the hallmark finding (appears in 60–80% of all cases).
    - ○ Painless, erythematous annular macular rash
  - Occurs usually about 7 days after the bite.
  - Lesion expands centrifugally over days to weeks.
  - 20% of cases develop multiple lesions.
  - Most patients develop viral-like symptoms, fatigue, myalgias, arthralgias, headaches, stiff neck, fever, and chills.
- ▶ Early disseminated phase
  - Occurs in untreated patients 1–2 months after bite.

- Patients have skin, musculoskeletal, neurologic, and cardiac involvement.
▶ Late or chronic phase
  - Occurs if the infection is untreated for > 1 year.
    ○ Lyme arthritis: painful swollen joints, usually the knee
  - Polyneuritis, encephalomyelitis, encephalopathy, cranial neuropathies, radiculopathies, and chronic meningitis may occur.

Emergency Department Management

▶ Doxycycline, 100 mg PO bid for 2–3 weeks.
▶ Pregnant/nursing women, children: amoxicillin, 500 mg tid or 25–50 mg/kg tid.
▶ Prophylactic treatment is not recommended because risk of infection is < 1%.

ROCKY MOUNTAIN SPOTTED FEVER

▶ Vector: *Dermacentor andersoni* (wood tick) and *Dermacentor variabilis* (dog tick).
▶ Organism: *Rickettsia rickettsii*.
▶ Most commonly seen in the southeastern, western, and south central U.S.
▶ Organisms multiply in the vascular endothelium with increased permeability and microinfarction of organs.
▶ Classic triad of fever, rash, and tick exposure appears in only 50% of cases.
▶ Diagnosis is clinical.

Clinical Presentation

▶ Onset of symptoms is non-specific; fever, nausea, vomiting, headache.
▶ Rash starts on the wrists, ankles, and forearms, blanching red macular, and progresses to form papules centrally to the arms, thighs, trunk, and face. Rash generally does not appear until day 4.
▶ Meningitis, focal neurologic deficits, myocarditis, pneumonitis, and GI symptoms are all possible.
▶ Death is the result of multi-organ failure with intracerebral hemorrhage, disseminated intravascular coagulation, and vascular collapse (~3%).

Emergency Department Management

▶ Doxycycline, 100 mg PO bid.
▶ In children, chloramphenicol, 50–100 mg/kg divided qid.
▶ Treatment course is 10–14 days.

HUMAN EHRLICHIOSIS

▶ Vector: *Amblyomma americanum* (*E. chaffeensis*), *Ixodes scapularis* [human granulocytic ehrlichiosis (HGE) agent], and *Dermacentor variabilis.*
▶ Organisms: *Ehrlichia chaffeensis* [human monocytic ehrlichiosis (HME)].
  • HGE agent similar to *Ehrlichia equi* and *E. phagocytophila.*
▶ Gram-negative bacteria that parasitize monocytes and granulocytes, and form characteristic morulae inside WBCs.
▶ Diseases are clinically indistinguishable.

Clinical Presentation

▶ Acute flu-like illness, with fever, malaise, myalgias, headache, nausea.
▶ Rash, if present, is fleeting.
▶ Labs show leukopenia, thrombocytopenia, mild elevation in transaminases.
▶ Wright's stain shows characteristic morulae in WBCs.

Emergency Department Management

▶ Treat patients with clinical and lab findings.
▶ Doxycycline, 100 mg PO bid, is the agent of choice.
▶ Chloramphenicol may also be used.
▶ Treatment course is 14 days.

Q FEVER

▶ Highly infectious, rickettsial agent.
▶ Organism is *Coxiella brunetti* transmitted by inhaling barnyard dust, where this organism is found in infected livestock, especially sheep.
▶ Presentation is an acute flu-like illness with fever, rigors, headache, malaise, myalgias.

▶ Pneumonia and hepatitis are primary infections.

▶ Doxycycline, 100 mg PO bid, for 14 days.

▶ Unrecognized endocarditis is the primary fatal complication years later.

TULAREMIA

▶ Tick-borne bacterial agent.

▶ Organism is *Francisella tularensis*, found in wild rabbits, mainly in the midwest.

▶ Presentation is acute onset of flu-like illness, with fever, chills, myalgias, fatigue.

▶ Painful, rapidly spreading regional lymphadenopathy may also be present.

▶ Labs show leukocytosis, elevated transaminases; patchy ill-defined areas on CXR.

▶ Serology testing is used to confirm the diagnosis.

▶ Treatment is streptomycin, 1 g IM q12h.

▶ Tetracyclines and chloramphenicol are alternatives.

▶ May be used as a biological weapon.

BABESIOSIS

▶ Tick-borne protozoan agent.

▶ Organism is *Babesia microti*.

▶ A malaria-like disease, caused by protozoan invasion of RBCs.

▶ Found mainly in Martha's Vineyard, Nantucket, eastern and south Long Island, and CT in the U.S.

▶ Presentation of high fever, drenching sweats, myalgias.

▶ Labs show hemolytic anemia, thrombocytopenia, hemoglobin-uria, elevated transaminases.

▶ Blood smear demonstrates "Maltese Cross" appearance of infected RBCs.

▶ May be confused with *P. falciparum*.

▶ Treatment is quinine, 650 PO mg tid, and IV clindamycin, 1200 mg IV bid for 7–10 days.

TICK PREVENTION

▶ Light-colored clothing helps identify ticks.

▶ Long-sleeved shirts tucked into pants.

▶ Twice daily "tick checks" while in the woods.
▶ DEET repellents.
▶ Awareness of seasonality of ticks.

TICK REMOVAL

▶ Use blunt instruments to grasp tick near the mouth parts, close to the skin.
▶ Pull in a steady, upward motion, away from the skin.
▶ Disinfect site with soap and water, rubbing alcohol, or peroxide.
▶ Record date and location of bite.
▶ **Do not** use sharp instruments, apply heat, or attempt to handle the tick with your bare hands.

CHAPTER 134

SCABIES AND PEDICULOSIS

Jacob MacKenzie

SCABIES

▶ Skin infestation with the mite *Sarcoptes scabiei* ($\frac{1}{3}$ mm, tortoise shaped).

▶ Requires direct skin-to-skin contact, as mites cannot jump or fly.

▶ 1-month lifespan, but can live only 2–3 days apart from host. Fomites (clothing or bedding) and pets may spread organism to humans.

▶ Female burrows into upper layers of skin and deposits eggs (hatch in 3–4 days) and feces.

▶ Symptoms begin after 2–4 weeks (1–4 days in those with prior infection).

▶ Scratching spreads the mites to other body locations.

Clinical Presentation

▶ Intense, generalized pruritus that begins gradually and is worse at night.

▶ Classic lesion is 2–15 mm, serpiginous, hair-width burrow with scattered papules and vesicles found on hands (especially finger webs), wrists, waist, axilla, and genitals. Infants often have face involved.

▶ Excoriations and secondary skin infection are common due to intense pruritus.

▶ Norwegian (crusted or hyperkeratotic) scabies is a variant afflicting immunocompromised, elderly, or mentally impaired, and is often only mildly pruritic.

Emergency Department Management

▶ Should be considered when more than one family members itches.

▶ Diagnosis is usually made clinically.

▶ Felt-tip pen can be used to highlight burrows (wipe off excess ink with alcohol wipe).

▶ Mites can be scraped from burrows and examined using a microscope.

▶ Treatment of choice is topical 5% permethrin (Elimite) cream applied from neck down and washed off 8–12 hours later. 30 g is usually sufficient for the average adult.

▶ Lindane 1% cream (Kwell) is no longer regarded as first-line treatment because of resistance, and it is also contraindicated in pregnancy, children, and seizure disorders.

▶ Precipitated sulfur 5% or 10% in petrolatum is recommended in infants < 2 months and pregnant or lactating women.

▶ Antihistamines and topical corticosteroids are useful adjuncts.

▶ Consider antibiotics for secondary bacterial infection (e.g., cephalexin).

▶ Treat all intimate/household contacts.

▶ Recommend washing or bagging (for 3 days) unwashed clothing and bedding.

▶ Educate that pruritus may take 1–2 weeks to subside, and, if it persists at this time, patient should seek further care.

PEDICULOSIS

▶ Infestation with lice that causes localized itching, usually without a rash.

▶ Pediculosis capitis (head), pediculosis corporis (body), and pediculosis pubis (pubic hair).

▶ Obligate human parasites and measure < 2 mm in length. Nits are lice eggs and are small, white, and densely adherent to base of hairs.

▶ Feed by piercing skin and sucking blood. Saliva and wastes can cause hypersensitivity reaction, and scratching can cause inflammation and secondary infection.

▶ Spread by close physical contact (most common route) or fomites.

▶ Lice have a 1-month lifespan and survive for several days separated from host.

Clinical Presentation

▶ Pediculosis capitis (head lice)
  • Pruritus without a rash is the most common presentation.

- Children most often affected and girls more frequently than boys. African Americans rarely affected.
- Lice and nits can be found anywhere on the head (including eyelids and beards) but are most often found in the back of the head/neck and behind the ears.
- Posterior cervical lymphadenopathy is common.
- Scratching or local reaction can cause a variety of lesions (e.g., papules or pustules) or secondary infection.
- Blepharitis or conjunctivitis can result from eyelid infestation.

▶ Pediculosis corporis (body lice)
  - Rarely encountered in the U.S.
  - Poor hygiene, overcrowding.
  - Body lice may serve as vectors for other disease (e.g., epidemic typhus and trench fever).

▶ Pediculosis pubis (pubic lice)
  - Most complain of pruritus in the groin and may have a "crawling" sensation.
  - Pubic lice ("crabs") and nits are found in the pubic hair but may also spread to the thighs or abdomen.
  - Very easily transmitted (up to 90% after a single encounter) and often (30%) are associated with other STDs.
  - Consider abuse in children with pubic lice.

Emergency Department Management

▶ Attempt to identify the louse. Fine-toothed comb ("nit comb") or woods lamp may assist.
▶ Nits (unlike dandruff or other conditions) are difficult to remove from the hair shaft.
▶ Topical insecticides are the mainstay of treatment. Similar to scabies, first-line treatment is permethrin.
▶ Eyebrow/lid infestations are treated with petrolatum (Vaseline) or baby shampoo applied to the eyelashes and eyebrows tid for 5 days.
▶ Resistance has been documented with all treatments and is suggested by multiple live lice of various sizes. In cases of re-infestation, a single, live adult louse is present.
▶ To prevent re-infestation, treat all close contacts and wash clothing/bedding.
▶ Nits may persist for months after successful treatment.
▶ Should re-examine at 10–14 days.

CHAPTER 135

HAND INJURIES

James Pribble

▶ Overall, 5% of ED visits are due to hand injuries.
▶ 19% of lost work time is due to injuries.

FRACTURE OF THE DISTAL PHALANX (TUFT FRACTURE)

▶ History often of crush injury with pain and swelling at tip of finger
▶ May have associated nail bed injury
▶ May have tendon injury if proximal portion of distal phalanx involved

Management

▶ None needed for isolated tuft fracture.
▶ May splint for comfort—avoid splinting the DIP.
▶ Proximal fracture, managed as tendon injury.
▶ If displaced and unable to reduce, refer to hand surgery.

MALLET FINGER

▶ Disruption of extensor tendon of proximal portion of the distal phalanx
▶ Common sports injury with forced flexion of extended finger
▶ Flexed position of distal phalanx with pain and weakness to extension of distal phalanx

Management

▶ Splinting for 6 weeks—immobilize the DIP
▶ Hand surgery referral

PROXIMAL AND MIDDLE PHALANX FRACTURES

▶ Most are stable and non-displaced.

▶ Neck fractures have volar angulation.
▶ Base fractures have dorsal angulation.
▶ Oblique X-rays may be needed to determine if condyle or neck of phalanx is fractured.

Management

▶ Depends on stability and alignment.
▶ Rotational alignment assessed by closed fist, four digits should point to the scaphoid.
▶ Transverse fractures usually stable.
  • Dynamic splinting: buddy taping
▶ Oblique/spiral fractures usually unstable.
  • Formal splinting that includes the wrist: outrigger splint
▶ Refer to hand surgery in 7–10 days.

THUMB METACARPAL FRACTURE

▶ Bennett's fracture
  • Intra-articular fracture at the base of first metacarpal with associated dislocation/subluxation of CMC joint
▶ Rolando's fracture
  • Comminuted intra-articular fracture at the base of first metacarpal
  • Mechanism similar for both: axial load on a flexed thumb

Management

▶ Closed reduction of Bennett's fracture
▶ Thumb spica
▶ Urgent hand surgery referral

METACARPAL FRACTURES

▶ Amount of angulation tolerated depends on mobility of CMC joints:
  • Index and middle fingers tolerate less angulation than ring and little finger.
  • Rotational deformity poorly tolerated; 5% can cause significant overlap.
▶ Head fractures: intra-articular—rare, usually from direct trauma and are comminuted.

- ► Neck fractures: most common fracture of the hand, common after a punch or load onto a clenched fist.
- ► Shaft fractures: commonly transverse, oblique, or comminuted.
  - Tolerate less angulation than neck fractures
  - No angulation acceptable for index and middle, 10 degrees for ring, and 20 degrees of angulation acceptable for little finger metacarpal shaft fractures
- ► Base fractures are rare.
  - Ring and little finger fractures can cause injury to motor portion of ulnar nerve and paralyze the intrinsic hand muscles.
- ► Clenched fist injury: open fracture after closed fist load, typically from human bite.

Management

- ► Head fractures: hand follow-up, place in "safe" position—wrist extension 20 degrees, MCP at 90 degrees, and digits extended
  - Needs urgent hand referral as complications are relatively high.
  - If laceration, consider clenched fist injury, antibiotics, and immediate hand consult in the ED to consider OR for washout.
- ► Neck fractures:
  - Displaced ring and little finger can be reduced in the ED (35% of angulation tolerated) then in gutter splint (little finger—boxer's fracture).
  - Index and long finger usually require surgical fixation; radial gutter splint and referral to hand surgery.
  - Splint to but not including PIP.
- ► Shaft fractures:
  - Splint to but not including the MCP if fracture does not involve the neck.
  - Hand referral.
- ► Base fractures: assess for neurovascular compromise; if none, volar splint and hand referral.

LIGAMENTOUS INJURIES

- ► DIP/PIP/MCP: have radial and ulnar collateral ligaments as well as a volar plate.
- ► Subluxation and dislocations are most commonly dorsal.
- ► Radial dislocations more common than ulnar dislocations.
- ► Usually from direct blow on extended finger.

▶ Test ligament stability actively and passively in both extended and slightly flexed position.

Management

▶ Closed reduction is often achieved after adequate anesthesia.
▶ If unable to reduce or open dislocation, hand surgery consult for operative reduction.
▶ Volar dislocations may require operative reduction.

GAMEKEEPER'S THUMB (OR SKIER'S THUMB)

▶ Injury to ulnar collateral ligament of thumb caused by forced radial abduction.
▶ 30 degrees of laxity suggests tear or > 15 degrees more laxity than contralateral side.

Management

▶ Thumb spica—referral to hand surgery. Complete tears usually need surgery.

TENDON INJURIES

▶ Extensor tendon more commonly injured.
▶ Most extensor and all flexor tendon injuries are referred to hand surgery for treatment.

EXTENSOR TENDON INJURY

▶ Maintain a high index of suspicion for extensor tendon injuries for any laceration or wound to the dorsum of the hand.
▶ Extensor tendon injury can also be caused by closed injury with no laceration.
▶ Extensor tendon zones of injury (Verdan):
  • Zone 1: DIP
  • Zone 2: middle phalanx
  • Zone 3: PIP
  • Zone 4: proximal phalanx
  • Zone 5: MCP
  • Zone 6: dorsum of hand
  • Zones 7 and 8: wrist and forearm

Management

▶ Complete laceration is repaired with non-absorbable sutures 4-0, 5-0 [polyester sutures (Ethibond) are preferred to nylon sutures].

▶ Partial lacerations are repaired with absorbable Vicryl.

▶ It is often appropriate to set up delayed closure by hand surgeon.

▶ Zones 1–2 can be treated in the ED (mallet finger).
  • May be with or without bony avulsion.
  • Closed injury: splint the DIP in extension for 6 weeks.
  • Open injury: usually repaired by hand surgery.

▶ Zone 3 injuries can cause boutonnière deformity due to injury to central slip (closed injury more common).
  • Closed injuries: splint PIP in extension for 6 weeks.
  • Open injuries: refer to hand surgery for repair.

▶ Zone 4 injuries can be primarily closed in the ED.
  • Injury mostly results from open wounds.
  • Splint hand with PIP in neutral position, MCP at 15–30 degrees flexion, and wrist at 30 degrees of extension.

▶ Zone 5 injuries usually repaired by hand surgery.
  • Can be caused by laceration or direct blow.
  • Open wounds: consider human clenched fist injury; this must be ruled out for patient to be sent out of the ED.
  • Splint with MCP in neutral position and wrist at 45 degrees of extension.

▶ Zone 6: repair can be done in the ED.
  • Splint wrist at 45 degrees of extension, affected digit at a neutral position, and remaining digits at 10 degrees of flexion.

▶ Zone 7–8 usually repaired by hand surgery.
  • Local wound management and skin closure.
  • Splint with volar splint with wrist at 35 degrees of extension and MCP at 15 degrees of flexion.

FLEXOR TENDON INJURY

▶ Although most flexor tendon injuries are caused by lacerations, closed mechanism can rupture the flexor digitorum profundus at the base of the distal phalanx.
  • Patient presents with inability to flex at the DIP.

▶ Flexor tendon lacerations repaired by hand surgeon usually within 12–24 hours.

▶ Examine tendon through entire ROM as lacerated end may have retracted.
▶ Test against resistance, as weakness and pain can indicate partial laceration.

NAIL BED INJURIES

▶ Commonly caused by direct blow and often associated with distal phalanx fracture.
▶ Subungual hematoma: > 50% chance of nail bed laceration. If associated fracture, 90% chance of nail bed laceration.

Management

▶ Controversy over trephination or nail removal and search for laceration
▶ Lacerations:
  • Repaired with 5-0, 6-0 absorbable sutures.
  • Nail needs to be replaced under nail fold or Vaseline/Xeroform gauze dressing to maintain space for new nail to grow.
▶ Fracture with nail bed laceration
  • Remove nail and repair laceration. Antibiotics controversial but usually given.

HIGH-PRESSURE INJECTION INJURIES

Pathophysiology

▶ Common occupational injury.
▶ Three factors affect severity of injury: force (lb/square in.), specific agent used, time since injury occurred.

Clinical Presentation

▶ Often present late as symptoms are minimal initially
▶ Severe pain and swelling
▶ May have signs of vascular compromise

Management

▶ IV antibiotics and tetanus.
▶ Pain control: avoid digital block as it can increase tissue pressure.
▶ Immediate orthopedic hand surgery consult in ED.
▶ Many need open debridement.

CHAPTER 136

HAND INFECTIONS

Joseph H. Hartmann

ACUTE PARONYCHIA

▶ *Staphylococcus aureus* most common, *Streptococcus* species, *Pseudomonas*, anaerobes (especially with exposure to oral flora)
▶ Often results from superficial "injury"—hangnail, nail biting, manicures, dishwashing, finger sucking

Clinical Presentation

▶ Erythema, tenderness, swelling of perionychium (epidermis adjacent to nail)
▶ Abscess with or without purulent drainage from nail fold margin

Management

▶ Early infection treated with frequent warm soaks and 3- to 5-day course of antibiotics.
▶ Abscess treated by incision and drainage: elevate eponychial fold from nail base, irrigate, and pack with gauze (remove 24 hours later).
▶ No antibiotics are needed for simple incision and drainage; however, if cellulitis is present, antibiotics are warranted.
▶ First-generation cephalosporin is drug of choice:
  • Cephalexin, 500 mg q6h for 7 days

FELON

▶ Infection in palmar distal pulp of fingertip usually associated with minor trauma.
▶ Abscess formation causes significant pain.
▶ Resultant swelling under pressure can lead to tissue necrosis, osteomyelitis, flexor tenosynovitis, or septic arthritis.
▶ Thumb and index finger most commonly involved.

Clinical Presentation

▶ Throbbing pain, erythema early with pointing of abscess possible later

Management

▶ Conservative care with frequent warm soaks and antibiotic therapy possible in early treatment without abscess.

▶ If abscess is seen, incision and drainage are required.

    • Single volar longitudinal incision or high lateral incision (avoid neurovascular bundle)—radial aspect of thumb, ulnar aspect of fingers

▶ Blunt dissection of septae, irrigate, pack loosely, dress, and splint.

▶ Avoid "fish-mouth" or "hockey-stick" incisions due to potential sensory loss and instability of finger pad.

▶ Consider X-ray to rule out presence of FBs or osteomyelitis.

▶ No antibiotics are needed for simple incision and drainage; however, if cellulitis is present, antibiotics are warranted.

▶ First-generation cephalosporin is drug of choice:

    • Cephalexin, 500 mg q6h for 7 days

HERPETIC WHITLOW

▶ HSV-1 or HSV-2 infection of distal finger

▶ More commonly occurs in children with gingivostomatitis and adults with or exposed to oral or genital herpes

Clinical Presentation

▶ Clear vesicular lesions with erythematous border on a single finger

▶ Pain disproportional to findings

▶ Tzanck test demonstrates multinucleated giant cells

Management

▶ Cover with dry dressing to prevent further viral transmission.

▶ Expect spontaneous resolution in 2–3 weeks.

▶ Analgesics as necessary.

▶ Acyclovir, famciclovir, or valacyclovir may lessen severity of symptoms if initiated early (first 48 hours)—no randomized trials to confirm.

► Do not mistake for felon and perform incision and drainage, allowing viral extension into healthy tissue (distal finger pulp is soft in HSV infection).

FLEXOR TENOSYNOVITIS

► Infection of tendon sheaths of digit(s).
► Puncture wounds and fight-bites are frequent causes.
► Typically staphylococcal or streptococcal species.

Clinical Presentation

► Four cardinal signs of Kanavel (1912):
  • Digit held in partial flexion
  • Symmetric, uniform swelling of entire digit
  • Marked tenderness directly over tendon sheath
  • Exquisite pain with passive extension of digit (may be earliest sign)

Management

► Hand surgeon should be notified immediately as surgical drainage may be needed.
► Antibiotics are started immediately.
  • Ampicillin/sulbactam, 3 g IV q6h, is drug of choice.
  • Vancomycin and gentamicin if penicillin allergic.
► Complications: tendon destruction, functional disability, extension of infection to deep fascial space.

DEEP FASCIAL SPACE INFECTION

► Potential spaces susceptible to infection by direct penetrating trauma, extension from neighboring structures (particularly from flexor tenosynovitis)

Clinical Presentation

► Commonly present with lymphangitis, fever, and lymphadenopathy.
► Web space infections: swelling and pain on both dorsal and palmar surfaces of hand predisposing to collar button abscess (due to hourglass shape).

▶ Mid-palmar space infection: swelling, pain, loss of palmar concavity, pain with movement of third and fourth digits. Dorsal swelling from extension into lymphatics.

Management

▶ Hand surgeon should be notified immediately for surgical drainage in OR.
▶ Antibiotics are started immediately.
  • Ampicillin/sulbactam, 3 g IV q6h, is drug of choice.
  • Vancomycin and gentamicin if penicillin allergic.

CHAPTER 137

WRIST INJURIES

Colin F. Greineder

▶ The wrist is a complex unit comprising eight carpal bones, the distal radius and ulna, the proximal metacarpals, and a mesh of ligaments stabilizing bones to each other.

▶ Loss of wrist mobility or strength due to unrecognized or improperly managed injury may have devastating functional impact.

▶ Eight carpal bones, arranged in two rows.

- Proximal row (radial to ulnar): scaphoid, lunate, triquetrum, pisiform.
- Distal row (radial to ulnar): trapezium, trapezoid, capitate, hamate.

▶ Scaphoid bone, which links the two carpal arches and has the largest radial articulation, has key role in stability of wrist and a greater propensity for injury.

EXAMINATION OF THE WRIST

▶ Physical exam is often limited by swelling and severe pain; consequently, main goal is to identify general area of tenderness.

▶ Landmarks:

- Anatomic snuff box: triangle formed by the extensor pollicis longus, extensor pollicis brevis, and the radial styloid—the scaphoid is palpable at base of snuff box.
- Lister's tubercle: bony prominence on dorsal surface of radius, ulnar to anatomic snuff box.

RADIOGRAPHIC INTERPRETATION

▶ PA view useful for evaluating *individual carpal bones* and *carpal bone fractures*

▶ Lateral view useful for evaluating *carpal alignment* and *forearm fractures*

SCAPHOID FRACTURE

▶ Most common carpal bone fracture and is easily missed without high index of suspicion

Clinical Presentation

▶ Mechanism of injury most often FOOSH with forced hyperextension.
▶ Exam usually reveals pain and swelling on radial side of wrist.
▶ Tenderness in the anatomical snuff box is the classical finding.
▶ Pain with axial loading of the thumb.
▶ Radiographs:
  • Standard wrist films may be normal in up to 10–20% of fractures.
  • Scaphoid view increases sensitivity but still may not demonstrate fracture acutely.
  • CT or MRI may detect fracture in radiograph-negative cases, but not often utilized in ED because management is the same.
  • Follow-up films at 4–6 weeks will usually reveal occult nondisplaced fractures.

Management

▶ Unstable fracture if as little as 1 mm of displacement or any rotation, angulation, or shortening.
  • Unstable fractures need immediate orthopedic consultation in ED.
▶ Stable fractures should be placed in long-arm thumb spica splint (extending to the thumb IP joint in neutral wrist position) with orthopedic follow-up in 5–7 days.
▶ Suspected fractures with normal X-rays should also be splinted (long- or short-arm thumb spica) with follow-up in 7–10 days—approximately 15% will have fracture.
▶ Major complications are AVN and non-union of fracture. More proximal and oblique fracture, the higher the risk of complications.

SCAPHOLUNATE LIGAMENT INSTABILITY/DISLOCATION

▶ Most common ligamentous injury of wrist

Clinical Presentation

▶ Mechanism most commonly FOOSH with impact on thenar eminence

▶ Pain usually dorsal, just distal to Lister's tubercle (see dorsal landmarks)

▶ May also present with clicking sound or sensation with wrist motion

▶ Radiographs

- Classic finding is diastasis of scapholunate joint up to 3 mm.
- Other radiographic finding in ligament injury is rotary subluxation of scaphoid, in which scaphoid rotates volarly as disruption of scapholunate ligament releases bone from stabilizing effect of lunate; scapholunate angle between two bones will be > 60 degrees on lateral film.
- PA view of rotary subluxation of scaphoid will display foreshortened bone with "cortical ring" sign as the bone and its circular cortex are viewed on end.

Management

▶ Scapholunate injury often treated surgically, so orthopedic consultation in ED or rapid referral is necessary.

▶ Can be acutely stabilized with radial gutter splint.

COLLES' FRACTURE

▶ Most common distal radius fracture; metaphysis is fractured and dorsally displaced.

Clinical Presentation

▶ Mechanism of injury is FOOSH.

▶ Wrist displays "dinner fork" deformity.

▶ May present with paresthesias in median nerve distribution.

▶ Radiographs

- Usually seen on both PA and lateral films.
- Important features are degree of dorsal angulation, intraarticular involvement, and extent of comminution, which determine relative stability of fracture.
- Associated ulnar styloid fracture should not be missed.

Management

▶ Closed reduction is generally indicated, with a goal of restoring the volar tilt and ulnar inclination of radius. If adequate reduction is obtained, plaster immobilization and referral are appropriate.

▶ Open or unstable fractures, in which marked comminution, inadequate reduction, or neurovascular compromise is present, require emergent orthopedic consultation.

SMITH'S FRACTURE

▶ "Reverse Colles' fracture," also a radial metaphyseal fracture, with volar displacement and angulation.

▶ Results from blow to dorsum of hand or FOOSH with palmar flexed wrist.

▶ Associated median nerve injury and ulnar styloid fracture should be assessed.

▶ Management similar to Colles' fracture, with closed reduction and plaster immobilization usually adequate, but more unstable cases requiring open fixation.

RADIAL STYLOID FRACTURE

▶ "Chauffeur fracture" results from twisting force along radial side of hand, formerly seen when automobile starting crank forcibly reversed direction, avulsing styloid.

▶ Notoriously subtle and unimpressive; usually appears as thin lucent line beneath radial styloid on radiograph, extending from scaphoid fossa to metaphysis.

▶ Considered unstable because of numerous extrinsic and intrinsic ligaments that originate at the radial styloid.

▶ Any displacement mandates orthopedic consultation for possible open fixation, due to risk of premature arthritis and loss of function.

CHAPTER 138

SHOULDER INJURIES

Matthew K. Hysell

CLAVICLE FRACTURE

▶ Fractures occur most commonly in middle third of clavicle, typically from lateral axial load injury from fall or sports injury.
▶ Proximal fractures usually occur from direct blow.
▶ Can be associated with coracoid or first rib fracture, subclavian vein injury, pneumothorax, brachial plexus injury.

Clinical Presentation

▶ History of injury leading to pain/disability
▶ Swelling, ecchymosis, bony tenderness, deformity, possible skin tenting

Management

▶ Proximal and middle third fractures typically treated with sling.
▶ Particularly comminuted or shortened middle third fractures may benefit from open repair.
▶ Fractures of distal third of clavicle subdivided between fractures distal to the coracoclavicular ligament (type I) and those proximal to coracoclavicular ligament (type II).
  • Type I treated with sling and swath.
  • Type II also treated with sling and swath but should be referred to orthopedics for 2–3 day follow-up to consider open repair.
  • Type III [rare fracture at acromioclavicular (AC) joint difficult to see without special radiographs] treated as in type I.

ACROMIOCLAVICULAR SEPARATION

▶ AC joint supported by ligaments strongest on superior aspect as well as by trapezius and deltoid muscles.

▶ Joint typically 1–1.5 cm in adults, symmetric within ~0.5 cm.
▶ Classic mechanism is downward force on point of shoulder with arm fully adducted, typically in contact sports.

Clinical Presentation

▶ Typically point tenderness at AC joint.
▶ Increasing degrees of pain with movement correlate roughly with severity of injury.

Management

▶ Films need to be underpenetrated for maximal radiographic evaluation of AC joint.
▶ AC separation graded from type 1 through type 6.
  • Type 1: radiographically normal as AC ligaments strained.
  • Type 2: AC joint can be mildly widened as AC ligaments torn and coracoclavicular ligaments strained.
  • Type 3: clavicle superiorly displaced and AC joint widened as AC and coracoclavicular ligaments torn as well as torn deltoid and trapezius insertions.
  • Type 4: same disruptions as type 3 but clavicle protrudes into or through trapezius on axillary view.
  • Type 5: same disruptions as Type 3 but clavicle in SC tissues.
  • Type 6: clavicle lies under coracoid or acromion.
▶ Types 1 and 2 placed in sling.
  • Pendulum exercises once pain-free
▶ Type 3 sometimes managed openly, especially if AC joint > 2 cm widened.
  • These should be referred to orthopedics within 72 hours.
▶ Type 4–6 managed in OR.

SCAPULAR FRACTURE

▶ Uncommon fracture generally caused by high-energy event often associated with other intrathoracic or cervical injuries.
▶ Scapular injuries classified by anatomic portion of scapula involved.

Clinical Presentation

▶ Many occur in context of multi-injured trauma victim.

▶ Painful with any movement of arm, also point tenderness, ecchymosis, crepitus.

Management

▶ High index of suspicion for other injuries.
▶ Surgical repair considered for displaced acromial fractures, displaced coracoid fractures, significantly displaced scapular neck, or glenoid fossa fractures.
▶ Scapulothoracic dissociation occurs when clavicle is disrupted, and scapula is displaced laterally with large soft tissue injury.
▶ Pendulum exercises and sling for uncomplicated scapular fractures.

SHOULDER DISLOCATION

▶ Anterior dislocation most common.
▶ Posterior dislocations most frequently follow seizures.
▶ Inferior dislocation rare with arm locked upward.
▶ Axillary nerve injury occurs in 25% of patients.
   • Test for sensation of lateral shoulder and ability to flex/contract deltoid.
   • Risk of permanent damage decreased by expeditious reduction.
▶ Fracture occurs in significant percentage, more common in elderly or first dislocation.
   • Hill-Sachs deformity is compression of humeral head.
   • Less commonly, fractures occur at anterior glenoid or greater tuberosity avulsions.
▶ Rotator cuff tears common in elderly.

Clinical Presentation

▶ Empty glenoid usually palpable and even visible on thin patients.
▶ Affected arm generally supported by good arm, slight external rotation.
▶ In posterior dislocation, arm cannot be externally rotated and abduction difficult.

Management

▶ Axillary view can help confirm anterior or posterior position; however, if too uncomfortable for patient, Y-view scapula view will demonstrate anterior dislocations as medial to scapula.

▶ Conscious sedation is usually necessary; however, local anesthesia probably under-utilized.

- Any hemarthrosis is aspirated from a posterior approach and then glenoid filled with 20 cc of 1% lidocaine and allowed to absorb over 15–20 minutes.

▶ Cooper maneuver: slowly flex shoulder to horizontal with gentle traction then abduct with outward traction.

▶ Stimson maneuver: patient lies prone with dislocated arm hanging off bed with 10-lb weight attached and allowed to self-reduce.

▶ Scapular manipulation: after failure of Stimson maneuver, brace medial and superior aspect while inferior tip is rotated medially; downward traction may be applied to humerus as well.

▶ Leidelmeyer maneuver: with patient sitting, elbow is flexed to 90 degrees, arm externally rotated, and then abducted.

▶ Traction-countertraction: bed sheet wrapped under dislocated shoulder's axilla and traction applied to sheet by assistant and to the dislocated arm until muscles eventually fatigue.

▶ Post-reduction film and neurologic exam to rule out fracture or neurologic injury.

▶ Once reduced, sling and swath, and follow-up in orthopedic clinic.

▶ Posterior and inferior dislocations: reduction should be discussed with orthopedics.

ROTATOR CUFF INJURY

▶ The rotator cuff initiates motion at shoulder and then stabilizes it as more powerful muscles take over.

▶ Frequently, overuse plays role in both acute and chronic injury.

Clinical Features

▶ Complete tear associated with inability to abduct arm without tilting body to side of lesion

▶ Frequently, point tenderness at insertion point at head of humerus

▶ Must be suspected in patients who cannot abduct arm following reduction of shoulder dislocation

Management

▶ Sling, analgesia, and refer to orthopedics for surgical repair

HUMERUS FRACTURE

▶ Humeral head fracture common, especially in the elderly following falls.
▶ Younger patients are more likely to have humeral shaft fractures.

Clinical Features

▶ Bony point tenderness, pain with arm movement
▶ Radial nerve in close proximity to proximal third of posterior humerus, necessitating careful neurologic exam
▶ Radial nerve sensation to lateral palm, motor for elbow/wrist/finger extension

Management

▶ Most fractures can be treated conservatively with sling and swath if minimally displaced.
▶ Fractures through greater tuberosity may require surgery.
▶ Most comminuted fractures of the head require surgery.
▶ Shaft fractures angulated > 20 degrees may require reduction.
▶ If splinting is necessary, a co-adaptation splint extends from axilla, down medial arm, around flexed elbow, and back up to shoulder. For maximal stability, a posterior splint may be added.

CHAPTER 139

PELVIC FRACTURES

Matthew J. Greenberg

► Pelvic fractures are most often associated with high-energy blunt trauma such as MVAs, motor vehicle–pedestrian accidents, motorcycle crashes, and falls from > 15 ft.
► Pelvic fractures are markers for high morbidity and mortality with a concurrent incidence of intra-abdominal or bladder injury in 11–20% of patients.

CLINICAL EXAMINATION

► Initial assessment and stabilization of ABCs with care taken to protect the spine.
► Standard fluid resuscitation utilizing two large-bore peripheral or central venous access is appropriate.
► Evaluation of pelvic stability should be assessed with both bilateral downward and lateral pressure applied to the iliac crests.
► Once a pelvis has been determined to be unstable, no further checks should occur.
► Rectal exam to determine the position of the prostate (if applicable) and presence of blood.
► Inspection of the gluteal cleft and perineum for evidence of a laceration, possibly indicating an open fracture.
► Ecchymosis and/or swelling of the scrotum should be documented in men as an indicator of pelvic bleeding.
► Evaluation of the urethral meatus for blood indicative of urethral injury.
► Bimanual exam should be performed in all women with suspected pelvic fracture to assess for possible bone fragments or blood, indicating an open fracture.

DIAGNOSTIC IMAGING

► Numerous classification schemes for pelvic fractures exist.

▶ Adequate description based on radiographic appearance is the most useful means for communicating with orthopedic colleagues.

▶ Initial radiograph is the AP view.
- Provides an overall appearance of the pelvis in regard to symmetry and disruption of the pelvic ring and rami

▶ Inlet-outlet views provide enhanced visualization of the pelvic ring.

▶ Judet views (45 degrees anterior and posterior oblique) provide enhanced view of the acetabulum.

▶ Lateral sacral radiographs delineate sacral fractures.

▶ CT with 3D reconstruction provides greatly enhanced details of the pelvic bones and is now considered standard for operative planning.

▶ Angiography can be utilized to determine the presence of pelvic arterial bleeding and provide therapeutic embolization of bleeding vessels.

▶ Retrograde urethrograms (RUGs): consider in any patient with outward signs of urethral injury such as blood at the meatus, high-riding prostate, or ecchymosis of the scrotum.

MANAGEMENT

▶ External stabilization of the pelvis
- Can be done utilizing a sheet wrapped around the pelvis and secured anteriorly.
- Other devices such as MAST, vacuum splints, and traction bands can also be employed.
- Should be done early in management of unstable pelvic fractures as it can help to reduce active bleeding.
  ○ Approximately 90% of bleeding in pelvic fractures is venous.
- Further management will be dictated by the type of fracture and is generally managed by an orthopedic surgeon.
  ○ Options include both internal and external fixation.
- Consider angiography for diagnosis and embolization of possible arterial bleeding in the persistently hypotensive patient.

▶ **Associated urethral injuries**
- Seen in 5% of pelvic fractures.
- At particular risk are men with combined pubic rami fractures and sacroiliac disruption.

- RUGs should be performed to exclude urethral trauma prior to catheterization. See Chap. 85 for technique.

EMERGENCY DEPARTMENT DISPOSITION

▶ Consult with orthopedic and/or trauma surgeons, as these patients are generally admitted.

CHAPTER 140

HIP AND FEMUR FRACTURES

Sanjeev Malik

► Hip fractures are associated with significant morbidity and mortality.
  • Nearly 20% of patients never regain ambulation.
  • High morbidity rate, including DVT, PE, and pneumonia due to immobility.
  • Only 50–60% of patients able to regain previous level of activity.
► Advanced age and associated osteoporosis are the biggest risk factors for hip injuries.

CLINICAL PRESENTATION
History

► Traumatic mechanism, which may be minor in elderly
► Hip pain
► Inability to bear weight

Physical Exam

► ABCs and full trauma evaluation.
► Tachycardia and hypotension may be present secondary to associated injuries or significant blood loss in the thigh.
► Inspection for pallor, abrasions, ecchymoses, and deformity.
► ROM can be deferred until after radiography in obvious fractures.
► Wounds near the fracture site should be considered part of an open fracture until proven otherwise.
► Assess for neurovascular status distal to injury.
  • Thorough neurologic exam including pinprick sensation
  • Assessment of pulses
  • ABI as needed
    ○ < 0.9 requires further evaluation.

▶ Position of the leg
  • Shortened, externally rotated, and abducted → femoral neck fracture
  • Shortened and internally rotated → intertrochanteric fracture
  • Flexed, adducted, and internally rotated → posterior hip dislocations

EMERGENCY DEPARTMENT MANAGEMENT

Diagnosis

▶ ABCs and initial evaluation as per ATLS protocol
▶ IV access and fluid/colloid resuscitation as indicated
▶ Pre-op labs (CBC, chem-7, PT/PTT, T&S), ECG, CXR
▶ Analgesia: opiates preferred
▶ Plain films: AP/lateral hip ± internal rotation view, AP pelvis, Judet views, and AP/lateral femur
  • Shenton's line: smooth, curved line drawn along superior border of obturator foramen and medial aspect of femoral metaphysis.
  • Angle of inclination between lines drawn through center of femoral neck and line drawn through the center of the femoral shaft should be 120–130 degrees.
  • Disruption of these normal radiographic features suggests fracture or dislocation.
▶ CT: helpful to evaluate acetabular fractures
▶ MRI
  • Indicated in patients with negative plain films who cannot ambulate
  • Should typically be done as an inpatient
  • Very sensitive for non-displaced femoral neck fracture

Types of Fractures

▶ Hip and femur fractures are classified by location.
▶ Fractures should still be described in regard to the following:
  • Open vs. closed (open is an orthopedic emergency), location, displacement, angulation, shortening, and type (e.g., transverse, oblique, spiral, or comminuted)
▶ Femoral head fractures.
  • Most commonly associated with hip dislocations.

- Reduction should be urgent due to risk of AVN.
- Reduction should be performed in consultation with orthopedics.
► Femoral neck fractures.
- Fractures through the neck of the femur proximal to trochanteric line.
- Often difficult to see on plain film if non-displaced (15–20%).
  - Internal rotation view can sometimes be helpful.
- High incidence of AVN of femoral head (20%) due to disruption of femoral neck blood supply.
- Impacted, non-displaced fractures can be treated by two methods:
  - Non-operative therapy and early ambulation
  - ORIF
    - Overall prognosis is good: 96% heal without complication.
- All other femoral neck fractures (displaced or non-impacted) require ORIF.
► Intertrochanteric fractures.
- Fracture line between greater and lesser trochanters
- Excellent blood supply
  - Lower risk of AVN
  - Much higher risk of hemodynamic instability due to hemorrhage
  - Up to 70% of patients under-resuscitated
- High association with other injuries (spinal compression fractures, upper-extremity fractures, and rib fractures).
- Recommended treatment is operative with internal fixation.
- Half of patients will not return to previous level of ambulation.
► Trochanteric fractures.
- Rare isolated fracture of either the greater or lesser trochanter.
- May result from fall or avulsion by iliopsoas.
- Treatment is non-operative with early ambulation and analgesic control.
► Subtrochanteric fractures.
- Fractures of the proximal 5 cm of the femoral shaft distal to intertrochanteric line.
- Typically result from high-impact trauma or underlying pathologic bone.

- Avascular cortical bone in this region leads to high rate of non-union.
- Hemodynamic instability may be associated secondary to blood loss.
- Recommended treatment is operative with internal fixation.

▶ Femoral shaft fractures.
  - Typically high-impact trauma in young individuals.
  - High association with hemorrhage and hemodynamic instability.
  - Pre-hospital traction devices should be removed on arrival to prevent neurovascular injury.
  - High association with ligamentous injury to the knee.
  - Treatment is operative with intra-medullary rod.

▶ Hip dislocations.
  - 80–90% posterior, 10–20% anterior.
  - High-speed MVA with flexed knee striking the dashboard is common mechanism.
  - High rate of associated traumatic injuries.
  - True orthopedic emergency due to time-dependent risk of AVN (6 hours).
  - Reduction techniques (posterior):
    ○ Stimson: patient in prone position with hip and knee flexed 90 degrees
      ▪ Downward traction in line with femur.
      ▪ Assistant stabilizes pelvis and applies pressure to greater trochanter toward the acetabulum.
    ○ Allis: patient in supine position with knee in 90 degrees flexion
      ▪ In-line traction as hip is slowly brought to 90 degrees flexion.
      ▪ Assistant stabilizes pelvis and applies pressure to greater trochanter toward the acetabulum.

Disposition

▶ Most patients with hip or femur fractures require admission to the hospital and operative repair.
▶ Isolated trochanteric fractures in reliable patients can be safely discharged home.
▶ Inability to ambulate with normal X-rays is an indication for admission and further imaging (MRI).

CHAPTER 141

KNEE PAIN

Rahul K. Khare

▶ Although most patients presenting with knee pain are non-emergent, knee dislocation is a true orthopedic emergency.

▶ Soft tissue injury to the knee represents a common musculoskeletal disorder presenting to the ED.

▶ Most knee injuries can be discharged from the ED with a knee immobilizer, crutches, and close follow-up.

  • Many will require additional testing, such as an MRI, if pain does not resolve within a week.

  • Good discharge instructions are key to patients' expectations and understanding of their injury.

▶ MCL is the most frequently injured ligament of the knee.

▶ ACL damage causes the highest incidence of pathological joint instability.

SOFT TISSUE INJURY OF THE KNEE: ANTERIOR CRUCIATE LIGAMENT, MEDIAL COLLATERAL LIGAMENT
Clinical Presentation

History

▶ ACL tears

  • Patients complain of immediate, severe pain made worse with movement and inability to ambulate.

  • Many patients report a popping sensation or sound at the time of injury.

  • Associated with blows to a hyperextended knee, excessive non-contact hyperextension of the knee, or extreme deceleration forces to the knee.

  • Disruption of the ACL may occur with other knee injuries, especially meniscal or MCL tears.

▶ MCL tears

  • Classic history is of young male playing football tackled from side with blow to lateral aspect of knee.

- Clinical findings may be subtle even with complete injury.
- MCL provides primary restraint to valgus stress.
  - Valgus stress/impact causes MCL tears.
- Patients may be able to ambulate, but with significant pain.

Physical Exam
▶ Knee effusion occurs in 50% of patients who sustain an acute ligament rupture.
▶ ACL tears:
- The Lachman maneuver (variant of anterior drawer test) confirms ACL integrity.
  - Knee placed in 15 degrees of flexion and external rotation.
  - Examiner grabs the inner aspect of the calf and the outer aspect of the distal thigh.
  - In millimeters, quantify degree of displacement, comparing this to the normal side.
    - 0–5 mm laxity: mild
    - 6–10 mm laxity: moderate
    - 11–15 mm laxity: severe, consider concomitant MCL tear
▶ MCL tears:
- Valgus stress test
  - Place patient supine with thigh resting on edge of table.
  - Provide valgus stress by pressing on lateral aspect of knee with one hand, while the other hand directs the ankle laterally.
  - If there is a significant gap in the medial aspect of the knee joint, MCL impairment may be the cause of injury.

Emergency Department Management
▶ X-rays of the knee may or may not be useful.
- Ottawa knee rules: when to order knee films
  - Age 55 and older
  - Tenderness at head of fibula
  - Isolated tenderness of patella
  - Inability to flex knee to 90 degrees
  - Inability to walk four weight-bearing steps immediately after injury or in the ED

▶ Knee immobilizer and crutches are essential for ligamentous injuries in order to minimize damage and reduce pain and inflammation.

Disposition

▶ Referral to an orthopedic surgeon within a week is essential for timely surgical intervention, if needed.
▶ Outpatient MRI referral, if possible, may be helpful in expediting care.
▶ Patients can be safely discharged home with a knee immobilizer, crutches, and instruction of RICE.

KNEE DISLOCATION

▶ True orthopedic emergency.
▶ Must be reduced as soon as possible; do not wait for your consultant.
▶ Amputation may be necessary in patients who fail to get timely care or who are subjected to inappropriate treatment.
▶ Classification described with tibia in relation to femur.

Pathophysiology

▶ Anterior dislocations occur from hyperextension of knee.
▶ Injury to popliteal artery and vein may occur with this injury.
▶ Peroneal nerve injury may also occur.
▶ Ligamentous injury is common.

Clinical Presentation

History

▶ Patients present with severe pain and inability to bear weight.
▶ Mechanisms include
  • MVAs
  • Auto vs. pedestrian impact
  • Falls
  • Athletic injuries

Physical Exam

▶ Knee usually grossly deformed with swelling and immobility

▶ Neurovascular exam
- Palpation of femoral, popliteal, dorsalis pedis, and posterior tibial arteries must be done.
- ABI should also be performed on both lower extremities.
  - A discrepancy of even 0.1 is an indication for the patient to get an arteriogram.
  - Some advocate an arteriogram on all acute, first-time knee dislocations despite a normal neurovascular exam.
- Peroneal nerve injury occurs in 25–35% of patients and manifests with decreased sensation at the first webspace of foot and impaired dorsiflexion.

Emergency Department Management

▶ ABCs, IV, and monitoring should be done for sedation.
▶ Adequate analgesia and conscious sedation required for reduction.
▶ Reduction of knee should be done emergently if vascular impairment occurs.
- Reduction is performed by longitudinal traction.
▶ X-rays may be done if vascular impairment is not present; this may help with diagnosing fractures.
▶ Arteriography may be done to rule out vascular injuries.

Disposition

▶ May go home if there is no need for operation and no vascular injury.
▶ After reduction, place patient in splint, crutches, RICE, and follow up with an orthopedic surgeon with referral for an MRI to help determine other ligamentous injures.

CHAPTER 142

ANKLE INJURIES

George M. Elliott

- ▶ Inversion (most common): due to relative weakness of lateral ligaments and the shorter medial malleolus.
- ▶ Eversion: generally more severe than inversion with greater joint instability.
- ▶ Other common fracture types are described in Table 142-1.
- ▶ The Weber classification (Table 142-2) can be used to classify fibular fractures according to their location and appearance.

CLINICAL PRESENTATION

- ▶ Recent injury with pain, swelling, deformity, and difficulty ambulating
- ▶ Decreased ROM

Physical Exam

- ▶ Obvious deformity.
- ▶ Malleolar tenderness: check anterior and posterior portions of both malleoli.
- ▶ ROM.
- ▶ Always do a complete neurovascular exam evaluating capillary refill and the dorsalis pedis and posterior tibial pulses.
- ▶ Always examine the entire extremity including ROM of the knee and hip. Beware referred pain from a knee or hip injury.

EMERGENCY DEPARTMENT MANAGEMENT

- ▶ Immobilization via Jones dressing or pillow splint while in the department.
- ▶ Ice and elevation to minimize swelling.
- ▶ Analgesia.

TABLE 142-1.
OTHER COMMON FRACTURES

Name	Description	Mechanism	Stable?	Notes
Pilon fracture	Distal tibial metaphysis fracture combined with disruption of the talar dome	Axial load	No	Immediate orthopedic consultation
Maisonneuve fracture	Proximal one-third fibular and medial malleolar fracture + disruption of syndesmosis	Eversion or external rotation	No	Cast if stable, OR repair if unstable. Immediate orthopedic consultation
Bimalleolar fractures	At least two elements of the ankle ring	—	No	Immediate orthopedic consultation
Trimalleolar	Medial, lateral, and posterior malleoli fractures	—	No	Immediate orthopedic consultation

▶ Imaging: three-view radiograph (AP, mortise, and lateral) of the affected joint; also consider films of the foot and knee.
  • CT, MRI, and bone scan are occasionally used but have limited utility in the ED.
▶ Ottawa ankle rules: obtain ankle/foot radiographs in patients with acute injury plus one of the following:
  • Tenderness at the posterior edge or tip of the medial malleolus
  • Tenderness at the posterior edge or tip of the lateral malleolus
  • Inability to bear weight both immediately and in the ED
  • Tenderness at the base of the fifth metatarsal, navicular, or cuboid
▶ IV antibiotics for open fracture.
▶ Immediate orthopedic consult for all unstable or open fractures or those needing operative repair; also consider vascular consult for pulseless fractures.

TABLE 142-2.
WEBER CLASSIFICATION ACCORDING TO LOCATION AND APPEARANCE OF FIBULAR FRACTURE

Name	Description	Mechanism	Stable?	Notes
Weber A	Transverse fibular avulsion fracture distal to tibiotalar joint.	Internal rotation and adduction	Yes	Non-operative management
Weber B	Oblique fracture of the lateral malleolus at level of the tibiotalar joint ± rupture of the tibiofibular syndesmosis and medial injury.	Supination and external rotation	± Depending on amount of medial involvement	Most common type of fibular fracture. Usually operative repair
Weber C	Fibular fracture above tibiotalar joint with rupture of the tibiofibular ligament and transverse fracture of the medial malleolus. Usually syndesmotic injury is more extensive than in type B.	Adduction or abduction with external rotation	No	Operative repair

▶ Reduction: usually performed by orthopedic consultants, but immediate reduction should be performed by the emergency physician for significant tenting or absent pulses; should be performed under conscious sedation.

▶ Splint vs. cast: generally performed via a non-circumferential splint such as a posterior splint or sugar tong to allow for swelling. Cast placed by orthopedist at a later date.

▶ Discharge planning: immobilization, crutches, non–weight-bearing, pain control, warning signs for compartment syndrome, and rest, ice, and elevation.

▶ Follow-up: be sure patient has close follow-up scheduled with orthopedics.

　• Special situations: elderly patients, those with many stairs who live alone, etc., may need extra assistance.

▶ Long-term complications include post-reduction arthritis (30%), chronic pain, reflex sympathetic dystrophy, and poor/malunion.

CHAPTER 143

THE PAINFUL JOINT

Candice A. Sobanski

► Septic joints are associated with significant morbidity and mortality and should be considered in all patients with joint pain.

SEPTIC ARTHRITIS

► Hematogenous spread is the most common etiology.
► Cartilage destruction begins as early as 20 hours after initial insult (residual joint damage is 30–50%).
► Patients with pre-existing joint disease, immunosuppression, IV drug abuse, or prosthetic joints are at an increased risk.
► Most common bacteria are *Staphylococcus aureus* followed by *Streptococcus* species.

Clinical Presentation

► Monoarticular joint pain, effusion, and erythema.
► Pain with active and passive ROM.
► Fevers and other constitutional symptoms.
► In the pediatric population, the parents will complain that a preverbal child is not ambulating or using an extremity pseudo-paralysis.
► May have more subtle presentation if immunocompromised.

Management

► Diagnosis is based on clinical exam and arthrocentesis results.
► If there is any suspicion for infection, a joint aspiration should be done for culture, Gram's stain, cell count, and crystal analysis.
  • A positive Gram's stain and/or culture is indicative of a septic joint.
  • A WBC count of the synovial fluid > 50,000 with a predominance of PMN cells suggests a bacterial infection, but this is not an absolute cut-off number. Many infected joints have < 50,000 WBC.

- Crystals indicate a crystal deposition process such as gout.
▶ Elevated WBC, ESR, and CRP may help support diagnosis.
▶ Blood culture should be sent to assist in organism identification.
▶ X-ray of the joint is usually not helpful for diagnosis, but baseline films are often requested by consultants.
  - Can be done to evaluate for osteomyelitis
▶ If there is a high suspicion for septic joint or a positive aspirate, patients should be admitted for IV antibiotic therapy and/or operative wash-out of joint.
  - IV antibiotics should be started.
    ○ Nafcillin, 1.5–2 g IV q4h, or cefazolin, 1 g IV q8h
  - An orthopedic surgeon should be consulted.

GOUT AND PSEUDO-GOUT

▶ Most commonly observed in men in their 40s–50s.
▶ Gout is the result of the deposition of uric acid crystals within the joint space.
▶ Pseudo-gout is from the deposition of calcium pyrophosphate crystals.
▶ Crystals lead to an inflammatory reaction within the joint space.
▶ Decreased clearance of uric acid by the kidneys or increased purine intake with certain foods can lead to hyperuricemia, which, over time, can cause crystal formation and deposition.
▶ Other risk factors include ETOH, diuretics, obesity, and FH.

Clinical Presentation

▶ Acute pain occurring over 12–24 hours, most commonly in great toe (classically at first MTP joint) or ankle.
▶ Edema and erythema at joint site.
▶ Pain with ROM of joint.
▶ Advanced gouty arthritis may have tophi present, which are nodules of uric acid deposition under the skin near joints and ear cartilage.
▶ May or may not have elevated blood uric acid levels (not sensitive or specific).

Management

▶ Diagnosis is based on history and clinical exam. Often patients with a history of gout can tell you that their pain is similar to previous episodes of gout.

- Must do a complete history and thorough joint exam to exclude other etiologies of acute joint pain, including septic arthritis.
- If uncertain about the diagnosis, joint aspiration should be done to evaluate for septic joint.
- Gout therapy: NSAIDs, such as indomethacin, ibuprofen, or naproxen, will decrease the joint inflammation.
- Indomethacin, 50 mg PO tid.
- Colchicine can be used for acute attacks if cannot tolerate NSAIDs.
  - Colchicine, 0.6 mg PO q1h, not to exceed 3 mg/day.
  - Side effects include diarrhea and abdomen pain or cramping.
- To reduce uric acid levels, allopurinol or probenecid may be used on a daily basis and may decrease future gouty attacks but should not be started in ED.
- Patients can usually be discharged to home with outpatient management and follow-up.

DISSEMINATED GONOCOCCAL ARTHRITIS

- In the U.S., approximately 600,000 new localized gonorrhea infections diagnosed every year.
- Approximately 1–2% of gonorrhea infections become disseminated with joint or tendon pain as the chief complaint.
- Always consider in young patients with new-onset arthritis and history of unprotected intercourse.

Clinical Presentation

- Polyarticular, migratory arthritis is present in 66% of patients.
- Fevers may be present.
- Diffuse rash in 25% of patients.
- May not have symptoms of local gonorrhea infection at time of disseminated symptoms.
- May have signs of meningitis or endocarditis if severe infection present.

Management

- Culture all possible sites of mucosal infection for both gonorrhea and chlamydia.
- Pain control with NSAIDs and narcotic medications.
- Joint aspiration is necessary for diagnosis; send for Gram's stain, culture, cell count, and crystals.

► Ceftriaxone, 1 g IV qd.
► Disseminated gonorrhea should be admitted for IV antibiotic therapy until symptom improvement.
► Partners should also be treated.

REACTIVE ARTHRITIS
► Either an acute or insidious systemic illness characterized by aseptic joint inflammation.
► Occurs in reaction to a prior bacterial illness of the GU or gastroenteric tract in genetically susceptible people.
► HLA-B27 present in 72–84% of cases of reactive arthritis.
► Typical infections that will lead to reactive arthritis include *Chlamydia*, *Salmonella*, *Shigella*, *Campylobacter*, and *Yersinia*.

Clinical Presentation
► Asymmetric, polyarticular joint pain with predominance in the lower extremities.
► Other symptoms such as skin lesions, conjunctivitis, cervicitis, urethritis, and cystitis are variably present.

Management
► Complete history and physical with special attention on preceding GI or GU illnesses within last 7–28 days.
► It is often difficult to determine a reactive arthritis from a septic arthritis.
► Consider joint aspiration for cell count, culture, Gram's stain, and crystals to evaluate for other etiologies of joint pain.
► If patient has history of recent diarrhea or cervical or urethral illness, obtain cultures of stool, cervix, and urethra, respectively.
► ESR and CRP to evaluate for systemic inflammation, variably elevated.
► Pain and inflammation control with NSAIDs: prolonged course often needed.
► Referral to rheumatologist for further evaluation and other arthritis disease–modifying therapies.
► Disposition is home with primary care physician and rheumatologic referral.

CHAPTER 144

COMPARTMENT SYNDROME

Jolie C. Holschen

► A true orthopedic emergency: limb- and potentially life-threatening

PATHOPHYSIOLOGY

► Increased pressure within a closed fascial space resulting in decreased perfusion pressure and eventual cell injury and death to neural and muscular tissues.
► Mechanism: hypoxia leads to cell injury, release of mediators, and increased endothelial permeability resulting in edema, further increasing compartment pressure, tissue pH falls, further necrosis, and release of myoglobin.
► Tissue pressure > capillary pressure; usually occurs at > 30 mmHg intra-compartmental pressure.
► Ischemic time: nerve < 4 hours, muscle < 4 hours; some say up to 6 hours.
► Locations: hand, forearm, upper arm, abdomen, buttock, thigh, leg, and foot.

CLINICAL PRESENTATION

► Pain out of proportion to injury
► Physical exam
  • Evidence of tense compartment
  • Decreased perfusion (capillary refill, pain)
  • Loss of tissue function (numbness and weakness: nerve and muscle involved in affected compartment)

DIFFERENTIAL DIAGNOSIS

► See Table 144-1.

TABLE 144-1.
DIFFERENTIAL DIAGNOSIS OF COMPARTMENT SYNDROME

Necrotizing fasciitis
Rhabdomyolysis
Neurapraxia
Arterial injury
Tenosynovitis
Gas gangrene
DVT

EMERGENCY DEPARTMENT MANAGEMENT
Diagnosis

▶ Acute/classic compartment syndrome:
- Examples: secondary to burn, soft tissue swelling, tight dressing, reperfusion ischemia, prolonged compression (lying on limb or improper casting), IV infiltration, hemorrhage, vascular injury, envenomation, seizures, and trauma: knee dislocation, long bone fracture (tibial plateau, supracondylar, hand), and crush injury.
- 5 Ps:
  - Pain (with passive extension or stretch)
  - Paresthesia (burning, etc.)
  - Pallor
  - Pulselessness
  - Paralysis
- Ischemia and necrosis can occur even in the presence of a pulse.
- Sensory nerves affected first, followed by motor.
- Timing: symptoms may develop hours to days after the insult.
▶ Consider clinical scenario: CBC, CPK, UA, X-ray, and ultrasound to rule out DVT.
▶ Definitive diagnosis is made by measuring compartment pressures.

Compartment Pressure Testing

▶ Needle techniques
- Simple needle (artificially high values)
- Stryker needle (preferred method)
- Arterial line transducer monitoring systems
▶ Procedure
- Sterilize skin, local anesthesia.

- Conscious sedation if patient unable to hold still or is unco-operative; muscle contraction falsely elevates pressure.
- Appropriate positioning: no external compression that may falsely elevate pressure readings.
- Place extremity at level of the heart, supine or prone.
- Introduce needle perpendicular and inject 0.3 cc sterile saline and note the pressure after equalization.
- Take compartment measurements close to injury site.
- Pay attention to position of extremity. Position should generally be neutral.
- Confirm placement of needle by seeing rise in pressure with digital compression of compartment, contraction of muscle, or passive stretch of muscle.

► Needle placement for lower leg
- Draw a line between proximal and middle one-third of tibia. About this line, all compartments will be tested. Patient is lying supine, with leg at level of heart.
- *Anterior compartment*: place needle 1 cm lateral to the anterior border of the tibia perpendicular to skin to depth of 1–3 cm.
- *Lateral compartment*: place needle anterior to posterior border of fibula directed toward the fibula to depth of 1 cm.
- *Deep posterior compartment*: place needle posterior to medial border of tibia and direct toward the posterior border of the fibula to depth of 2–4 cm.
- *Superficial posterior compartment:* place patient prone for this compartment. Place needle 3 cm lateral to midline of calf on either side to depth of 2–4 cm.

► Results
- Normal: resting pressure < 4 mmHg
- Abnormal: pressure > 30 mmHg

Treatment

► Remove offending compression.
► O$_2$.
► Keep extremities level with heart.
► Urgent orthopedic or surgery consultation.
► Fasciotomy:
- Indications (acute compartment syndrome): compartment pressure > 30 mmHg.

- A surgeon should do the fasciotomy; however, in limbs in which pressures increase or there is a delay to surgery, emergent fasciotomy may need to be performed in the ED.
▶ Complications:
  - Permanent nerve damage, myonecrosis, deformity, infection, loss of limb, rhabdomyolysis, ARF, Volkmann's ischemic contracture, and death

Disposition

▶ All patients with compartment syndrome should be admitted to a surgical service.

CHAPTER 145

LOW BACK PAIN

Jacob MacKenzie

- 90% of LBP is musculoskeletal, and patients recover in 4–6 weeks.
- Serious causes of LBP are uncommon, and usually red flags in either history or exam alert the physician (Table 145-1).
- LBP is acute when present for < 6 weeks, subacute when present for 6–12 weeks, and chronic when present for > 12 weeks.

DIFFERENTIAL DIAGNOSIS
- See Table 145-2.

MUSCULOSKELETAL LOW BACK PAIN
- Most common diagnosis for back pain.
- Definitive diagnosis is rarely reached, and the exact pathophysiology is often unclear.
- Usually attributable to musculoligamentous injury and/or degenerative changes.

Clinical Presentation
- History usually yields trauma or some mechanical history.
  - Lifting/twisting while holding heavy object
  - Operating machine that vibrates
  - Prolonged sitting (e.g., long-distance truck driver)
  - MVA in recent history
- Classically a fairly acute onset of pain described as a dull aching made worse with movement and better with rest.
- Patients often have a previous history of LBP.
- May radiate to buttocks or thighs but should not extend below the knee.

TABLE 145-1.
RED FLAGS IN THE HISTORY OF LBP

Fever/chills, recent bacterial infection, IV drug abuse, diabetes/immunocompromised
Pain that worsens with rest or supine position
History of cancer, weight loss
Progressive neurologic deficits, including bowel/bladder incontinence, urinary retention, major motor weakness, perianal/perineal sensory loss

▶ Review of system is crucial in ruling out other causes.
- Bowel or bladder dysfunction, weakness
- Medical history (recent diagnosis of cancer)
▶ Physical exam should include a full neurologic exam with strength, sensory, gait, palpation of spine, and documentation of anal sphincter tone and sensation.

Management

▶ Analgesia may require parenteral therapy if severe pain or spasm.
- Ibuprofen, 600 mg PO q8h PRN pain
- Acetaminophen (APAP)/hydrocodone, 500 mg/5 mg 1–2 tabs PO q6h PRN pain
- Diazepam, 5 mg PO q6h PRN muscle spasm
▶ Indications for radiographic imaging:
- Trauma

TABLE 145-2.
DIFFERENTIAL DIAGNOSIS OF LBP

Musculoskeletal
Sciatica/lumbosacral radiculopathy
Fracture
Infection (osteomyelitis, discitis, epidural abscess)
Spinal cord compression (cord compression, cauda equina syndrome, conus medullaris syndrome)
Spinal stenosis
Herpes zoster
Abdominal pathology (AAA, renal colic, appendicitis, pancreatitis, biliary disease)
Pelvic disease (PID, ovarian cyst or torsion)
Prostatitis
Pulmonary disease (pneumonia, PE)
Bony metastasis
Inflammatory arthritis

- Age > 60 years, < 15 years
- History of cancer, immunocompromise, or fever
- Duration > 6 weeks

▶ Heat or ice application may be helpful and can be used to manage symptoms.

▶ Most patients can be discharged home with outpatient follow-up in a primary care setting to ensure recovery.

▶ Rarely, patients with severe pain that does not respond to IV narcotics are admitted for pain control.

SCIATICA

▶ Sciatica is a term used to describe LBP with symptoms of lower lumbar/sacral nerve root irritation (radicular pain or sensory deficits below the knee).

▶ Usually due to disc disease; rarely due to tumor or infection.

Clinical Presentation

▶ Leg symptoms often more prominent than back pain.

▶ Severity of pain variable but often worse than in other causes of LBP.

▶ As 95% of disc herniations occur at the L4-L5 (L5 nerve root) and L5-S1 (S1 nerve root) levels, pain typically extends below the knee in a dermatomal distribution.

▶ SLR (80–95% sensitivity) and crossed-SLR testing (25% sensitive, 90% specific) generally positive with disc herniation.

▶ Anal sphincter tone and bowel and bladder control should be normal.

▶ Decreased sensation in a dermatomal distribution, altered deep tendon reflexes, and motor weakness may be present (Table 145-3).

TABLE 145-3.
NERVE ROOT INVOLVEMENT AND EXAM FINDINGS

Nerve root	Motor exam	Functional test
L3	Extend quadriceps	Squat down and rise
L4	Dorsiflex ankle	Walk on heels
L5	Dorsiflex great toe	Walk on heels
S1	Stand on toes	Walk on toes

Management

▶ Most patients can be discharged home with outpatient follow-up, as 80% will improve with conservative treatment.

▶ Sciatica accompanied by significant or rapidly progressive neurologic deficits will need an MRI and should have urgent specialty referral.

▶ Treatment is similar to that for musculoskeletal LBP.

LUMBAR SPINAL STENOSIS

▶ Most often caused by spondylosis of the lumbar spine

▶ Usually disease of the elderly female (onset late 50s to early 60s)

▶ Most often occurs at the L4-L5 (L5 root) and L3-L4 (L4 root) levels

Clinical Presentation

▶ Early in natural history, pain is like non-specific LBP but more insidious in onset.

▶ Later, pain is usually present in the low back, buttocks, and thighs and is described as an ache and stiffness that worsens with lumbar extension and is relieved with flexion.

▶ Can progress to cauda equina syndrome (CES).

▶ Back is usually non-tender and SLR testing negative.

▶ Atrophy, weakness, or sensory deficits may be present.

Management

▶ In the absence of serious neurologic deficits or significant findings on plain films, most patients can be discharged home with symptomatic treatment and outpatient follow-up.

INFECTION: OSTEOMYELITIS, DISCITIS, AND EPIDURAL ABSCESS

▶ Usually result from hematogenous source but can be due to local procedures.

▶ Originates in the disc in children and the vertebral body in adults.

▶ Causative organisms: *Staphylococcus aureus* (most common), gram-negative rods (post-operative/procedure or immunocompromised), *Pseudomonas* (IV drug abuse), *Mycobacterium tuberculosis* (rare in U.S.).

▶ Risk factors include diabetes (18–25% of those with pyogenic spinal infection), immunocompromise, elderly age, dialysis, IV drug abuse, malignancy, spinal fracture, paraplegia, endocarditis, pneumonia, UTI, urogenital procedures, spinal surgery, and sickle cell disease.

Clinical Presentation

▶ Pain (97%) that is localized and has gradually progressed is most consistent symptom.
▶ 50% of diagnosed cases have had > 3 months of pain.
▶ Post-operative infection usually occurs after 14–30 days.
▶ Fever (50% of osteomyelitis and 83% of epidural abscess) is often present.
▶ Spinal tenderness and limited ROM are usually present.
▶ Neurologic deficit present in ≤ 15% at presentation.

Management

▶ In the patient with concern for spinal infection, orthopedic consult and imaging with MRI are indicated.
▶ Epidural abscess treated with emergent surgery.
▶ Antibiotics should be started if suspicious for infectious etiology.
▶ Any patient with evidence of spinal infection should be admitted.

CAUDA EQUINA SYNDROME

▶ Caused by compression of the cauda equina (herniation of disc, spinal stenosis, trauma, tumor, hematoma, or abscess)

Clinical Presentation

▶ Classic symptoms are mild to moderate back pain with bilateral sciatica, saddle anesthesia or hypoesthesia, and lower-extremity weakness and sensory changes associated with bowel or bladder dysfunction.
▶ Urinary retention is 90% sensitive and 95% specific for CES.
▶ Absence of large (> 100 ml) post-void residual has 99.9% negative predictive value for CES.
▶ Exam is variable (especially in early disease), but weakness, sensory, and reflex deficits are usually present bilaterally (can also be unilateral).

► Decreased anal sphincter tone is often present due to compression of multiple sacral roots.

Management

► Patients with suspected CES require early spine surgery consultation and an emergent MRI (scan the entire spine if neoplasm suspected).
► Disposition is per the results of the MRI.
► Post-void residuals may be helpful in borderline cases but should not be relied upon if suspicion for CES is high; always obtain imaging.

CHAPTER 146

APPROACH TO PSYCHIATRIC EMERGENCIES

Marc Olson and Sara Chakel

▶ Psychosis is an alteration of mental status characterized by abnormal thought processes and behavior. Patients have difficulty recognizing reality.
  • This can involve a variety of symptoms, including delusions, hallucinations, and disordered patterns of thought and behavior.
  • Patients have little or no insight or understanding of their abnormal behaviors.
▶ **Delusion:** an idea or belief that is maintained despite irrefutable evidence to the contrary.
▶ **Hallucination:** false perception.
  • Visual hallucinations more common in delirium
  • Auditory hallucinations more common in primary psychiatric disorders
▶ **Psychosis** is usually divided into two broad categories:
  • **Organic psychosis (or delirium):** dysfunction resulting from an abnormality of the anatomy, physiology, or biochemistry of the brain
    ○ Organic etiology is suggested by new onset of symptoms in a patient > 35 years old, rapid onset of symptoms in a previously normal person, visual hallucinations, abnormal vital signs, and lethargy or disorientation.
  • **Functional psychosis:** dysfunction in which no chemical, structural, or physiologic abnormality of brain function can be identified

DIFFERENTIAL DIAGNOSIS
▶ See Table 146-1.

TABLE 146-1.
DIFFERENTIAL DIAGNOSIS OF PSYCHIATRIC EMERGENCIES

Mnemonic for differential of acute psychosis: **TOD'S TIPS**
  Trauma: head injury, intracranial hemorrhage
  Organ dysfunction/failure: thyroid disease, DKA, porphyria,
    pneumonia, MI/ACS
  Drugs: illicit drugs, anticholinergics, anti-emetics, antibiotics, many
    others
  Structural lesions: brain tumor, cerebral abscess
  Toxins: CO toxicity, heavy metals, plants, herbal medications
  Infection: meningitis, encephalitis, HIV/AIDS, tertiary syphilis
  Psychiatric: depression with psychotic features, schizophrenia
  Substrate deficiency: hypoxia, hypoglycemia, B_{12} or folate
    deficiency

CLINICAL PRESENTATION

History

▸ Obtain from patient, family members, caregivers, paramedics,
  and past medical records.

- History of present illness: gradual/abrupt onset of symptoms, duration and fluctuation of symptoms, history of
  trauma, suspected toxic ingestion.

- Ask about hallucinations and delusions.

- Past history: baseline mental status, prior similar symptoms, and underlying medical and psychiatric disease.

- Medications: recent changes in medications or dosage; psychoactive medications.

- Social history: functional status, support system, and substance use.

Physical Exam

▸ General appearance and behavior.

▸ Vital signs are usually normal. Transient tachycardia or HTN
  caused in acutely agitated, but persistent abnormalities need to
  be explained.

▸ Mental status: affect and mood, thought content and process,
  perceptions, insight and judgement, and suicidal or homicidal
  ideation.

▶ Neurologic exam: orientation, mini-mental state examination, cranial nerves, motor and sensory function, reflexes, coordination, and gait.

DIAGNOSIS

▶ Based primarily on history and exam
▶ **Laboratory tests**
  • CBC with platelets, serum electrolytes, BUN, creatinine, ethanol level, UA, and urine drug screen
▶ **Radiographic tests**
  • Non-contrast head CT: obtain on all patients with suspected traumatic injury or focal neurologic findings.

TREATMENT

▶ Begin with the ABCs, including C-spine immobilization if history of trauma.
▶ Removal and storage of personal effects are essential for safety of the patient and staff.
▶ All staff members should approach the patient with a calm and reassuring demeanor.
▶ Patients who are agitated or violent may require restraints to assure safety of staff and themselves.
  • Physical restraints have a high rate of morbidity for ED patients.
  • Strict adherence to a protocol including frequent re-evaluation of the restrained patient is critical to prevent complications from restraint devices.
  • Restrained patients should be on continuous monitoring, including pulse oximetry, to minimize risk.
▶ Medical therapy: antipsychotics and benzodiazepines may be used separately or together for treatment of the acutely agitated patient.
  • Antipsychotics: haloperidol, risperidone, and olanzapine.
  • Benzodiazepines: lorazepam.
  • Common initial dosing for agitated patient:
    ○ Haloperidol, 5 mg IM × 1, **with**
    ○ Lorazepam, 1–2 mg IM × 1, **or**
    ○ Olanzapine, 10–20 mg IM alone
  • Known psychiatric patients may only need a dose of their antipsychotic medication if non-compliance is suspected.

DISPOSITION

▶ Discharge: patients with known psychiatric illness for whom follow-up can be arranged and who do not pose a risk to themselves or others.

▶ Psychiatric consultation: obtain if uncertain of safety, diagnosis, disposition, or follow-up in patients with a known or suspected primary psychiatric disorder.

▶ Medical admission: delirious patients require admission for further diagnosis, treatment, and frequent re-evaluation.

  • Definitive treatment of delirium results from identification and correction of the underlying disorder.

◖ **PEARLS AND PITFALLS**

  • The most common pitfall is failure to consider and carefully evaluate organic etiologies of psychosis, especially in patients with a known history of psychotic symptoms and in patients with co-existing substance abuse.

    ○ Infection, electrolyte abnormalities, and medication complications are all common.

  • Patients with psychosis have a high rate of suicide.

    ○ Nearly half will attempt, and 10% succeed.

    ○ Attempts often come when patients are improving and recover some insight into the gravity of their illness.

CHAPTER 147

DEPRESSION

Ellen C. Walkling

▶ Depression:
- Nearly 20% of the population will have an episode of major depression during their lifetime.
- 30% of adults over 60 have symptoms.

▶ Suicide:
- Third most common cause of death in those aged 15–24.
- Up to two-thirds of patients who commit suicide had visited a physician in the prior month.

▶ Primary risk factors for major depressive disorder include
- Female gender
- History of depression in first-degree relatives
- Prior episodes of major depression
- Remote FH of depressive disorder
- Lack of social support
- Significant stressful life events
- Current alcohol and/or substance abuse
- Chronic pain and/or chronic disease

CLINICAL PRESENTATION

▶ Vague physical symptoms
- Weakness, headache, non-specific complaints of pain

▶ Recurrent negative thoughts
- Depressed mood, sleep disturbance, change in appetite, altered level of activity, anhedonia

DIFFERENTIAL DIAGNOSIS

▶ See Table 147-1.

TABLE 147-1.
DIFFERENTIAL DIAGNOSIS OF DEPRESSION

Hypothyroidism	Hypokalemia
Adrenal insufficiency	Hyponatremia
Cushing's syndrome	Anxiety
Hypocalcemia	Medications, multiple
Substance abuse	Steroids
Alzheimer's disease	Beta-blockers

EMERGENCY DEPARTMENT MANAGEMENT
Diagnosis

▶ To make the *Diagnostic and Statistical Manual of Mental Disorders*, 4th edition, diagnosis of depression (IN SAD CAGES), at least five (including either depressed mood or loss of interest) of the following symptoms must be present daily for a minimum of 2 weeks:
  - **In**terest (diminished interest or pleasure in almost all activities)
  - **S**leep (insomnia or hypersomnia)
  - **A**ppetite (significant weight loss or gain)
  - **D**epressed mood
  - **C**oncentration (impaired concentration, indecisiveness)
  - **A**ctivity (psychomotor agitation or retardation)
  - **G**uilt (feelings of worthlessness or guilt)
  - **E**nergy (fatigue or loss of energy)
  - **S**uicide (recurring thoughts of death or suicide)
▶ These symptoms must not be due to
  - Effects of a substance (medication, alcohol, or illegal drugs)
  - Any medical condition or within 2 months of the loss of a loved one
▶ **Suicide risk factors (SAD PERSONS):**
  - All patients who are being evaluated for depression should also be evaluated for suicidality.
  - ≥ Six positive answers and patient should be considered at increased risk of suicide.
    ○ **S**ex (male)
    ○ **A**ge (< 19 or > 45)
    ○ **D**epression
    ○ **P**revious suicide attempt
    ○ **E**xcessive drugs or alcohol
    ○ **R**ational thinking loss

- ○ **S**eparated, divorced, or widowed
- ○ **O**rganized attempt at suicide (as opposed to gesture)
- ○ **N**o social support
- ○ **S**tated future intent
- ▶ Be direct in questioning about mood and suicidality.
- ▶ Gather visual as well as verbal information.
- ▶ Interview family members (alone if needed), EMS, and others.
- ▶ Prediction of suicide risk: SAD PERSONS mnemonic.
- ▶ If admission likely, many inpatient units will want screening of CBC, chemistries, drug screen, and alcohol level.

Treatment and Disposition

- ▶ Identify and treat any physiological factors that may be contributing.
- ▶ Assess for suicidality and for ability to function at home.
  - • If patient has suicidal ideations, patient should be hospitalized with his or her consent or via emergency commitment unless a clear-cut means to assure the patient's safety exists while outpatient treatment is begun.
  - • May require legal certification that the patient is in need of emergency evaluation and protective observation.
  - • A child who is suicidal should be admitted until medical and social services can evaluate situation.
- ▶ Patients should be told that depression is a treatable illness.
- ▶ Antidepressant therapy is not usually started by the ED physician.
- ▶ Set up close follow-up for non-suicidal depressed patients.

CHAPTER 148

ANXIETY DISORDERS

Marc Olson

▶ Anxiety is a complex feeling of apprehension, fear, and worry often accompanied by pulmonary, cardiac, and other physical symptoms.

▶ Lifetime prevalence of anxiety disorder is 1.5–3.5%.

▶ Nearly 50% of patients thought to have anxiety disorders are later found to have organic disease.

- Careful assessment of the anxious patient is crucial to prevent morbidity.

▶ Common anxiety disorders include

- Panic attacks
  - ○ Recurrent episodes of spontaneous, intense periods of anxiety, usually lasting < 1 hour.
  - ○ A patient with a classic panic attack experiences at least four of the following symptoms: palpitations, diaphoresis, tremulousness, SOB, chest pain, dizziness, nausea, abdominal discomfort, fear of injury or going crazy, derealization (perception of altered reality), and depersonalization (perception that one's body is surreal).
- Generalized anxiety disorder
  - ○ Defined as persistent fear, worry, or tension in the absence of panic attacks. The disabling persistent worry usually is out of proportion to the impact of the feared event.
- Post-traumatic stress disorder
  - ○ Recurrent experiences of a traumatic event accompanied by symptoms of increased anxiety and avoidance of stimuli associated with the trauma.
- Substance-induced anxiety disorder
  - ○ Anxiety symptoms that occur as a direct consequence of drug abuse, medications, or toxins

TABLE 148-1.
DIFFERENTIAL DIAGNOSIS OF ANXIETY DISORDERS

Diseases	Drugs
Dysrhythmias	Alcohol withdrawal
ACS	Benzodiazepine withdrawal
Hyperthyroidism	Theophylline
Pneumonia	Steroids
PE	Stimulants
Pheochromocytoma	Cocaine
	Amphetamines

CLINICAL PRESENTATION

▶ Most common presentation in the ED is panic disorder.

▶ Typical history includes sudden profound anxiety symptoms, including physiologic symptoms such as palpitations, sweating, tremulousness, SOB, chest pain, GI distress, near-syncopal episodes, and paresthesias. This is combined with psychological symptoms of fear and a sense of impending doom.

▶ Physical exam findings include vital signs consistent with a hyper-adrenergic state (tachypnea, tachycardia, and HTN). Notably, temperature and pulse oximetry are normal, and abnormalities of either should prompt evaluation for other illnesses. The remainder of the physical exam is usually normal.

DIFFERENTIAL DIAGNOSIS

▶ See Table 148-1.

EMERGENCY DEPARTMENT MANAGEMENT
Diagnosis

▶ History, physical exam, and focused work-up to rule out concomitant medical conditions.

▶ Additional work-up is tailored to each patient's presentation and risk stratification.

▶ Consider work-up for metabolic, cardiac, and pulmonary conditions.

▶ If indicated, labs: glucose, thyroid profile, and electrolytes, including calcium, toxicology screen, and cardiac marker testing.

▶ Cardiac monitoring and ECG for arrhythmia.
▶ CXR, V/Q, or CT angiogram.

Treatment

▶ ED physicians should provide a reassuring encounter.
  • Place patient in calm, quiet room.
  • Breathing exercises.
  • Verbal reassurance.
▶ Titrated doses of oral or IV benzodiazepines are effective for acute episodes.
  • Lorazepam, 0.5–1 mg PO/IV

Disposition

▶ Most patients can be discharged after symptoms are controlled and medical evaluation is complete.
▶ Short-term prescriptions for benzodiazepines are safe and effective; abuse potential is very low. Urgent follow-up with a psychiatrist for medication management is optimal.

◗ **PEARLS AND PITFALLS**
  • The most serious pitfall is diagnosing anxiety without a careful work-up to exclude organic and life-threatening causes of symptoms.
  • Under-treatment of acute anxiety is common. Benzodiazepines are safe and effective for short-term treatment.

CHAPTER 149

NEUROLEPTIC MALIGNANT SYNDROME

William E Lew

▶ Idiosyncratic drug reaction of high-potency neuroleptic agents (e.g., haloperidol and thiothixene).
▶ Affects approximately 0.2% of those treated with neuroleptics.
▶ Most common in first 3–9 days of therapy but can occur at any time.
▶ Syndrome develops over 24–72 hours.

CLINICAL PRESENTATION

▶ Hyperthermia, encephalopathy, skeletal muscle rigidity, and autonomic instability.
▶ Associated clinical findings include tachycardia, HTN/hypotension, tachypnea/hypoxia, diaphoresis/sialorrhea, tremor, and incontinence.
▶ Lab findings may include elevated CPK, myoglobinuria, metabolic acidosis, sodium imbalance, leukocytosis, and coagulopathy.
▶ Complications include
  • Renal failure due to rhabdomyolysis
  • Respiratory failure due to aspiration pneumonia
  • Hematologic/hepatic dysfunction due to hyperthermia

DIFFERENTIAL DIAGNOSIS

▶ See Table 149-1.

EMERGENCY DEPARTMENT MANAGEMENT
Diagnosis

▶ High index of suspicion.
▶ Diagnosis of exclusion (evaluate for trauma and infection with head CT and LP).

TABLE 149-1.
DIFFERENTIAL DIAGNOSIS OF NEUROLEPTIC MALIGNANT SYNDROME

CNS disorders (infection, hemorrhage, vasculitis, tumors, stroke, trauma)
Systemic disorders (infection, metabolic, hyperthyroidism, autoimmune)
Status epilepticus
Heat stroke
Tetanus
Lethal catatonia/psychosis
Acute dystonic reactions
Serotonin syndrome
DTs
Tetanus
Drugs (MAOI, anticholinergic, sympathomimetic, lithium toxicity)

▶ Lab evaluation is non-specific but may reveal rhabdomyolysis
  (elevated CPK, myoglobinuria, renal failure) or evidence of
  severe hyperthermia (hepatic failure).

Treatment

▶ Withdrawal of neuroleptic medication.
▶ Supportive care: aggressive hydration to support renal failure
  due to rhabdomyolysis and active cooling to treat hyperthermia.
▶ Benzodiazepines decrease extrapyramidal neuromotor effects.
  • Lorazepam or midazolam, 1–2 mg IV PRN
▶ Non-depolarizing neuroparalytics decrease muscular rigidity.
  • Avoid depolarizing (succinylcholine) agents due to possible
    hyperkalemia from rhabdomyolysis.
▶ Dantrolene sodium, 3–5 mg/kg IV divided tid/qid.
  • Blocks calcium release from muscular sarcoplasmic reticu-
    lum resulting in skeletal muscle relaxation
▶ Dopamine agonist.
  • Bromocriptine, 5 mg PO qid
  • Amantadine, 100 mg PO bid

Disposition

▶ ICU admission.
▶ Duration of syndrome 7–10 days.
▶ < 10% mortality.
▶ Avoid neuroleptics for at least 2–3 weeks.

CHAPTER 150

EATING DISORDERS

Manya Faith Newton

- ▶ Prevalence: 0.5–2.0%, mean age of onset ~15 years old.
- ▶ Female to male ratio of roughly 10:1.
- ▶ Often presents with very vague, non-specific symptoms; have a high index of suspicion in at-risk population.

ANOREXIA NERVOSA

- ▶ Severe limitation of caloric intake for the purpose of reshaping one's body or controlling one's weight
  - Patients are unaware that behavior is unhealthy or that the ideal for which they are striving may be unachievable.
- ▶ Associated with participation in sports or activities that promote thinness: distance running, ballet, gymnastics, modeling, etc.

Pathophysiology

- ▶ Lack of caloric intake leads to muscle wasting, loss of hair, dehydration, electrolyte abnormalities, alterations in female reproductive functions (including infertility), delayed wound healing, and peripheral edema secondary to hypoalbuminemia.
- ▶ Electrolyte abnormalities can lead to fatal arrhythmias, osteoporosis, and seizures.
- ▶ Changes in fat and nutrient absorption and metabolism can lead to neuropathies, constipation, and pancreatitis.

Clinical Presentation

- ▶ Cases usually present with non-specific symptoms: asthenia, lack of energy, or dizziness.
- ▶ Physical exam may be entirely normal in the early stages or in mild cases.
- ▶ Other signs include emaciation, dry skin, brittle nails, thinning scalp hair, hypotension (postural or static), loss of female fat pattern, and loss of menses.

Management

▸ Fluid resuscitation: 2–3 L NS IV if tachycardic, orthostatic, or hypotensive.

▸ Exclude other causes of weight loss.

▸ Lab evaluation:
- CBC for anemia, thrombocytopenia, and leukopenia.
- Metabolic panel for alkalosis, dehydration, hypocalcemia, hypokalemia, hypomagnesemia, and/or hypophosphatemia.
- LFTs and coagulation studies.
- Beta-hCG.
- Tests to confirm diagnosis or to rule out other entities on differential may be considered.
  - TSH/free T_4 and cortisol

▸ ECG should be done on any patient suspected to have anorexia nervosa since sudden death caused by ventricular arrhythmias related to QT interval prolongation has been reported.

▸ Risk assessment for suicide.

▸ Society for Adolescent Medicine guidelines for hospitalization (strongly consider hospitalization with one; more than one should definitely be hospitalized):
- Weight < 75% of average body weight for age, sex, and height
- Dehydration requiring IV hydration
- Electrolyte disturbances requiring correction
- Dysrhythmias
- Severe bradycardia (< 50 BPM)
- Hypotension (< 80/50 mmHg)
- Hypothermia (< 96° F)
- Orthostatic changes in pulse (> 20 BPM) or BP (> 10 mmHg)
- Arrested growth and development
- Acute psychiatric emergency (e.g., suicidal ideation)
- Acute medical complications of severe malnutrition (syncope, seizures, cardiac failure, pancreatitis, neuropathy)

BULIMIA NERVOSA

▸ Defined by binge eating and then purging to control weight.

▸ Binging: eating a large number of calories in a discrete period of time.

▸ Purging: self-induced vomiting, use of laxatives or diuretics, fasting or strict dieting (< 800 calories a day), or rigorous exercise done for the purpose of ridding oneself of calories eaten during a binge.

▶ Most bulimics are not underweight.

▶ To meet *Diagnostic and Statistical Manual of Mental Disorders*, 4th edition, criteria for bulimia, the patient must have a minimum of two binge-eating episodes a week for at least 3 months.

▶ Use of alcohol is far more common among bulimics than in other types of eating disorders, and bulimic patients should additionally be screened for alcohol abuse.

Clinical Presentation

▶ Physical exam may be entirely normal in early stages/mild cases.

▶ Cases usually present with non-specific symptoms (asthenia, lack of energy, dizziness, non-healing wounds on the fingers, tooth pain).

  • Russell's sign: scars on the back of the hand or knuckles from rubbing against the teeth during induced vomiting

▶ Parotid and salivary glad swelling/infection.

▶ Enamel erosion on lingual surface of teeth.

▶ Petechial hemorrhages on the soft palate, periorbital region, or cornea (including subconjunctival hemorrhage).

Management

▶ Lab evaluation
  • CBC for acute anemia or indications of infection
  • Metabolic panel for electrolyte abnormalities secondary to vomiting or laxative abuse (e.g., hypokalemia, hyperchloremic metabolic acidosis); may also show hyponatremia, hypocalcemia, hypomagnesemia
  • LFTs, amylase, and lipase to evaluate for pancreatitis
  • Beta-hCG
  • Tests to confirm diagnosis or to rule out other entities on differential
    ○ TSH/free T_4, cortisol, and head CT, if appropriate

▶ Screening
  • "Are you satisfied with your eating habits?" and "Do you ever eat in secret?"
  • Answering "no" to the first question and "yes" to the second question has 100% sensitivity and 90% specificity for bulimia.

CHAPTER 151

CONJUNCTIVITIS

Richard G. Taylor

- ▶ Most commonly caused by viruses and usually is self-limiting.
- ▶ Allergic conjunctivitis is an IgE-mediated hypersensitivity to seasonal and environmental antigens.
- ▶ The majority of viral conjunctivitis cases are caused by adenovirus. Coxsackie and enterovirus may also cause local epidemics. The common causes of bacterial conjunctivitis are listed in Table 151-1.

CLINICAL PRESENTATION

- ▶ Hyperemia and edema of conjunctiva, FB sensation, tearing, and ocular discharge; photophobia and vision loss are not present.
- ▶ Allergic conjunctivitis is characterized by pruritus, tearing, and often concomitant nasal congestion. Papillae under eyelids frequently observed. It may be associated with systemic inflammatory disorders.
- ▶ Acute bacterial conjunctivitis classically begins unilaterally with mucopurulent discharge that collects at the bases of the lids. Discharge can collect overnight with crusting of the lids on awakening. Symptoms may spread to the contralateral eye in 24–48 hours.
- ▶ Hyperacute bacterial conjunctivitis classically has an abrupt onset, rapid progression, and copious purulent discharge and is

TABLE 151-1.
PATHOGENESIS OF BACTERIAL CONJUNCTIVITIS

Acute	Hyperacute	Chronic
Staphylococcus aureus *Streptococcus pneumoniae* *Haemophilus influenzae* *Chlamydia trachomatis* *Pseudomonas aeruginosa* (contact lens wearers)	*Neisseria gonor-rhoeae* *Neisseria menin-gitides*	*Staphylococcus aureus* *Moraxella lacunata* *Chlamydia tra-chomatis*

most often associated with gonococcal or chlamydial infection in a sexually active patient. Untreated infection may progress to corneal involvement. Chlamydial infection typically is not as clinically acute as gonococcal infection.

▸ Hyperacute, purulent conjunctivitis during the first 28 days of life is usually caused by vertical transmission of gonococci.

▸ Viral conjunctivitis classically involves the eyes bilaterally and is accompanied by watery discharge. Preauricular adenopathy is common. The patient frequently has other viral symptoms, such as fever and myalgias, or concomitant URI.

▸ Herpetic conjunctivitis often occurs in children and usually resolves spontaneously. Herpetic keratitis often occurs after immunosuppression with topical corticosteroids.

▸ Irritative or toxic conjunctivitis frequently occurs secondary to topical ocular medications such as aminoglycosides; may occur in the first few days of life in neonates given prophylactic silver nitrate.

DIFFERENTIAL DIAGNOSIS OF THE RED EYE

▸ FB, abrasion, or corneal ulcer: recognize on slit-lamp exam
▸ Keratitis: eye pain, decreased vision, and corneal defects
▸ Iritis: eye pain, perilimbic injection, anterior chamber cells, and flare
▸ Uveitis
▸ Orbital trauma history
▸ Acute-angle glaucoma: eye pain, halos/blurred vision, hazy cornea, mid-dilated pupil, and increased IOP
▸ Orbital cellulitis: erythema soft tissues with pain on EOM

EMERGENCY DEPARTMENT MANAGEMENT
Diagnosis

▸ Diagnosis is primarily based on clinical findings and history.
▸ Culture is indicated in cases of suspected infection with *Neisseria gonorrhoeae* or *Chlamydia trachomatis*, neonatal conjunctivitis, or unusual presentations of conjunctivitis.

Treatment

▸ Most infections are self-limiting; however, there is an expectation by the public that this is treated. Children in daycare may not be allowed back without being treated.

▶ Broad-spectrum topical antibiotic drops or ointments will speed the time to recovery while limiting discomfort of the disease.

▶ Erythromycin, 0.1% ointment qid.

▶ Avoid contact lens wear.

▶ Avoid use of corticosteroids.

Disposition

▶ Follow-up for uncomplicated viral or bacterial conjunctivitis should be with primary care physician.

▶ Refer to ophthalmologist if corneal involvement or if chlamydial, gonococcal, or herpetic infection is suspected.

◑ **PEARLS AND PITFALLS**

- Pain, photophobia, and vision loss are not associated with conjunctivitis and should prompt further evaluation.
- Contact lens wearers are at greater risk for pseudomonal infections as well as progression to keratitis.
- Consider gonococcal or chlamydial infection in the sexually active patient.
- Patients may present with toxic/irritative conjunctivitis following course of aminoglycosides.

CHAPTER 152

CORNEAL DISORDERS

Joanne Torres

CORNEAL ABRASIONS

- ▸ Traumatic erosion of the corneal surface, usually confined to epithelium.
- ▸ Most heal spontaneously in 48 hours.
- ▸ Infection is rare.

Presentation

- ▸ Patients complain of FB sensation, possible blurring of vision, pain, redness, tearing, and/or photophobia.
- ▸ Ask about a history of trauma or contact lens use.
- ▸ Exam reveals conjunctival injection. Decreased visual acuity can occur if the abrasion involves the visual axis or is very large.
- ▸ After application of topical anesthetic, a slit-lamp examination (SLE) should be performed. Fluorescein staining/cobalt blue light assist with demonstrating the lesion. A Wood's lamp can be used when a slit lamp is not available.

Management

- ▸ Diagnosis is made clinically. Remember to always check visual acuity and evert eyelid to evaluate for retained FB.
- ▸ Have a high index of suspicion for ruptured globe in high-velocity impact.
- ▸ Despite low risk of infection, most prescribe topical antibiotics as they provide lubrication.
    - Erythromycin ophthalmic ointment 0.5%, 1 cm ribbon tid
    - Tobramycin ophthalmic 0.3% drops, 1–2 gtt qid
- ▸ Consider infection with *Pseudomonas* in contact lens wearers.
    - Ciprofloxacin ophthalmic 0.3% solution, 1–2 gtt tid

▶ If in significant pain/spasm, consider a cycloplegic agent.
- Cyclopentolate ophthalmic 1% solution, 1–2 gtt.
- Avoid atropine because of long duration of action.

▶ Discharge the patient with narcotic pain medication or topical non-steroidal for 48 hours.

▶ Arrange a follow-up exam in 1–2 days. Patients who have had an abrasion caused by farm equipment or vegetable material require closer follow-up.

▶ Patching has not been shown to improve healing time or mitigate pain. Steroids are contraindicated in patients with corneal abrasions.

▶ Advise the patient not to use contacts for at least a week.

▶ Instruct patients on preventing eye injuries.

▶ Corneal abrasions should receive tetanus prophylaxis if needed.

CORNEAL FOREIGN BODY

▶ Usually airborne debris that blows into eye

Clinical Presentation

▶ Consists of pain, FB sensation, injected conjunctiva, tearing, and blepharospasm.

▶ Diagnosis occurs with a slit lamp; always evert eyelid as part of the eye exam.

Management

▶ Most FBs can be removed in ED.

▶ Apply a topical anesthetic.
- Proparacaine hydrochloride 0.5%, 2 gtt

▶ Attempt removal with saline solution; if unsuccessful, try using moistened cotton-tipped applicator, ophthalmologic burr, or 25-G needle held tangential to cornea. Stabilize hand on zygoma. A slit lamp should be used for removal.

▶ After removing FB, eye should be stained with fluorescein. Patients with corneal epithelial defects should be placed on topical antibiotics and, if having significant spasm, a cycloplegic agent.

▶ A rust ring may form with metallic FB. Removal of the rust ring should be done by the ophthalmologist at follow-up in next 24 hours and not attempted in the ED.

▶ If FB is very large, perforation is suspected, or removal is impossible, then immediate ophthalmology consultation is required; otherwise, patient follow-up in 24 hours.

CORNEAL ULCER

▶ Vision-threatening if not recognized and appropriately treated.
▶ Break in the epithelial barrier secondary to trauma, contact lens use, dessication, or direct microbial invasion.
▶ Always consider *Pseudomonas* in contact lens wearers.

Clinical Presentation

▶ Presents with pain, FB sensation, photophobia, and blurred vision.
▶ Exam reveals conjunctival hyperemia and localized white corneal defect. A hypopyon (WBCs in anterior chamber) may be present.

Treatment

▶ Topical ofloxacin or ciprofloxacin, q1h.
▶ Topical cycloplegic.
▶ Ophthalmology referral for evaluation within 24 hours.
▶ Do not patch eye.

KERATITIS

▶ Inflammation of the cornea caused by infection, trauma, dry eyes, ultraviolet exposure, contact lens, or immunogenic states.
▶ Radiation burns result in direct corneal epithelial damage from sun lamps, tanning booths, welder's arc, or high-altitude environments. There is normally a latent period of 6–10 hours.
▶ Contact lens use is the most common cause of infectious keratitis in the U.S. *Acanthamoeba* is associated with contact lens use.
▶ Infectious keratitis is one of the leading causes of blindness in the world and represents a preventable and treatable ophthalmic disease. Herpes simplex is a common corneal pathogen.
▶ Keratitis can also occur from air bags being deployed. This can result in a thermal, friction, or chemical burn.

Clinical Presentation

▶ History: FB sensation, blurred vision, tearing, intense pain, photophobia, and blepharospasm.
▶ Physical exam: may have decreased visual acuity and conjunctival hyperemia concentrated around the cornea or limbal region, called ciliary flush.
▶ Herpes simplex appears as a dendritic ulceration of the cornea.

▶ Herpes zoster ophthalmicus: unilateral vesicular eruption in dermatome supplied by the ophthalmic branch of the trigeminal nerve; ocular involvement ranges from conjunctivitis to keratitis. Lesions on the tip of the nose (Hutchinson's sign) signal high likelihood of ocular involvement.

▶ Ultraviolet keratitis shows superficial punctate keratitis (SPK), which appears as dots on the corneal surface.

Management

▶ Herpes simplex
  • Prompt referral to ophthalmology
  • Topical antiviral, q1h
  • Cycloplegic
▶ Herpes zoster ophthalmicus
  • Ophthalmology consult
  • Oral acyclovir
  • Cycloplegic
▶ Ultraviolet keratitis
  • Topical cycloplegic.
  • Topical broad-spectrum antibiotic.
  • Oral antibiotic.
  • Consider eye patch for comfort.
  • Next-day follow-up with ophthalmology.

CHEMICAL BURNS

▶ True ocular emergency that requires immediate irrigation.
▶ Alkali burns tend to be more devastating.
▶ Alkali burns cause a liquefactive necrosis that penetrates deeply and dissolves tissues (e.g., drain cleaners, chemical detergents, industrial solvents, and lime in plaster and concrete).
▶ Acidic burns cause a coagulation necrosis that causes precipitation of tissue proteins, which limit the depth of the injury (e.g., sulfuric acid in car batteries).

Clinical Presentation

▶ Presents with eye irritation, pain, corneal cloudiness, and scleral whitening.

Treatment

- ► Irrigate immediately with 2 L of NS for at least 30 minutes.
- ► The pH should then be checked with Nitrazine paper dipped in the inferior conjunctival fornix.
- ► If the pH is neutral, complete eye exam and follow with a cycloplegic, topical antibiotics, and pain management.
- ► If the pH continues to be abnormal, continue irrigation and recheck the pH every 10 minutes.
- ► Record IOP in alkali burns.
- ► Ophthalmologic consultation is indicated with all severe alkali burns.

CHAPTER 153

OCULAR TRAUMA

Richard G. Taylor

- ► > 2 million eye injuries in the U.S. annually.
- ► Majority of injuries occur at < 30 years of age.

ORBITAL BLOWOUT FRACTURE

- ► Blunt force to eye and orbital rim → increased intra-orbital pressure → fracture of medial wall and floor.
- ► Limitation of ocular motility results from entrapment of ocular muscles, most commonly the inferior oblique and inferior rectus muscles. This may result in diplopia.
- ► Approximately 40% of orbital fractures are associated with ocular injury.

Clinical Presentation

- ► Typically present following blunt trauma with swelling and ecchymosis of soft tissues, pain, and bony tenderness.
- ► Restriction of ocular motility, diplopia with upward gaze and ipsilateral hypoesthesia of cheek (infra-orbital nerve), or SC emphysema may be present.

Management

- ► Blunt ocular trauma and suspicion for injury warrant imaging studies.
- ► X-rays: Water's view may reveal air-fluid level or tear drop sign (herniation of muscle and fat through orbital floor).
- ► CT scan with axial and coronal cuts is regarded as imaging modality of choice.
- ► Surgical intervention is indicated for herniation of orbital contents with persistent diplopia. Surgical repair is usually delayed 7–10 days to allow swelling to reduce.
- ► Patients are usually discharged with broad-spectrum oral antibiotics, ophthalmology follow-up, and advice not to blow nose.

HYPHEMA

► Blood in the anterior chamber of the eye
- Microhyphema is RBCs floating in the anterior chamber of the eye and is best appreciated on slit-lamp exam (SLE).
- Gross hyphema may be detected by visual or pen light exam.
- "Eight-ball" hyphema refers to a total hyphema with dark-colored clots.

► Results from direct or concussive trauma to the vasculature of the iris and angle

► May result in compromise of the outflow of aqueous humor and progress to glaucoma

Clinical Presentation

► Blurred vision, pain, and photophobia following blunt or concussive injury to the eye

► ± Decreased visual acuity

Management

► Non-traumatic hyphema warrants consideration of systemic coagulopathy.

► Hospitalization for all patients is controversial. Most patients with microhyphema and uncomplicated small hyphemas may be managed as outpatients.

► If discharged from the ED, must be asked to avoid ASA, other NSAIDs, and any strenuous activity.

► IOP must be monitored and controlled.

► Ophthalmology consultation and serial follow-up.

► Major complication is re-bleeding. Occurs most commonly at 3–5 days. Risk factors include hyphema > one-third, decreased visual acuity, and increased IOP. Patients should avoid ASA and NSAIDs.

► Other complications include synechiae formation, staining of cornea, and glaucoma.

RETINAL DETACHMENT

► Involves the sensory retina dissecting from the underlying pigmented epithelial layer

Clinical Presentation

▶ Painless, visual blurring, visual field cuts, abrupt loss of vision, floaters, and flashes of light.

▶ Unilateral retinal detachment may result in afferent papillary defect.

▶ May observe hazy gray membrane of retina on ophthalmoscopy but often difficult to visualize in ED.

▶ IOP may be reduced.

Management

▶ All patients with symptoms of retinal detachment must have dilated funduscopic exam.

▶ Patients should have ophthalmology consultation.

▶ Prognosis depends on involvement of macula.

RUPTURED GLOBE

▶ Blunt or penetrating injury to the eyeball with extrusion of orbital contents

Clinical Presentation

▶ Traumatic injury, eye deformity, pain, reduced or absent vision, diplopia, hyphema, chemosis, lens displacement, and vitreous hemorrhage

Management

▶ Immediate ophthalmology consultation for surgical repair.

▶ Avoid pressure on globe; metal eye shield and make patient NPO.

▶ Analgesia and antiemetics to prevent vomiting and Valsalva movements by the patient.

▶ Broad-spectrum IV antibiotics.

▶ Imaging may be indicated in suspected FBs or concern about concomitant injuries.

EYELID LACERATIONS

▶ Complex lid lacerations are those involving the lid margins, canalicular or lacrimal drainage system, lacrimal sac, levator aponeurosis, canthal tendons, and laceration through the orbital septum.

Clinical Presentation

▶ Blunt or penetrating injury to the eyelid.

▶ Eyelids do not contain SC fat. Protrusion of fat through an eyelid laceration should raise suspicion for injury to the orbital septum.

Management

▶ A complete eye exam must be performed on every patient with eyelid or periorbital lacerations to exclude other ocular injuries.

▶ Lacerations of the medial and inferior portion of the eyelid merit high suspicion for canalicular injury.

▶ Complex lid lacerations need immediate referral for repair by an ophthalmologist.

▶ Superficial, simple horizontal, or oblique partial thickness lacerations can be repaired under local anesthesia in the ED. 6-0 or 7-0 interrupted sutures should be used to close simple lacerations. Sutures should never be in direct contact with the eye.

RETROBULBAR HEMATOMA

▶ Hemorrhage into potential space around the globe following blunt trauma

▶ Causes increased IOP, which is transmitted to globe, optic nerve, and eventually blood supply

Clinical Presentation

▶ Proptosis, limited movement, vision loss, and increased IOP

Emergency Department Management

▶ Diagnosis may be obvious clinically but can be confirmed by CT scan.

▶ Treatment consists of ophthalmology consult for surgical decompression.

▶ Indications for urgent ED lateral canthotomy: significant proptosis with decreasing visual acuity.

▶ Lateral canthotomy:
  • Lateral canthus is anesthetized with 2–4% lidocaine with epinephrine.

- Small hemostat is used to crush canthus for 1–2 minutes.
- Canthus is then incised using small iris scissors.

TRAUMATIC IRITIS

▶ Inflammation of iris and ciliary body may be secondary to trauma or systemic illness.

Clinical Presentation

▶ Symptoms: deep-seated pain that is unrelieved by topical anesthetic and photophobia; may have blurred vision
▶ Exam findings: ciliary flush (circumcorneal hyperemia), cellular debris, and flare in anterior chamber on SLE; may have small sluggish pupil

Treatment

▶ Ophthalmology referral.
▶ Cycloplegic and topical steroids if confirmed no corneal defect; always prescribe in conjunction with ophthalmologist to ensure timely follow-up.

SUBCONJUNCTIVAL HEMORRHAGE

▶ Caused by rupture of conjunctival vessels, most commonly associated with trauma, but can also be secondary to increased IOP, HTN, or coagulopathies.
▶ The hemorrhage is limited to the bulbar conjunctiva and demarcated at the limbus.

Clinical Presentation

▶ Patients present with conjunctival erythema. If the patient has complaints of pain, photophobia, or change in vision, consider alternative diagnoses.

Treatment

▶ No referral is necessary unless diagnosis is uncertain.
▶ Recommend cold compresses to patient for 24 hours. If no obvious insult per history, check for blood dyscrasias and check BP.
▶ Signs of hemorrhage should resolve within 14 days.

CHAPTER 154

VISION LOSS

Joanne Torres and Christopher R. H. Newton

▶ History serves a primary role in the evaluation of vision loss. Crucial points to the history are onset of symptoms, acuity, whether the loss has been transient or persistent, history of trauma, and any systemic symptoms.

▶ Monocular complaints are usually associated with anterior pathologic conditions such as the optic nerve, retina, or media; central lesions produce binocular loss.

▶ Pain is usually associated with anterior pathology except in the case of the retina, which does not have nociceptive fibers.

▶ Nine-step evaluation includes
  • External visualization (always evert the eyelid to look for FB).
  • Test pupils looking for APD.
    ○ Swinging flashlight test for APD: pupil dilates in response to light
  • Check visual fields to confrontation.
  • Visual acuity (use pinhole if without glasses).
  • Extraocular movements and alignment.
  • Slit-lamp exam (SLE).
  • Stain eye with fluorescein for rupture or corneal abrasion.
  • IOP for glaucoma.
  • Funduscopic exam of retina.

OPTIC NEURITIS

▶ Autoimmune inflammatory process causing acute demyelination of the optic nerve.

▶ Typically in females 15–45 years old.

▶ Long-term vision loss occurs in 20–40%.

▶ Inflammatory disorder observed in multiple sclerosis, sarcoidosis, and systemic lupus erythematosus.

▶ Between 25% and 60% of patients who develop optic neuritis develop multiple sclerosis within 15 years.

Clinical Presentation

▶ Presents as progressive, painful monocular vision loss; pain with extraocular movements.

▶ Decreased central vision with preservation of peripheral vision and an APD; may have elevation/swelling of optic disc.

▶ Red vision desaturation specific for optic neuritis: color red perceived as less intense in affected eye.

Management

▶ Urgent ophthalmologic consult.

▶ Admission for IV steroids.

  • Methylprednisolone, 250 mg IV qid for 3 days, followed by prednisone, 1 mg/kg for 11 days

▶ Steroids do not improve visual outcome but can reduce new neurologic events.

TEMPORAL (GIANT CELL) ARTERITIS

▶ Inflammatory process of medium and large arteries that can cause optic nerve infarction and permanent vision loss.

▶ Affects patients over the age of 60 with a female predominance of 3:1.

▶ It is associated with polymyalgia rheumatica.

Clinical Presentation

▶ Presents as sudden onset of painless, monocular vision loss usually associated with unilateral headache; may also complain of myalgias, malaise, fever, jaw claudication, and pain over temporal artery.

▶ Physical findings include tenderness over temporal artery and APD; may observe optic nerve edema.

Management

▶ Obtain ESR (usually elevated from 50–100 mm/hour) and CRP. Usually elevated but, if normal, does not exclude the diagnosis.

▶ Temporal artery biopsy confirms diagnosis.

▶ Treatment should be initiated when diagnosis is suspected; consists of high-dose corticosteroids.

  • Prednisone, 2 mg/kg/day PO, if no vision loss and low suspicion

- Methylprednisolone, 250 mg IV q6h, if highly suspicious or vision loss present
▶ All should have ophthalmology consultation.
▶ Patients with high probability of disease should be admitted for IV steroids.

UVEITIS/IRITIS

▶ Inflammation of the iris, ciliary body, or choroids.
▶ It may be caused by trauma, Reiter's syndrome, ankylosing spondylitis, sarcoidosis, TB, or collagen vascular diseases.

Clinical Presentation

▶ Presents as painful red eye with blurred vision and photophobia; ciliary flush common clinical exam finding. A small or irregular pupil may be present secondary to adherence of the iris to anterior lens. IOP is variable.
▶ Classically, pain is unrelieved by topical anesthetic and may have consensual photophobia.
▶ May have prior history of iritis or similar undiagnosed pain in the past.
▶ SLE diagnostic, revealing cells and flare in the anterior chamber.

Treatment

▶ Long-acting cycloplegic for comfort; also prevents formation of synechiae.
- Homatropine ophthalmic 5%, 1–2 gtt
▶ Topical steroids in consultation with ophthalmology.
▶ Follow up with ophthalmology within 24 hours.

CENTRAL RETINAL ARTERY OCCLUSION

▶ Caused by emboli from carotid plaques, cardiac valves, fat emboli, arteriosclerosis, collagen vascular disease, hypotension, sickle cell disease, or temporal arteritis
▶ Most commonly affects elderly males

Clinical Presentation

▶ Presents as sudden painless monocular vision loss.
▶ On exam, have markedly reduced visual acuity and APD.

▶ Funduscopy may demonstrate pallor of retina with cherry red macula.

Treatment

▶ Full vision may be restored if treatment instituted within 2 hours.
▶ The goal is to restore retinal artery flow.
▶ Treatments include digital massage (moderate pressure for 5 seconds then release for 5 seconds and repeat for 5–10 minutes), anterior chamber paracentesis, acetazolamide IV, and inhaled carbogen.
▶ Obtain an emergency ophthalmology consult; they may offer urokinase or tPA.
▶ Response to treatment is rare.

CENTRAL VEIN OCCLUSION

▶ Thrombosis of central retinal vein.
▶ Patients are generally over the age of 50 and have significant cardiovascular disease, HTN, vasculitis, coagulation disorders, or glaucoma.

Clinical Presentation

▶ Presents as sudden painless monocular vision loss
▶ Sluggish pupil, retinal exam reveals classic "blood and thunder fundus" caused by retinal hemorrhages, venous dilation, and optic disc edema

Treatment

▶ No treatment is really effective, but because of the difficulty of making the diagnosis, patients should have ophthalmology consult to confirm the diagnosis.

VITREOUS HEMORRHAGE

▶ Associated with diabetes, trauma, malignancy, leukemia, anemia, and thrombocytopenia
▶ Caused by ruptured retinal vessels

Clinical Presentation

▶ Sudden painless unilateral loss of vision; patients may have floaters or "cobwebs" prior to vision loss.

▶   Red reflex is absent, and there is decreased view of fundus.

Treatment

▶   Urgent ophthalmologic consult to rule out retinal detachment and treat underlying disorder, especially BP

RETINAL DETACHMENT

▶   Caused by the separation of the pigment epithelium and the neurosensory retina
▶   Associated with age, male gender, diabetes, trauma, and/or sickle cell disease

Clinical Presentation

▶   Presents as painless monocular vision changes. Early symptoms include flashes of light (as retina begins to separate), floaters, or a curtain obscuring the visual field. Visual acuity is affected if the fovea is involved.
▶   On exam, the detached portion of the retina may appear opaque or translucent.

Treatment

▶   Diagnosis requires dilated indirect exam by ophthalmology because it can be easily missed.
▶   Emergent ophthalmology consult where the patient may receive diathermy or laser photocoagulation.
▶   Prognosis is determined by whether the macula is affected. Percentage of patients retaining 20/50 or better is 85% vs. 50% if the macula is involved.

MACULAR DEGENERATION

▶   It is the most common cause of permanent blindness in the elderly.
▶   This is a slowly progressive disease causing binocular loss of vision secondary to the deterioration of the retinal pigment in the macula.
▶   The incidence is 2.2% in individuals older than age 65.
▶   It is of unknown etiology. The incidence is associated with age, smoking, being Caucasian and female, and if there is an FH.

Clinical Presentation

▸ Presents as blurred vision, scotoma, or central vision loss. On exam, the physician may see yellow/white deposits beneath the pigment epithelium, called drusen.

Treatment

▸ Laser photocoagulation and vision aids

AMAUROSIS FUGAX

▸ Emboli from a proximal carotid plaque embolize to the ophthalmic artery causing transient vision loss.
▸ Associated with HTN, carotid artery disease, AF, sickle cell disease, or hypotension.

Clinical Presentation

▸ Patients complain of a loss of vision lasting several minutes; can also be described as curtain drawn over the visual field.
▸ Exam is usually normal.

Treatment

▸ ASA, 325 mg PO.
▸ Consider admission for work-up similar to stroke, including ECG, carotid studies, and cardiac echo.
▸ Ophthalmology consult is indicated.

CYTOMEGALOVIRUS RETINITIS

▸ Caused by infectious invasion of the macula seen primarily in patients who are immunocompromised (most commonly in advanced AIDS).

Clinical Presentation

▸ Initially may be asymptomatic; scotomas and vision loss develop.
▸ Retinal hemorrhage along with retinal necrosis resulting in an appearance of red and white areas ("cheese and ketchup" fundus).

Treatment

▶ IV antiviral therapy with foscarnet or ganciclovir
▶ Ophthalmology consult

GLAUCOMA

▶ Major cause of blindness.
▶ Open-angle glaucoma affects elderly and causes about 70% of all glaucoma cases; results in chronic painless loss of peripheral vision. Patients have moderate elevations in IOP. If present to the ED, should be referred to ophthalmologist for definitive care.
▶ Acute-angle closure is caused by the iris blocking drainage in shallow anterior chamber. The rest of this section refers to presentation and treatment of acute-angle glaucoma.

Clinical Presentation

▶ Patients classically present with nausea/vomiting, eye pain, and blurred vision after moving from daylight to a darkened room.
▶ On exam, they have decreased visual acuity, mid-dilated fixed pupil, and hazy cornea.
▶ IOP is elevated (> 50 mmHg).

Treatment

▶ Ophthalmology consult is indicated.
▶ Medications include
  • Topical pilocarpine 2%, 1 gtt q15min × 5
  • Timolol 0.5%, 1 gtt q10min × 2
  • Pred Forte 1%, 1 gtt q5min × 4
  • Acetazolamide, 500 mg IV/PO
  • Analgesia
▶ Functional vision loss is a diagnosis of exclusion. Test to check a patient feigning blindness by passing a piece of paper with vertical lines in front of the patient. If there is presence of optokinetic nystagmus, vision is present. A patient feigning blindness may also demonstrate the inability to approximate the opposing outstretched forefingers, which should not be affected by blindness.

CHAPTER 155

PERIORBITAL AND ORBITAL CELLULITIS

Richard G. Taylor

▶ More common in winter months due to increased incidence of sinusitis.
▶ More common in children than adults.
▶ Complications of orbital cellulitis include vision loss, cavernous sinus thrombosis, and CNS or bony involvement. It is, therefore, imperative to have high suspicion in unilateral eye swelling.

PATHOPHYSIOLOGY

▶ The orbital septum is a layer of fascia separating eyelids from orbit.
▶ Periorbital (pre-septal) cellulitis is confined to the superficial tissues anterior to the orbital septum. Orbital cellulitis is infection of tissues posterior to orbital septum.
▶ Occurs as a result of bacteremic spread of infection, direct seeding of organisms secondary to trauma or surgery, or extension of infection from sinuses.
▶ Majority of orbital cellulitis cases (90%) caused by paranasal sinusitis.
▶ Decreasing incidence of *Haemophilus influenzae* secondary to HIB vaccine, typically *Staphylococcus* and *Streptococcus* species. Fungal infection with *Mucor* and *Aspergillus* species may occur.

CLINICAL PRESENTATION

▶ **Periorbital cellulitis:** erythema, swelling, warmth, and tenderness of eyelid ± fever. Visual acuity and EOM are normal.
▶ **Orbital cellulitis:** has similar external appearance to periorbital cellulitis. Patient is usually febrile with ocular pain, and the hallmark feature used to differentiate between the disease enti-

ties is pain with EOMs (ophthalmoplegia). May have chemosis, proptosis, decreased visual acuity, and increased IOP.

EMERGENCY DEPARTMENT MANAGEMENT
Diagnosis

▶ Based on history and exam findings.
▶ CT with thin-cut axial and coronal views of orbits should be used liberally in those with ocular pain or pain with EOMs.
▶ CBC, blood cultures, and nasal swab for culture. Consider soft tissue aspirate for Gram's stain and culture.

Treatment

▶ Periorbital cellulitis without any concerning features can be started on oral antibiotics with good staphylococcal/streptococcal coverage.
  • Cephalexin, 500 mg PO qid 10 days
▶ Orbital cellulitis is treated with broad-spectrum IV antibiotics, again covering staphylococcus/streptococcus.
  • Unasyn, 3 g IV q6h
▶ Urgent ENT/ophthalmology consultation for any patient with orbital cellulitis.

Disposition

▶ Patients with periorbital cellulitis can be discharged with next-day follow-up. They should have strict warnings to come back if they become febrile or have ocular pain.
▶ All patients with orbital cellulitis should be admitted for close observation. Many hospitals use the ICU setting for this.

CHAPTER 156

OTITIS EXTERNA

Marc Olson

▶ OE is inflammation and infection of the external auditory canal.
▶ The protective layer of the ear canal is disrupted by prolonged exposure to moisture combined with local trauma (e.g., cleaning with Q-tips). This leads to maceration and inflammation of the canal, predisposing to infection.
▶ The most common causative organisms are *Pseudomonas* and *Staphylococcus* species.
▶ Malignant or necrotizing OE may be observed in diabetics and the immunocompromised. It involves bacterial spread to the cartilage of the external ear and the bony portion of the external canal, resulting in osteomyelitis and mastoiditis.

CLINICAL PRESENTATION
History
▶ Typical presentation is 1–2 days of increasing ear pain, often associated with gradual unilateral hearing loss from canal edema.
▶ Recent exposure to water (typically swimming) is common.
▶ Pruritus of the canal may precede pain.
▶ Occasionally, otorrhea is present.

Physical Exam
▶ Vital signs are usually normal. Fever > 101° F, tachycardia, or hypotension should prompt careful evaluation for alternate source of infection or consider possibility of systemic toxicity from malignant OE.
▶ On inspection, the external ear often appears normal; edema and/or otorrhea may be observed.
▶ The classic physical finding is pain with traction on the external ear.

▶ Examination of the canal reveals erythema, edema, and debris in the canal.
▶ The TM may be difficult to visualize because of canal edema but is typically without erythema or effusion.
▶ Periauricular adenitis may be present.

DIFFERENTIAL DIAGNOSIS
▶ OM
▶ FB, especially in children
▶ Herpes zoster oticus (Ramsay Hunt syndrome): viral infection causing pain, erythema, swelling, and vesicular eruption
▶ Cholesteatoma

EMERGENCY DEPARTMENT MANAGEMENT
Diagnosis
▶ Evaluation usually requires only thorough history and physical exam.
▶ Lab evaluation is not indicated for routine OE; however, a bedside glucose test should be considered if occult diabetes is a concern.
▶ Culture of drainage or canal epithelium is indicated only in patients who fail initial standard treatment.
▶ If mastoiditis or osteomyelitis from malignant OE is a concern, CT scan is the best technique for defining bone involvement and extent of disease.

Treatment
▶ Consists of gently removing debris from ear canal and application of topical antibiotics.
▶ Canal edema can impede application of topical medications. A foam (Pope) or gauze ear wick may assist with application of drops and help reduce the swelling.
▶ Commonly used preparations include
  • Neomycin polymyxin-B hydrocortisone (Corticosporin otic), 4 drops qid
  • Ciprofloxacin hydrocortisone (Cipro HC otic), 3 drops bid
▶ Topical preparations should be applied for 3 days after cessation of symptoms (average 7–10 days total).

▶ Oral analgesics are often needed, as pain can be severe.
▶ Systemic antibiotics should be considered in diabetics and immunocompromised patients with OE.
  • Ciprofloxacin, 750 mg PO bid for 10 days
▶ Diabetics with evidence of systemic toxicity or severe otitis should be admitted for IV antibiotics.

Disposition

▶ Patients with OE are usually managed as outpatients with primary care physician follow-up in 1–2 days to assess improvement. If a wick is placed, it should be changed within 48 hours.
▶ Patients with malignant OE should be hospitalized for IV antibiotics and have ENT consultation.

CHAPTER 157

DISORDERS OF THE SALIVARY GLANDS

David Renken

SIALOLITHIASIS

▶ Hardened intraluminal deposits form stones.
▶ Stone formation associated with decreased flow of saliva, high calcium content, increased viscosity, and increased alkalinity.
▶ Not correlated with serum calcium level.
▶ Sialolithiasis occurs at submandibular gland (80%) > parotid (19%) > SL (1%).
  • Length and orientation of Wharton's duct as well as salivary characteristics responsible for this
▶ 75% of patients are 50–80 years old.

Clinical Presentation

▶ Classic history is pain and swelling of gland exacerbated by eating or anticipation of eating.
▶ Painless swelling present in 30% of submandibular stones.
▶ Stone may be visible at opening of duct or be palpated over duct.

Emergency Department Management

Diagnosis
▶ History and physical are usually diagnostic.
  • Palpation of gland and course of duct may reveal presence of stone.
▶ May be able to "milk" stone from duct if it can be palpated (< 3 mm size generally removable), but avoid probing of duct for stone, may precipitate inflammatory response or infection.
▶ Ancillary testing usually not needed unless concern for infection.

Treatment
▶ Hydration, analgesia, moist heat, massage, and sialogogues (e.g., lemon drops).

- ▶ Stop anticholinergic medications, if possible (e.g., Benadryl).
- ▶ Antibiotics, if question of infection.
- ▶ ENT referral for persistent pain/stone or multiple recurrence.
  - • May need procedure for removal or breakup of stones

PAROTITIS

- ▶ Acute bacterial causes relate to decreased salivary production and ascending bacterial contamination.
  - • Decreased salivary production may be related to dehydration, Sjögren's syndrome, chemotherapy, radiation, medication side effects, prolonged anorexia.
  - • Incidence increased over age 50 years, immunocompromised (e.g., diabetes, HIV), and poor oral hygiene.
  - • *Staphylococcus aureus,* frequently penicillin resistant, is most common; *Streptococcus*, *Haemophilus influenzae,* and anaerobic bacteria also found.
- ▶ Chronic bacterial parotitis is generally related to obstruction of salivary flow related to calculus, stricture, or mucous plug; similar bacterial causes.
- ▶ Atypical infectious and inflammatory causes are rare but include sarcoidosis, TB, actinomycosis, cat-scratch disease, toxoplasmosis, and tularemia.
- ▶ Viral is usually bilateral (90%), and most common etiology is mumps (paramyxovirus), but is now much less frequently observed with advent of immunization.
  - • 2- to 4-week incubation period, droplet spread, primarily in children
  - • Rarely, may be complicated by orchitis, pancreatitis, or meningoencephalitis

Clinical Presentation

- ▶ Acute bacterial infection presents with painful swelling and induration of the skin overlying gland (usually unilateral) with associated fever, chills, and malaise.
  - • Frequently will see purulent discharge from ductal orifice.
  - • Patients are often systemically ill with tachycardia, hyperpyrexia, and possible sepsis.
- ▶ Chronic infection has previous history, and presentation may range from mild to severe (less common) symptoms and exam findings.

▶ Viral illness presents with prodrome of low-grade fever, malaise, anorexia, and headache, followed by bilateral swelling and tenderness of parotid glands, which lasts 7–10 days.

Emergency Department Management

Diagnosis

▶ Is generally clinical, but some ancillary testing may be needed.
▶ In toxic patients, lab studies may include CBC, cultures of drainage/blood, and chemistries for glucose/hydration status.
▶ CT is test of choice for suspected abscess (10× more sensitive for detecting stones than plain X-rays).

Treatment

▶ Bacterial
  • ENT consult for abscess treatment and ongoing management.
  • Beta-lactamase–resistant penicillin or first-generation cephalosporin for acute bacterial presentation, parenteral if toxic.
  • Clindamycin or vancomycin if penicillin allergic.
  • Fluid and electrolyte replacement as needed, oral hygiene, and sialagogues.
  • Analgesics and heat for pain control.
  • External massage may aid duct drainage.
▶ Viral
  • Rest, hydration, and analgesia.
  • Modify diet to minimize secretory activity (may be more painful).

Disposition

▶ Admission usually required for acute bacterial infection.
▶ Outpatient treatment is usually appropriate for other causes.
  • ENT follow-up for chronic infection and suspected atypical causes.
  • Simple mumps will not need referral but needs instruction about spread of disease, communicable for 1 week prior to 10 days post-onset.

CHAPTER 158

ADULT EPIGLOTTITIS

Trac Xuan Nghiem

- More commonly found in adults than in children (due to widespread use of *Haemophilus influenzae* vaccine)
- 2:1 male to female ratio
- Mortality around 7% (children < 1%)

PATHOPHYSIOLOGY

- Swelling and edema of supraglottic structures, including base of tongue, vallecula, aryepiglottic folds, arytenoids, and epiglottis.
- If unrecognized, can progress to airway compromise/obstruction and death.
- Complicated by aspiration of secretions, laryngospasm, and abscess formation.
- Often no culture-proven bacteria; when positive, responsible organisms commonly include *H. influenzae* (25%), beta-hemolytic streptococci, and *Streptococcus pneumoniae*.

CLINICAL PRESENTATION

- See Table 158-1.
- Usually have abrupt onset of symptoms although can have viral URI prodrome for 1–2 days.
- Sore throat is usually severe and classically out of proportion to findings on clinical exam.
- Signs of imminent airway compromise include respiratory compromise, stridor, drooling, and patient in the sniffing or tripod position.

DIFFERENTIAL DIAGNOSIS

- See Table 158-2.

TABLE 158-1.
CLINICAL PRESENTATION OF ADULT EPIGLOTTITIS

Signs and symptoms	Range of patients (%)
Sore throat	91–95
Odynophagia	82–94
Hoarseness/muffled voice	54–79
Anterior neck tenderness	50–79
Cervical adenopathy	32–55
Fever	26–42
Drooling	22–30
Stridor	12–27

EMERGENCY MEDICINE MANAGEMENT
Diagnosis

▶ Severe cases are usually obvious, but diagnosis is missed on initial presentation in up to one-third.

▶ CBC may reveal leukocytosis (non-specific and non-sensitive), blood cultures.

▶ Lateral neck X-rays: overall, approximately 80% sensitive, vallecula sign (loss of vallecula space between hyoid bone and epiglottis), and thumbprint sign (edematous epiglottis).

▶ CT scan used in stable patients with fever, sore throat, and dysphagia without significant exam findings. Gives information on deep spaces in neck in addition to supraglottic region.

▶ Fiberoptic laryngoscopy: considered most sensitive and specific, generally considered safe in adult patients without significant respiratory distress.

TABLE 158-2.
DIFFERENTIAL DIAGNOSIS OF ADULT EPIGLOTTITIS

Infectious	Non-infectious
Pharyngitis	Angioedema
Tonsillitis	FB
Peritonsillar or retropharyngeal abscess	Epiglottic hematoma
	Thermal injury/inhalation injury
Mononucleosis	Tumor

Treatment

▶ Patients who exhibit signs of respiratory distress should go to the OR with ENT and anesthesia to perform direct laryngoscopy and secure airway.

▶ If patient does not show evidence of respiratory distress, then can be worked up in ED. Should be on monitor with airway equipment at bedside (including cricothyrotomy kit).

▶ IV antibiotics: second- or third-generation cephalosporin (cefuroxime, cefotaxime, ceftriaxone, etc.) or broad-spectrum penicillin with beta-lactamase inhibitor (ampicillin-sulbactam or ticarcillin-clavulanate).

▶ IV steroids: controversial, may reduce airway angioedema but lacking supportive scientific data that reveal true benefit.

Disposition

▶ Even if no need for emergent airway management, patients should be admitted to ICU for close monitoring with ENT/anesthesia service involvement.

CHAPTER 159

PERITONSILLAR ABSCESS

Paige W. Archey

▶ Infection in the tonsillar crypts or Weber's mucous glands in the superior tonsillar pole results in acute tonsillitis and local cellulitis.
▶ An abscess then forms, usually located between the tonsillar capsule, palatopharyngeus muscle, and superior constrictor muscle. Most commonly at the upper pole of the tonsil.
▶ Usually polymicrobial.

CLINICAL PRESENTATION
History

▶ Sore throat, odynophagia, fevers, headache, dysphagia, drooling, dehydration, "hot potato voice."

Exam

▶ May be limited by trismus.
▶ The patient may have purulent tonsillar exudates, tonsillar enlargement and erythema, cervical lymphadenopathy, and, classically, deviation of the uvula with inferomedial displacement of the tonsil and/or soft palate.
▶ Palpation of the tonsillar region may reveal a fluctuant site suggestive of abscess.

EMERGENCY DEPARTMENT MANAGEMENT
Diagnosis

▶ Diagnosis is made clinically.
▶ Major entity in differential is peritonsillar cellulitis. Trismus and uvular shift are uncommon with peritonsillar cellulitis.
▶ FNA is a safe and cost-effective means of diagnosis and treatment. Needle aspiration is diagnostic if purulent material is

obtained—a negative aspirate, however, does rule out a peritonsillar abscess.

▶ If the patient cannot tolerate FNA, a CT scan or intra-oral ultrasound is an effective means of diagnosis. CT or intra-oral ultrasound can also be used to guide the direction of FNA.

Treatment

▶ Consists of drainage, antibiotics, and analgesia.

▶ **Drainage of abscess** requires a cooperative patient without severe trismus.
- FNA is the mainstay of treatment.
  - Anesthetize area topically with Cetacaine spray and then with lidocaine/epinephrine intramucosally in an attempt to blanch the area.
  - Use an 18-gauge needle. Cut off 1 cm at the end of the needle guard and replace it onto the needle to prevent deep penetration of the needle into the tonsil and adjoining structures.
  - Insert the needle into the most fluctuant area, usually superior pole of tonsil. If no pus obtained, attempt second and then third aspiration at medial and then inferior pole of tonsil.
  - Care should be taken to avoid the carotid artery, which is located approximately 2.5 cm posterolateral to the tonsil.
  - Cure rate 94%, reoccurrence 10%.
- Open I&D.
  - Anesthetize as described above.
  - Using No. 11 blade scalpel (with tape guard at 0.5 cm), make stab incision at area of maximum fluctuance.
  - Suction pus and expect the area to bleed.
  - May benefit to gargle with saline following procedure.
  - Should be watched in ED for about 1 hour following drainage.
- Failure to obtain pus should prompt antibiotics and follow-up at 24 hours to re-evaluate. Some have advocated a more conservative approach with admission for IV antibiotics, but assuming the patient is tolerating PO and is non-toxic appearing, this is usually unnecessary.

▶ **Antibiotics:**
- Penicillin, 250 mg PO qid for 7 days.

- For penicillin allergy, use erythromycin or clindamycin.
- Consider single dose of dexamethasone, 10 mg IM; shown to be beneficial in symptomatic relief of acute pharyngitis.

Disposition

▶ Most may be discharged home with 24-hour follow-up at oto-laryngology clinic or, if not available, back in ED.

▶ Admit those patients who are unable to tolerate PO intake, are dehydrated or toxic appearing, have complications of FNA, or have other underlying disease.

▶ Otolaryngology evaluation is recommended in those patients who have diabetes; age > 60; severe trismus, sepsis, or laryngeal edema; CT showing abscess unreachable by FNA; as well as those who do not tolerate FNA, as these patients may need abscess tonsillectomy.

CHAPTER 160

RETROPHARYNGEAL AND PARAPHARYNGEAL ABSCESS

Paige W. Archey

RETROPHARYNGEAL ABSCESS

▶ Initial infection in the pharynx, sinuses, or dental region spreads to the retropharyngeal lymph nodes and then extends to the retropharyngeal space.

▶ Begins as a cellulitis, progressing to phlegmon, and then to abscess formation.

▶ The disease is most common in children due to the infectious etiology and the fact that children have more retropharyngeal lymph nodes.

▶ Usually polymicrobial with mixture of aerobes and anaerobes.

▶ Risk factors include AIDS, diabetes, lymphadenitis, pharyngitis, poor dentition, sinusitis, and tonsillitis.

Clinical Presentation

▶ Sore throat, odynophagia, fevers, headache, dysphagia, drooling, dehydration, neck pain, torticollis, or dysphonia (like a duck "quack" or *cri du canard*).

▶ These patients usually appear ill and may prefer to hyperextend the neck and lie in the supine position, preventing the edematous posterior pharynx from compressing the airway.

▶ Physical exam findings include cervical lymphadenopathy and trismus, which may limit the pharyngeal exam. Pharynx may appear surprisingly normal given the degree of pain and dysphagia.

Differential Diagnosis

▶ See Table 160-1.

TABLE 160-1.
DIFFERENTIAL DIAGNOSIS OF RETROPHARYNGEAL ABSCESS

Cervical osteomyelitis	Meningitis
Epiglottitis	Parapharyngeal abscess
FB aspiration	Retropharyngeal tumor
Local inflammation or hematoma	Retromolar abscess
Internal carotid artery aneurysm	Ludwig's angina

Emergency Department Management

Diagnosis

▶ Must have high index of suspicion, particularly when there is paucity of findings on exam with suggestive symptoms.

▶ Lateral neck X-rays may reveal increased depth of pre-vertebral tissue (> 7 mm in adults and children at C2, > 22 mm adults and > 14 mm children at C6). Can also show air-fluid levels and reversal of normal lordosis. Taken in inspiration with neck in slight extension.

▶ CT scan usually regarded as imaging modality of choice, as it not only aids in the diagnosis and differentiation between cellulitis and abscess but also determines the extent of the disease process and the presence of complications.

Treatment

▶ Airway equipment at bedside and be prepared for difficult airway
▶ IV antibiotics
   • Ampicillin-sulbactam (Unasyn), 3 g IV q6h
   • High-dose penicillin and metronidazole IV
▶ ENT consultation to consider drainage in OR

Disposition

▶ Admit these patients to a monitored bed for observation and IV antibiotics.

▶ Any patient with airway compromise should have an I&D performed immediately in the OR.

PARAPHARYNGEAL ABSCESS

▶ Initial infection of dental or pharyngotonsillar origin, or seeding from IV drug abuse, spreads to the parapharyngeal space.

Clinical Presentation

▶ Classically presents with severe neck pain, swelling associated with odynophagia.

▶ Sore throat, fevers, headache, dysphagia, drooling, dehydration, neck pain, torticollis, ear pain, or dysphonia.

▶ On exam, there may be edema of the lateral pharyngeal wall or edema of the lateral neck, below the mandible. Trismus may limit the physical exam.

Emergency Department Management

Diagnosis

▶ High index of suspicion based on history and physical exam.

▶ X-rays may reveal pre-vertebral swelling but are often non-diagnostic.

▶ CT or MRI of the neck regarded as gold standard for making diagnosis.

Treatment

▶ IV antibiotics.

▶ ENT consult to consider drainage of abscess.

▶ Admit to monitor/ICU setting.

CHAPTER 161

LUDWIG'S ANGINA

George M. Elliott

- First described in 1836 by Wilhelm Friedrich von Ludwig
- Rapidly progressing, gangrenous cellulitis that originates in the submandibular space
- Most commonly caused by dental disease

PATHOPHYSIOLOGY

- Initial event can be tooth extraction/infection, oral neoplasm, or penetrating injury to the floor of the mouth.
- Periapical abscesses of the second or third molars penetrate into the mandibular cortex extending deep into the area of the submandibular space, giving the infection a direct route to spread.
- Inferior surface of mandible, hyoid, and deep cervical fascia act as a firm border, so, as the infection progresses, the path of least resistance is caudally, which results in the superior and posterior displacement of the tongue and floor of the mouth.
- Displacement of these structures leads to progressive airway compromise.
- Infection is polymicrobial. Most commonly isolated organisms include streptococci, staphylococci, and *Bacteroides* species.
- Predisposing factors include diabetes, poor nutrition, poor dental hygiene, immunocompromised state.

CLINICAL PRESENTATION

- Common symptoms include dysphagia, neck swelling and pain, "hot potato" voice, and drooling.
- Ask about recent dental extraction/disease.
- Vitals: febrile, tachycardic, ± hypotension.
- Physical exam:
  - Neck swelling: tense edema and brawny induration "bull neck"

- Tongue protrusion and elevation
- Also may have facial swelling and trismus
- Markedly tender to palpation and may have SC emphysema

DIFFERENTIAL DIAGNOSIS

▶ Retropharyngeal or peritonsillar abscess
▶ Cellulitis confined to the superficial soft tissue of the neck without extension
▶ Parotitis
▶ Angioedema

EMERGENCY DEPARTMENT MANAGEMENT

▶ Airway compromise suggested by stridor, inability to handle secretions, dyspnea, and agitation:
  - Call ENT and anesthesia.
  - Nebulized epinephrine may assist when assembling airway equipment.
  - Fiberoptic nasotracheal intubation with anesthesia in OR is the preferred method to secure airway; nebulized lidocaine may assist.
  - Should have surgical option available.
▶ Without impending airway compromise:
  - Airway equipment at bedside.
  - Sitting upright and on monitor.
  - CBC, blood cultures.
  - Involve consultants early: ENT, anesthesia.
  - Consider imaging with soft tissue X-ray of neck or CT scan.
  - Broad-spectrum antibiotics to cover oral flora.
    ○ High-dose penicillin and metronidazole
    ○ Ampicillin-sulbactam, 3 g IV q6h
  - Steroids: dexamethasone, 10 mg IV, may help reduce edema.
  - Surgical I&D considered for those who do not respond to conservative management.
▶ Admit all to ICU setting where they can be monitored closely for deterioration.

CHAPTER 162

EPISTAXIS

Kerry L. Kikuchi

- ▶ Most cases occur in children and elderly.
- ▶ Incidence of posterior epistaxis increases in elderly patients.
- ▶ More common in colder seasons and in northern climates because of low humidity.
- ▶ Vast majority stop with pressure alone and do not require ED care.

PATHOPHYSIOLOGY

- ▶ 90% anterior involving Kiesselbach's plexus on the anterior-inferior nasal septum.
  - • Etiology includes URI, blunt or digital trauma, FB, HTN, anti-coagulant medication, coagulopathy, tumors, and cocaine abuse.
- ▶ 10% posterior involving the posterior branch of the sphenopalatine artery.
  - • More common in elderly, thought to be secondary to atherosclerosis and HTN.

CLINICAL PRESENTATION

- ▶ Inquire about onset, duration, and severity. Which side did bleeding start? Does patient have HTN, take anti-coagulants, have recent surgery, or use cocaine?
- ▶ Anterior epistaxis:
  - • Unilateral and usually no blood in the posterior oropharynx
- ▶ Posterior epistaxis:
  - • Bleeding is more profuse, and often seen in posterior oropharynx and from both nares

EMERGENCY DEPARTMENT MANAGEMENT

▶ Lab tests usually not required, except when there is a clinical suspicion of co-existing coagulopathy or anemia, or patient is hemodynamically unstable.

▶ Have patient apply continuous pressure to bilateral nasal septum by compressing cartilaginous portion of nose for 10–15 minutes. It is important to teach this technique to patients so they can perform at home if bleeding recurs.

▶ Assemble all necessary equipment:
- Gown, gloves, eye-shield, emesis basin, light source
- Suction, nasal speculum, bayonet forceps, topical anesthetic and vasoconstrictor, cotton swabs, 4×4 gauze
- Silver nitrate sticks, Gelfoam, nasal packs

▶ Aspirate all clots from the nose.

▶ Insert large cotton pledget dampened with topical anesthetic and vasoconstrictor (e.g., lidocaine 4% solution–epinephrine 1:1000 or cocaine 4%) for 5–10 minutes.

▶ Attempt to identify site of bleeding, examine posterior pharynx.

▶ Options for anterior source of bleeding:
- Cautery with silver nitrate stick.
  ○ Will not work on active bleeding vessels.
  ○ Avoid prolonged or bilateral application to avoid septal necrosis.
- If large area oozing, can try hemostatic material (e.g., Gelfoam) applied directly to the bleeding site.
- If bleeding continues despite initial attempts to stop it, then need to place anterior nasal pack/tampon (often bilateral nasal packing required to create enough pressure). Pack must be kept in place for 24–48 hours, and prescribe antibiotics to prevent sinusitis as well as possibility of toxic shock syndrome (e.g., cephalexin, amoxicillin-clavulanate).

▶ If patient continues to bleed despite anterior nasal pack, or if a posterior source of bleed is suspected, then a posterior nasal pack may be necessary (as well as consultation with otolaryngology). Commercially available epistaxis balloons are available, or a standard Foley catheter may be used.
- Anesthetize the pharynx and soft palate (e.g., nebulized 4% lidocaine).
- Lubricate catheter with antibiotic ointment and pass in naris until visible in oropharynx. Inflate balloon as indicated.

- Firmly pack petroleum gauze into nose anteriorly against catheter.
▶ If above techniques do not control epistaxis, consult otolaryngology, as patient may require internal maxillary artery ligation or embolization, or posterior endoscopic cautery.

DISPOSITION

▶ Patients with posterior packs should be admitted to the hospital, as they are at risk for hypoxia and cardiac dysrhythmias.
▶ Hospital admission rarely needed for anterior epistaxis if good control of bleeding attained. Should follow up with primary physician or otolaryngology in 2–3 days.
- Instruct patient not to blow nose forcefully or manipulate nose for several days.
- If bleeding recurs and no nasal packing, instruct patient to re-apply pressure as taught in the ED for 10–15 minutes continuously. If, after three repeated attempts, bleeding continues, patient should return to ED.
- If bleeding recurs around anterior nasal pack, patient should return to ED and not remove nasal pack.

CHAPTER 163

SINUSITIS

Kerry L. Kikuchi

▶ An estimated 31 million people in the U.S. are affected by sinus disease each year; it accounts for 16 million physician visits each year.
▶ Fifth most common diagnosis for which an antibiotic is prescribed.
▶ Inflammation of paranasal sinuses (frontal, maxillary, ethmoid, and sphenoid).
▶ Classifications:
  • Acute sinusitis: > 3 weeks
  • Chronic sinusitis: > 3 months

PATHOPHYSIOLOGY

▶ Obstruction of the ostia with decreased ventilation and mucus drainage predisposes to the development of sinusitis.
▶ Most commonly caused by viral URI.
▶ Other predisposing factors include allergic rhinitis, dental procedures, facial trauma, mechanical ventilation, NG tubes, nasal packing, nasal septum deviation, nasal polyps, hypertrophy of the adenoids/tonsils, immunocompromised host, and mucociliary dysfunction.
▶ *Streptococcus pneumoniae*, *Haemophilus influenzae*, and *Moraxella catarrhalis* most common pathogens in acute sinusitis.
▶ Anaerobic bacteria and *Staphylococcus aureus* more common in chronic sinusitis.
▶ *Pseudomonas aeruginosa* associated with HIV and cystic fibrosis.
▶ *Aspergillus* species can cause acute sinusitis in immunocompromised and diabetic patients.

CLINICAL PRESENTATION

▶ Symptoms include
  • Headache, nasal congestion, pain over the involved sinus, maxillary toothache, fever, mucopurulent nasal discharge;

TABLE 163-1.
DIFFERENTIAL DIAGNOSIS OF ACUTE SINUSITIS

Protracted URI	Migraine, tension headache, or
Rhinitis	cluster headache
Periorbital cellulitis	Temporal arteritis
Dental disease	Temporomandibular disorders
Nasal FB	Meningitis
	Cavernous sinus thrombosis

    aggravated by bending forward, coughing, or sneezing, biphasic illness (original URI improves, then congestion and pain return), failure to improve with decongestants or antihistamines

▶ Signs include

   • Tenderness to percussion over the involved sinus, abnormal transillumination of the infected sinus, injected and swollen turbinates

DIFFERENTIAL DIAGNOSIS

▶ See Table 163-1.

EMERGENCY DEPARTMENT MANAGEMENT
Diagnosis

▶ Acute sinusitis is typically a clinical diagnosis.

▶ Imaging studies are not usually necessary in the assessment and treatment of patients with clinical findings suggestive of acute sinusitis.

▶ Radiographs, however, may be helpful in uncertain or recurrent cases, which may reveal sinus opacity, air-fluid levels, or ≥ 6 mm of mucosal thickening.

▶ CT scan best for suspected ethmoid/sphenoid sinusitis, chronic sinusitis, or possible extension of infection beyond paranasal sinuses.

Treatment

▶ There is scant evidence that antibiotics are beneficial in acute sinusitis. Despite this, standard treatment consists of a course of oral antibiotics.

▶ Patients with a high probability of having bacterial sinusitis may be considered for antibiotic treatment.
  • Amoxicillin, 500 mg PO tid 14 days
               or
  • SMX-TMP DS 1 tablet PO bid 14 days
▶ Chronic sinusitis may require longer courses of antibiotics and, possibly, operative irrigation and drainage by otolaryngology.
▶ Adjunctive therapies include steam, saline nasal rinses, topical decongestants, oral decongestants, and, possibly, mucolytic agents or intranasal corticosteroids.
  • Phenylephrine nasal 0.25%, 2 sprays/nostril q4h
▶ Use of topical decongestants should be restricted to 2–3 days because of the concern for rebound rhinitis.
▶ There is no rationale for using antihistamines in treating acute sinusitis (may dry the mucous membranes and block the ostia).
▶ Most patients can be treated as outpatients with follow-up with their primary physician or otolaryngology. Those with complications of spread beyond the sinus cavity, septic patients, or those with neurologic signs should be given IV antibiotics, otolaryngology consult, and admission to the hospital.

CHAPTER 164

PERIODONTAL DISEASE

J. Jeff Downie and Stephen P. R. MacLeod

- ▶ Periodontal disease is an infection of the tissues that support the teeth.
- ▶ Teeth are supported by the gingiva. A tooth's root is anchored to its socket by fibers called periodontal ligaments. Periodontitis is the inflammation of these fibers.
- ▶ Gingivitis is the mildest form of periodontal disease. It causes the gums to become red, swollen, and bleed easily. Gingivitis is reversible with good oral care.
- ▶ If left untreated, gingivitis may progress to periodontitis, abscess formation, and subsequent tooth loss.
- ▶ The flora at different oral sites varies. Anaerobes usually outnumber aerobes and facultative anaerobes.

CLINICAL PRESENTATION

History

- ▶ Intra-oral, throbbing pain and swelling may progress over a few hours to days. May have increased sensitivity to hot or cold.
- ▶ This may be associated with fever and general malaise.
- ▶ Halitosis is often present with the patient complaining of a bad taste.
- ▶ Intra-oral exam may reveal
  - Inflamed gingivae that bleed easily
  - Swelling or a fluctuant mass
  - Tooth mobility and percussion tenderness
  - More severe infections associated with trismus, facial and neck swelling, regional lymphadenopathy, difficulty swallowing, and even respiratory difficulty

DIFFERENTIAL DIAGNOSIS

▶ **Periodontal abscess:** involves the supporting structures of the teeth (periodontal ligaments, alveolar bone). This is the most common dental abscess in adults but may occur in children following impaction of an FB in the gingiva.

▶ **Periapical abscess:** originates in the dental pulp and is usually secondary to dental caries. This is the most common dental abscess in children. Dental caries erode the protective layers of the tooth (i.e., enamel, dentin) and allow bacteria to invade the pulp, producing a pulpitis. Pulpitis can progress to necrosis with bacterial invasion of the alveolar bone, forming an abscess.

▶ **Acute necrotizing ulcerative gingivitis:** acute ulcerating condition affecting the marginal gingivae leading to grayish pseudomembrane formation. Usually associated with smoking. Pain is a significant feature.

▶ **Acute herpetic gingivostomatitis:** characterized by vesicular lesions, which occur on the gingivae and rapidly rupture to form small irregular superficial ulcers with erythematous halos.

▶ **Pericoronitis:** inflammation around the crown of a tooth usually associated with a partially erupted tooth such as an impacted third molar.

▶ **Alveolar osteitis (dry socket):** loss of clot and localized osteomyelitis. Usually pain free for 3–4 days following extraction, followed by the abrupt onset of severe dental pain.

EMERGENCY DEPARTMENT MANAGEMENT
Diagnosis

▶ Diagnosis is based on clinical exam findings and only rarely needs to be augmented by lab or radiologic evaluation.

▶ Imaging studies:
  • Plain radiography (Panorex) may be helpful to indicate whether bone or teeth are involved. Rarely used for this indication in the ED.
  • CT scan with IV contrast is the most accurate method to determine the location, size, extent, and relationship of the inflammatory process. This is particularly valuable if involvement of the fascial spaces or airway is suspected.

Treatment

▶ Consists of analgesia and PO antibiotics. Penicillin or clindamycin is good first-line therapy against oral flora.
  • Penicillin, 250 mg PO qid 7 days
  • Clindamycin, 300 mg PO qid 7 days
▶ A supraperiosteal infiltration (tooth block—contraindicated when abscess involves injection site) or regional nerve block using a long-acting anesthetic should be considered, as this provides immediate, long-lasting relief and reduces need for oral narcotics.
▶ Abscesses that are obvious on clinical exam should be drained in the ED after local anesthetic. An attempt at needle aspiration can be made or a 0.5- to 1-cm incision can be made using a No. 11 blade scalpel.
▶ If unable to aspirate pus, manage medically until a more localized infection develops.

Disposition

▶ Usually can be discharged to home on PO antibiotics to follow up with dentist.
▶ Consult oral maxillofacial surgeon if the patient has a complicated abscess.

◑ **PEARLS AND PITFALLS**
  • Infective endocarditis: any dental procedures involving manipulation that causes bleeding and a bacteremia may result in endocarditis. The presence of gingivitis increases this risk by making the gingiva more likely to bleed with simple manipulation.

CHAPTER 165

DENTAL TRAUMA

Rahul Rastogi

- ► 50% of children with peak incidence at 2–5 years old—usually from falls and collisions.
- ► In adults, most commonly occurs in MVAs and fights.
- ► Male to female ratio is 2:1.
- ► Most common injury is fracture of crown of maxillary central incisor > maxillary lateral incisor > mandibular central incisors.
- ► Low-velocity injuries are associated with tooth support injuries, while high-velocity injuries are associated with crown fractures.

ANATOMY

- ► 32 teeth in normal adult, 20 teeth in the child (by age 3).
- ► Crown is the visible portion and is covered by the enamel.
- ► Dentin underlies the enamel and is similar to bone in its micro-tubular structure.
- ► Pulp in center carries the nerves and blood vessels and makes the dentin.
- ► Three structures hold the tooth into the bone:
  - • Cementum, periodontal ligament, and alveolar bone.
- ► Cementum connects the ligament to the bone.

EXAM

- ► Need accurate history of event and must exclude other facial injuries.
- ► After stabilization and primary survey, secondary survey permits proper evaluation of oral cavity.
- ► Inspect jaw and all soft tissues both inside and outside the mouth.
- ► Assess bite alignment.
- ► Percuss each tooth with tongue depressor and then assess mobility.

IMAGING

▶ Panoramic radiograph (Panorex): look for dental fractures and also may assist in diagnosis of mandibular and maxillary fractures.

▶ Dental intra-oral radiographs provide more accurate information but are usually not performed in the ED.

DENTAL FRACTURES

▶ Injuries divided into those involving the crown or the root.

▶ Ellis classification divides crown injuries:
  - **Ellis class I:** fracture through enamel only
    ○ Treatment entails dulling of sharp edges of enamel.
  - **Ellis class II:** through to the dentin visualized as yellow center
    ○ May be painful to touch with sensitivity to air.
    ○ Dentin should be covered with calcium hydroxide paste and aluminum foil.
    ○ Should see dentist within 24 hours.
  - **Ellis class III:** fracture into pulp layer
    ○ Exposes the nerves and blood vessels of tooth and will show small amount of bleeding or redness.
    ○ Painful and very sensitive to air.
    ○ **Dental emergency that requires immediate referral.**
    ○ Tooth should be covered by moistened cotton wool and aluminum foil.

▶ Root injuries are divided into horizontal fractures (commonly occur in the anterior teeth due to direct forces) and vertical fractures (occur in the posterior teeth due to clenching forces).
  - Horizontal fractures have a good prognosis if they are reduced and splinted in place for about 10–12 weeks.
  - Vertical fractures are more difficult to identify and, hence, are more likely to have worse prognosis.
  - Referral to maxillofacial surgeon.
  - Patients should be prescribed prophylactic antibiotics (e.g., penicillin) and have tetanus updated.

DISPLACED TEETH

▶ Displacements of tooth > 5 mm usually result in pulp necrosis, while those < 5 mm heal 50% of the time.

▶ Gentle repositioning and prompt splinting with referral to dentist are recommended.

▶ Concussion is injury to support structures without significant displacement of tooth. If movement > 2 mm, the tooth should be splinted.

▶ Avulsion results in complete tear of support structures. Tooth must be replaced immediately into socket (within 30 minutes for best prognosis).

▶ Avulsed tooth handling:
  • Handle by crown only.
  • If tooth is dirty, may rinse in saline, milk, or—last option— tap water.
  • Do not scrub or sterilize the root.
  • After rinsing, replace tooth immediately into socket.
  • If unable to replace tooth into socket, store in pre-made solution, e.g., Hank's solution (increases tooth viability up to 6 hours), or milk, for transport to dentist. Do not allow tooth to air dry.
  • May use splinting material (e.g., COE-PAK) to temporarily splint tooth.
  • Prophylactic antibiotics and update tetanus.
  • Primary teeth should not be replaced—they should all be referred to the dentist.

CHAPTER 166

APPROACH TO THE SOLID ORGAN TRANSPLANT PATIENT

James A. Freer

▶ 25,464 solid organ transplants in 2003 with 82,884 on waiting list

▶ Kidney > liver > heart > lung > kidney/pancreas > intestine > heart/lung

COMMON PROBLEMS

▶ **Rejection**
  - Hyperacute: antibody-mediated, PMN reaction [e.g., amino-levulinic acid (e.g., blood type) mismatch]
  - Acute: cell-mediated, lymphocyte reaction (i.e., graft vs. host)
  - Chronic: antibody-mediated, cytokine and tissue growth factor reaction

▶ **Infection** (66% of patients; most common cause of transplant-related mortality)
  - Pre-transplant acquired
    ◦ Viral: CMV, EBV, hepatitis B and C, HSV, VZV
    ◦ Bacteria: TB
    ◦ Fungal: blastomycosis, coccidioidomycosis, histoplasmosis
    ◦ Parasitic: *Strongyloides stercoralis*
  - Post-transplant acquired (temporally can class 0–1, 1–6, > 6 months)
    ◦ Community-acquired
    ◦ Viral: CMV, EBV, influenza, primary varicella
    ◦ Bacteria: *Mycobacterium, Legionella, Salmonella*
    ◦ Fungal: see pre-transplant; add cryptococcosis, nocardiosis
    ◦ Parasitic: *Pneumocystis carinii*
  - Nosocomial
    ◦ Bacteria: gram-negative (e.g., *Pseudomonas, Legionella*)
    ◦ Fungal: *Aspergillus*

▶ **Medication** (immune system modifiers)
- Azathioprine (Imuran®)
  - Adverse reactions: GI, infection, hematologic
  - Drug interactions: allopurinol, ACE inhibitors, live vaccines
- Corticosteroid (prednisone, methylprednisolone)
  - Adverse reactions: psychosis, adrenal insufficiency
  - Drug interactions: antifungals, phenobarbital, phenytoin, rifampin (RIF)
- Cyclosporine (Neoral®, Sandimmune®)
  - Adverse reactions: nephrotoxicity, hepatotoxicity, refractory HTN, neuropathy, malignancy
  - Drug interactions:
    - Increased: antifungals, macrolides, CCBs, methylprednisolone, allopurinol, colchicine
    - Decreased: nafcillin, RIF, carbamazepine, phenytoin, phenobarbital
- Mycophenolate mofetil (MMF; CellCept®)
  - Adverse reactions: nausea, vomiting, and diarrhea; leukopenia, opportunistic infection
  - Drug interactions (avoid live vaccines):
    - Increased: acyclovir, ganciclovir
    - Decreased: antacids, iron, *Echinacea*
    - Variable: oral contraceptives
- Sirolimus (Rapamune®)
  - Adverse reactions: HTN, lipid disorder, rash; at higher doses: anemia, thrombocytopenia, arthralgia, diarrhea, hypokalemia
  - Drug interactions (avoid live vaccines):
    - Increase: antifungal, CYP34A inducers
- Tacrolimus (Prograf®)
  - Adverse reactions: nausea, vomiting, and diarrhea; tremor; headache; hyperglycemia; hyperkalemia; hypermagnesemia
  - Drug interactions, effect (avoid live vaccines):
    - Increased: antifungal, CCBs, cimetidine, macrolide antibiotics, phenytoin, and many others
    - Decreased: grapefruit, St. John's wort
    - Variable: CYP34A active agents

CLINICAL PRESENTATION

▸ Fever → infection, acute rejection
▸ Medication change → drug interaction
▸ Vomiting → infection, rejection, medication, bowel obstruction/perforation
▸ Dehydration → poor organ perfusion and electrolyte abnormality
▸ Tender liver or kidney transplant → rejection
▸ Creatinine elevated from baseline → rejection, medication, dehydration, anatomic
▸ Headache, altered mental status → meningitis, encephalitis
▸ Seizure → CNS infection, electrolyte abnormality, drug
▸ Hypotension, vomiting, paucity of bowel sounds → consider perforated viscus
▸ Heart transplant with hypotension, tachycardia, cyanosis → rejection
▸ Skin rash, fever, constitutional and joint complaints, diarrhea → consider graft vs. host disease
▸ Fever, abdominal pain/mass, lymphadenopathy → post-transplantation lymphoproliferative disorder, more common in children

DIAGNOSIS

Laboratory

▸ Urine with pyuria, bacteria → UTI/outflow tract problem
▸ CBC → leukocytosis (infection), hematotoxicity
▸ Electrolytes → dehydration, renal failure, drug toxicity
▸ BUN/creatinine → to monitor renal function, dehydration
▸ LFT → to monitor liver function, hepatotoxicity
▸ Blood, urine, sputum cultures/studies → useful for potential infection
▸ Fungal culture/studies → immunomodulation increases risk
▸ Cyclosporine/other drug levels → trough level; generally not useful in ED

Imaging

▸ Plain film radiography → pneumonia, bowel obstruction, stent location.

- ► CT → IV contrast with caution! Consider consulting transplant service.
- ► Ultrasonography → to evaluate organ blood flow, anatomy (GI, GU).

ECG/Monitor

- ► Electrolyte abnormality → changes with abnormal potassium
- ► Heart transplant rejection → may display low voltage

TREATMENT/DISPOSITION

- ► Stabilization → treat volume depletion, shock, hypoxemia with appropriate measures.
- ► Continuity → consider early contact with the transplant service following the patient.
- ► Drug therapy → after appropriate initial care, coordinated with transplant service.
- ► Disposition → coordinate with transplant service after condition stabilized.

CHAPTER 167

APPROACH TO BLEEDING DISORDERS

Swagata Mandal

- ▶ Hemostasis depends on the presence and proper function of the vasculature, platelets, and coagulation cascade.
- ▶ Disorders of hemostasis can be inherited or acquired (e.g., drug-related, secondary to co-existing disease, or iatrogenic).
- ▶ Platelets are responsible for primary hemostasis, and the clotting cascade is responsible for secondary hemostasis.
  - Platelet disorders: usually acquired, more common in women, and present as petechiae, purpura, and mucosal bleeding
  - Bleeding disorders: usually congenital, more common in men, and present as delayed deep muscle or joint bleeding

PATHOPHYSIOLOGY

- ▶ The coagulation cascade (Fig. 167-1)
- ▶ Clotting factors associated with abnormalities
  - Factors II, VII, IX, X: vitamin K–dependent clotting factors affected by warfarin, liver disease
  - Factor VIII: deficiency associated with hemophilia A
  - Factor IX: deficiency associated with hemophilia B
  - Factor Xa: affected by LMWH
  - Factors IIa, IXa, Xa, XIa, platelet factor 3: affected by unfractionated heparin

CLINICAL PRESENTATION
History

- ▶ Type of bleeding: petechiae, purpura, ecchymosis, and major bleeding episodes
- ▶ Sites of bleeding: skin, mucous membranes, muscle, GI or GU tracts, joints

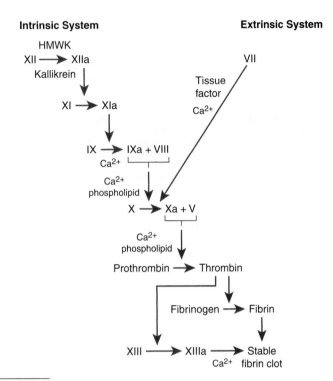

FIGURE 167-1.

The coagulation cascade. HMWK, high molecular weight kininogen.

▶ Patterns of bleeding: recent in onset vs. lifelong, frequency and severity, spontaneous vs. post-injury, prior challenges (tooth extraction, surgery)

▶ Co-existing diseases: uremia, liver disease, sepsis, malignancy

▶ Transfusion history, FH, and medications

Physical Exam

▶ Vital signs: evidence of hemodynamic instability.

▶ The skin exam provides many clues:
  • Presence of pallor
  • Petechiae, purpura, ecchymosis
  • Signs of liver disease: spider angiomata, palmar erythema, telangiectasias

▶ The abdominal exam helps determine the presence or absence of ascites, hepatomegaly, or splenomegaly.

TABLE 167-1.
COAGULATION STUDIES

Elevated PT	Factor VII deficiency	Inherited: rare, autosomal-recessive transmission	Defect in extrinsic pathway
		Acquired: warfarin use, vitamin K deficiency, liver disease	
Elevated PTT	Factor VIII, IX, and XI deficiencies	Account for 99% of inherited bleeding disorders	Defects in intrinsic pathway
		Factor VIII deficiency: hemophilia	
		Factor IX deficiency: hemophilia B, Christmas disease	

▶ Lymphadenopathy may be a clue to an underlying or undiagnosed malignancy.
▶ Examine other sites of possible blood loss: GI and GU tracts.
▶ Examine the joints for hemarthrosis.

DIAGNOSIS

Blood Tests

▶ CBC with differential and smear
  • HCT and Hgb may not reflect true blood loss in acute hemorrhage.
  • Schistocytes or fragmented RBCs: disseminated intravascular coagulation, TTP.
  • Teardrop-shaped or nucleated RBCs: myelophthisic disease.
  • Platelets < 20,000 associated with spontaneous hemorrhage.
▶ Coagulation studies (Table 167-1)
  • PT
    ○ Assesses function of the extrinsic clotting pathways
    ○ Usually reported using the INR
    ○ Abnormal in patients on warfarin therapy and with liver disease
  • PTT
    ○ Assesses function of the intrinsic clotting pathway
    ○ Abnormal in patients on heparin therapy
▶ Electrolytes, including BUN and creatinine
▶ LFTs

TABLE 167-2.
FACTOR VIII COAGULANT SEVERITY

Factor VIII: C activity (%)	Severity	Risk of spontaneous bleeding	Rate of complications with surgery or trauma
< 1	Severe	High	High
1–5	Moderate	Rare	Increased
5–10	Mild	Low	Moderate
> 10	Very mild	Very low	Low

▶ Other tests that are not as useful in the ED
  • Bleeding time, platelet function studies
  • Specific factor levels

HEMOPHILIA A

▶ 70% of cases are sex-linked recessive in inheritance.
▶ Intracranial hemorrhage major cause of death in all age groups.

Pathophysiology

▶ Abnormal clot-promoting property of factor VIII
▶ Severity based on level of factor VIII coagulant (factor VIII: C) activity (Table 167-2)

Presentation

▶ Antecedent history of trauma or surgery
▶ Delayed bleeding after 1–3 days possible, but usually occurs by 8 hours
▶ Bleeding into deep muscles, joints, GU tract, and intracranial

Diagnosis

▶ FH
▶ Elevated PTT
▶ Abnormal factor VIII: C activity (usually not available to the ED)

Treatment

▶ In life-threatening active bleeding:
  • FFP, 15 ml/kg
▶ Recombinant factor VIII (Recombinate, ReFacto):
  • Treatment of choice

- Comparable to plasma-derived factor VIII in action
- No side effects
▶ Factor VIII concentrate:
  - Freeze-dried, plasma-derived anti-hemophilic factor
▶ Dosage of factor VIII calculated based on bleeding risk, patient's plasma volume, and desired factor activity level.
▶ Cryoprecipitate:
  - Past mainstay of hemophilia A therapy
  - Derived from FFP
▶ Cryoprecipitate and factor VIII concentrate administration carry a small risk of hepatitis B, hepatitis C, and HIV.

Disposition

▶ Patients with a significant bleeding episode should be admitted for further observation and monitoring.
▶ Other hemophiliacs with injuries to areas where development of bleeding or hematoma (head, eye, airway, spine) is potentially life-threatening should be admitted as well.

HEMOPHILIA B (CHRISTMAS DISEASE)

▶ Deficiency of factor IX activity

Presentation

▶ Identical to hemophilia A

Diagnosis

▶ FH
▶ Elevated PTT with normal factor VIII: C activity
▶ Abnormal factor IX assay

Treatment

▶ Recombinant factor IX preferred.
▶ Purified factor IX concentrate available.
▶ Plasma prothrombin complex (factors II, VII, IX, X) or FFP may be used.
▶ Human-derived products carry risks of hepatitis B, hepatitis C, and HIV.
▶ Factor IX replacement dosing is based on bleeding risk from injury, patient's plasma volume, and desired factor activity lev-

el, but repeated doses are administered less frequently because of the longer half-life of factor IX.

Disposition

▶ Similar to patients with hemophilia A

VON WILLEBRAND DISEASE

▶ Most common hereditary bleeding disorder with a prevalence of 1%
▶ Autosomal-dominant inheritance with variable penetrance
▶ Generally milder than hemophilia A

Pathophysiology

▶ Disorder of primary hemostasis caused by abnormal interaction between platelets and endothelium

Clinical Presentation

▶ Usually severe bleeding only with a history of trauma or surgery.
▶ Patients may give a history of epistaxis, easy bruising, or menorrhagia.
▶ Prolonged bleeding after minor trauma.
▶ Evidence of bruising or bleeding on exam.
▶ Women with vWD may have a normal labor and delivery but can develop post-partum bleeding.

Diagnosis

▶ FH.
▶ Normal PT.
▶ Elevated PTT in 50% of patients with vWD.
▶ Factor VIII, vWF antigen, and ristocetin cofactor levels vary depending on the type of vWD.
  • vWF levels increase during pregnancy and other physiologic stress.
  • Not useful in the ED setting.

Treatment

▶ Desmopressin (DDAVP) given IV or intranasally causes release of stored vWF in patients with type I vWD with peak effect in 30–60 minutes.
  • Patients with type II vWD have variable responses to DDAVP.

- ▶ Purified plasma-derived factor VIII is the therapy of choice in patients with type III vWD.
  - • Recombinant and monoclonal factor III concentrates do not contain enough vWF.
- ▶ Cryoprecipitate or FFP may be used if necessary, but carries the risk of viral transmission.
- ▶ Estrogens may be helpful in controlling menorrhagia.

Disposition

- ▶ Similar to hemophilia A

CHAPTER 168

SICKLE CELL ANEMIA

Jonathan Shenk

EPIDEMIOLOGY

- ▶ Autosomal-recessive disorder, most common in people of African descent.
- ▶ One in 600 African-Americans has SCD.

PATHOPHYSIOLOGY

- ▶ Valine substituted for glutamic acid in position 6 of the Hgb beta chain.
- ▶ Hgb S polymerizes in deoxygenated state, causing RBCs to sickle.
- ▶ Sickled cells are less pliable and cannot easily pass through capillary beds.
- ▶ Local tissue ischemia leads to micro-infarctions and pain.
- ▶ Sickling causes RBCs to be fragile, causing shorter RBC life expectancy, 17 days.
- ▶ Recurrent micro-infarctions cause functional asplenia.
  - Often occurs by age 3; 90% have functional asplenia by age 5.
  - Decreased resistance to encapsulated organisms.

APLASTIC ANEMIA

- ▶ Generally secondary to infection by parvovirus B-19.
- ▶ Infection causes transient (5–10 days) bone marrow suppression.
- ▶ Also can be nutritional, secondary to decreased folate.
- ▶ Since RBC lifespan only 17 days in SCD, transient marrow suppression can cause severe anemia.
- ▶ Fatigue and dyspnea are common presenting complaints.
- ▶ Identified by severe anemia and concurrent decreased reticulocyte count.
- ▶ Management:
  - Admission for observation and serial CBCs, possible transfusion.

- Give folate: will help nutritional causes and will not hurt other causes.
- Must be considered an infectious etiology with strict isolation from other SCD patients and pregnant women.
  - Parvovirus B-19 causes hydrops fetalis/miscarriages.

HYPERHEMOLYTIC ANEMIA

▶ Anemia due to accelerated hemolysis.
▶ Often associated with severe pain crisis or infection.
▶ Pain, fatigue/weakness, and scleral icterus are common presenting complaints.
▶ Lab evaluation:
- Increased anemia compared with patient's historical baseline
- High reticulocyte count
- Elevated indirect bilirubin and LDH
▶ Management:
- Admission for drop in Hgb > 1 g/dl from baseline
- Pain control
- Supportive care: hydration to euvolemia
- Transfusion if severely anemic

ACUTE SPLENIC SEQUESTRATION CRISIS

▶ Occurs in children before auto-infarction—generally before 3 years of age.
▶ 15% mortality per episode, 50% recurrence rate.
▶ Syncope is often the presenting complaint.
▶ Characterized by
- Severe anemia with thrombocytopenia, often hypovolemic shock
- Generally, toxic-appearing child
- Massive splenomegaly
- Often associated with abdominal pain
- Brisk reticulocytosis
▶ Management:
- Hypovolemia much more dangerous than anemia.
  - 20–40 cc/kg NS bolus immediately
- Blood transfusion: like all severe anemias, want to match cc/kg PRBC with Hgb (g/dl).
  - I.e., if Hgb is 3 g/dl, want to give 3 cc/kg PRBC initially

- Monitor size of spleen.
  - Once transfusion initiated, blood often released from sequestration.
  - If spleen shrinking, evaluate for volume overload, diuretics PRN.
- After acute event, surgical evaluation for possible splenectomy.

ACUTE CHEST SYNDROME

▶ Chest pain, fever, SOB with new infiltrate on CXR (absent 30% on initial ED presentation)
▶ Respiratory findings (common cough, wheeze, hypoxia, tachypnea)
▶ Most common in older children, adolescents; most serious in adults
▶ Children, adolescents:
  - Usually due to infection
  - Fever, cough typically present
  - Chest pain often absent
▶ Adults:
  - Often multilobar disease
  - Fever often absent
  - Chest pain generally present
  - High mortality
▶ Management:
  - Supplemental O_2
  - Hydration to euvolemia: caution not to overhydrate
  - Broad-spectrum antibiotics in children *and* adults
  - Incentive spirometry
  - Exchange transfusion if toxic appearance

FEVER/INFECTION

▶ Leading cause of death in SCD patients.
▶ Poor resistance to encapsulated organisms.
  - *Streptococcus pneumoniae* and *Haemophilus influenzae*
▶ In addition to sources of fever common to other patients, be sure to consider
  - Osteomyelitis (*Salmonella* species, *Staphylococcus aureus*)
  - CSF infections
  - Joint infections
  - Bacteremia

- Basic work-up includes CXR, UA, CBC with differential, blood cultures.
  - LP, joint aspiration, bone scan, CT abdomen/pelvis as indicated by clinical exam
- Management:
  - Adults with fever typically treated like non-SCD patients with fever
  - Children with fever
    - Empiric broad-spectrum parenteral antibiotics
      - Ceftriaxone, 50 mg/kg IV.
      - Clindamycin, 25–40 mg/kg/day divided q8h.
      - Antibiotics may be held for blood cultures, but otherwise should be given prior to further evaluation.
    - Admission criteria
      - Temp > 40° C
      - WBC > 30 or < 5
      - Pulmonary infiltrates (acute chest syndrome)
      - Infants < 12 months
      - Toxic appearing
      - Unable to contact primary care physician/hematologist to assure 24-hour follow-up
      - Questionable social situation

ABDOMINAL PAIN

- Difficult because abdomen is often involved in a typical pain crisis.
- Not all abdominal pain is a simple pain crisis.
  - Biliary.
    - Increased incidence of gall stones, even in pediatrics
    - Calcium bilirubinate stones from hemolysis
  - Acute hepatic crisis.
    - Characterized by fever, severe RUQ pain, often hepatomegaly
    - Due to hepatic ischemia
    - Labs: leukocytosis, markedly elevated bilirubin and transaminases
    - Progression to fulminant liver failure common with high mortality
    - Management
      - Supportive
      - Exchange transfusion often helpful

- Acute splenic sequestration syndrome: see Acute Splenic Sequestration Crisis.
- SCD patients have typical abdominal pathology.
  - Appendicitis, intussusception, pancreatitis, ischemic bowel, diverticulitis, volvulus, bowel obstruction, etc.
- Strongly consider a pathologic source of pain when exam shows
  - Focal pain
  - Hypoactive bowel sounds
  - Fever
  - Hepatomegaly or splenomegaly
  - Absence of simultaneous pain elsewhere in the body
  - Peritoneal signs on abdominal exam
  - Toxic appearance of patient

ACUTE PAIN CRISIS

▶ Most common ED diagnosis in SCD patients.
▶ Diagnosis of exclusion.
▶ Common mistake is to attribute all pain to "pain crisis" without excluding abdominal pathology, acute chest, osteomyelitis, joint infections, etc.
▶ Pain from acute pain crisis:
- Often involves long bones, ribs, sternum, vertebrae, abdomen
- Is often identifiable by adults as their typical pain pattern
- Can be migratory
- Is often associated with leukocytosis and low-grade fevers, even in the absence of infection
▶ Several well-defined triggers, but often, no trigger can be identified.
- Dehydration, infection, altitude/hypoxia, stress, cold, menses, alcohol
▶ Management:
- Rule out infection and more pathologic causes of pain.
- Aggressive analgesia with narcotics.
- NSAIDs controversial: because pain is hypoxic rather than from PG excess, NSAIDs theoretically should not be very beneficial.
- Admit patient if unable to control pain with narcotics.
- Fluids when evidence of dehydration: target is euvolemia.
- O_2 for hypoxia only. Caution: prolonged O_2 administration can decrease reticulocytosis and lead to worsening anemia.

CHAPTER 169

ONCOLOGIC EMERGENCIES

Rahul K. Khare

▶ As more patients are getting aggressive cancer treatment, EM physicians are seeing more complications of malignancy.

PATHOLOGIC FRACTURES

▶ Pathologic fractures are secondary to diseased bones in which fractures result from normal activity.
▶ Most common pathologic fracture locations: vertebra, pelvis, and femur.

Clinical Presentation

▶ Patients complain of moderate to severe pain at the fracture site.
▶ Patients often can walk on a pathologically fractured hip.
▶ Plain radiographs are sufficient for screening vertebral deformity. If negative with high suspicion of fracture, then CT is warranted to evaluate bone integrity and soft tissue extension.
▶ If cord compression is suspected, then MRI will identify the degree of compression.

Management

▶ Radiation therapy significantly reduces pain and shrinks tumor.
▶ Treatment is pain control with narcotic analgesia, immobilization of fracture, and discussion of the probable metastatic lesion.
▶ Criteria for admission to the hospital include pathologic fractures that involve hip or femur, comminuted fractures, fractures causing hemodynamic compromise, fractures causing neurologic deficits, or fractures that cause significant pain with need for IV narcotics.

ACUTE SPINAL CORD COMPRESSION

▶ 5–10% with metastatic cancer develop spinal cord compression.
▶ Most common cancers that metastasize to bone: prostate, breast, and lung.
▶ Metastatic cancer to vertebrae then into the spinal canal causes gradual symptoms but requires rapid intervention to minimize irreversible dysfunction.

Clinical Presentation

▶ Back pain (97%), weakness (74%), autonomic dysfunction (52%), sensory loss (53%).
  • Patients complain of significant, constant back pain that progressively gets worse.
  • Patients often state that supine position makes back pain worse.
  • Motor deficits usually occur at the proximal extremity musculature.
  • Although late findings, bladder and bowel incontinence may occur.
▶ Plain films can identify level of vertebral involvement; MRI of entire spine is warranted as an emergent test to find the site and extent of cord compression.
▶ Patients with high suspicion of compression, any neurologic deficit, or known history of compression should get MRI.
▶ CT can be used if MRI is not accessible or contraindicated.

Management

▶ IV narcotics for pain control.
▶ IV corticosteroids: studies show either high or moderate doses useful.
▶ Consultation with the patient's oncologist or radiation oncologist (if available) due to imminent disability.
▶ Spinal surgery for patients with
  • Unstable spine
  • Bony compression of spinal cord
  • Patients previously irradiated
▶ Early diagnosis and treatment relieve 90% of cases.
▶ Admission to the ICU with frequent neurologic assessment may be warranted.
▶ Transfer to facility if treatment (radiation or surgery) is unavailable.

SUPERIOR VENA CAVA SYNDROME

▶ Compression of the SVC.
▶ 90% occur by tumor or mediastinal nodes compressing SVC.
▶ 65–80% secondary to lung cancer.
▶ May be caused by thrombus due to indwelling catheter.

Clinical Presentation

▶ Venous engorgement of the neck (66%) and trunk (54%), due to collateral vessels, as well as facial swelling (50%).
▶ Symptoms include dyspnea (63%), cough (24%), orthopnea, or hoarse voice.
▶ Diagnosis made with histology; however, clinical suspicion can lead to CXR and chest CT showing mediastinal mass.

Management

▶ Initial treatment: supplemental O_2, head elevation, and cautious use of fluid.
▶ Glucocorticoids (dexamethasone, 20 mg IV) and diuretics (furosemide, 40 mg IV) should be administered for immediate ED management.
▶ Radiation and/or chemotherapy should be done urgently, both of which usually relieve symptoms.
▶ Secondary treatments include surgical procedures, vena caval stents, and anticoagulants.
▶ If an indwelling catheter is the etiology, treatment is removal of catheter and a short course of anticoagulation.
▶ Should be admitted to the ICU if SOB or airway concerns occur.

HYPERCALCEMIA

▶ Hypercalcemia: most common metabolic complication of malignancy.
▶ Up to 20% of patients with metastatic cancer have hypercalcemia.
  • 40% with metastatic myeloma and breast cancer get hypercalcemia.

Clinical Presentation

▶ Symptoms: nausea, vomiting, anorexia, altered mental status, mania, bone pain (arthritis), constipation, and polyuria.

▶ ECG findings: shortened QT intervals, prolonged PR interval, or bradycardia.

▶ Calcium level (ionized or non-ionized) should be drawn for screening.

▶ PTH level may be added later to help differentiate cause of hypercalcemia.

Management

▶ Treatment: rehydration, as many of these patients are dehydrated.

▶ Diuresis with furosemide, 40–60 mg, promotes excretion of the calcium and should be used after adequate rehydration.

- Should only be used when patient is symptomatic (significant weakness, ECG changes, etc.).

▶ For profound mental status change, renal failure, or patients unable to tolerate fluids, dialysis is indicated.

▶ Mitramycin, bisphosphonates, and glucocorticoids can be used in conjunction with the admitting team.

▶ Disposition is to the ICU for altered level of consciousness or to a monitored bed (watch for hypokalemia due to the diuretics) for those without mental status change.

SYNDROME OF INAPPROPRIATE ANTIDIURETIC HORMONE, HYPONATREMIA

▶ May occur in malignancy from variety of etiologies: malignancy secreting antidiuretic hormone (ADH), chemotherapy releasing ADH, carbamazepine, or narcotics.

▶ SIADH occurs in the absence of diuretics or renal failure.

Clinical Presentation

▶ Early symptoms: nausea, anorexia, and malaise

▶ Late findings: headache, confusion, lethargy, seizures, and coma

▶ Hyponatremia: most common electrolyte disorder in SIADH

▶ Life-threatening symptoms: sodium levels < 105 mEq/L

▶ SIADH diagnosed by urine sodium > 30 mEq/L, decreased serum osmolality (< 280 mOsm/kg), and dilute urine

Management

▶ Patients who have a sodium of 125–134 mEq/L should be placed on fluid restriction (500 ml per day).

▶ More severe hyponatremia gets NS, 1 L, with furosemide, 40 mg IV, for free water clearance.

▶ One must be careful with 3% hypertonic saline due to rapid correction and subsequent central pontine myelinolysis.
  • Indication for 3% hypertonic saline is seizure or lethargy.
  • In general, 300–500 ml of 3% hypertonic NaCl in adult patients.
  • In seizing patients, give enough to stop seizure, then discontinue.

▶ Rate of correction should be no more than 0.5 mEq/L per hour, with only 12–15 mEq in the first 24 hours.
  • If patients are symptomatic, correction rate can be 1–2 mEq/L per hour for the first 1–3 hours only.

▶ For mental status changes or severe hyponatremia, admit to ICU.

▶ For patients without severe hyponatremia, admit to monitored bed.

CHAPTER 170

HIV/AIDS EMERGENCIES

Keith E. Kocher

▶ CDC estimates that 900,000 people in the U.S. currently live with HIV.

▶ Since the introduction of antiretroviral drugs and highly active antiretroviral therapy (HAART), mortality and hospitalizations have decreased.

▶ HIV infection is acquired through sexual intercourse, exposure to contaminated blood, perinatal transmission, and, rarely, through organ/tissue donation.

▶ HIV is a retrovirus of the lentivirus family that kills infected cells.

▶ HIV selectively attacks host cells involved in immune function, primarily CD4 T cells.

CLINICAL PRESENTATION

▶ Symptoms of acute HIV infection are reported to occur in 50–90% of patients:

- Diagnosis is missed in up to 75% of cases due to its non-specific presentation.
- Most common presentations of acute HIV infection are fever (> 90%), fatigue (70–90%), pharyngitis (> 70%), rash (40–80%), headache (30–70%), and lymphadenopathy (40–70%).

▶ Seroconversion occurs 3–8 weeks after infection, followed by a long asymptomatic period (with generally no findings on physical exam except for possibly a persistent generalized lymphadenopathy). Incubation time from exposure to development of AIDS in untreated patients is approximately 8 years in adults, and 2 years in children under 5.

▶ AIDS is defined by the CDC as the appearance of an indicator condition or a CD4 count < 200. Mean survival time after the

CD4 count drops below 200 is 3.7 years, after an AIDS-defining condition, it is 1.3 years.

- Indicator conditions include esophageal candidiasis, cryptococcosis, cryptosporidiosis, CMV retinitis, HSV, Kaposi's sarcoma (KS), brain lymphoma, *Mycobacterium avium* complex (MAC), *Pneumocystis* pneumonia, progressive multifocal leukoencephalopathy (PML), brain toxoplasmosis, HIV encephalopathy, HIV wasting syndrome, disseminated histoplasmosis, isosporiasis, disseminated *Mycobacterium tuberculosis* disease, recurrent *Salmonella* septicemia, pulmonary TB, recurrent bacterial pneumonia, invasive cervical cancer (CDC definition).

▶ Advanced HIV infection occurs with a CD4 count < 50.

▶ Majority of HIV-related ED presentations consist of systemic symptoms such as fever, weight loss, malaise.

▶ It is important to remember that patients with later stage HIV and AIDS may not manifest the typical symptoms, signs, and lab findings associated with systemic infections.

MANAGEMENT

▶ Universal/standard precautions should always be used.

▶ Diagnosis of an HIV infection is made by detecting antibodies to the virus after seroconversion. Typically, this involves an ELISA (sensitivity 98.5%, specificity 99%) followed by a Western blot assay (nearly 100% sensitive and specific).

▶ Diagnosis of an acute infection cannot be made with serologic testing and requires less standardized techniques to detect DNA, RNA, or HIV antigens.

▶ In cases of health care worker exposures, there are two rapid HIV tests: single-use diagnostic system (SUDS) and a saliva- or blood-based rapid assay that can provide results in < 20 minutes.

▶ Testing for HIV in the ED has been generally considered of limited utility.

▶ Recent CD4 T-cell counts and HIV viral load are helpful when evaluating HIV-infected patients.

- CD4 counts < 200 and viral loads > 50,000 are associated with increased risk of developing AIDS-defining illnesses.

▶ If this information is unavailable, then a total lymphocyte count < 1000 is strongly predictive of a CD4 count < 200.

▶ Work-up in the ED must include exclusion of systemic infection and malignancy and may include any or all of the following:

electrolytes, CBC, blood cultures (aerobic, anaerobic, fungal), UA and culture, LFTs, CXR, serologic testing (syphilis, cryptococcosis, toxoplasmosis, CMV infection, coccidioidomycosis), LP.

▶ Ill-appearing patients should receive resuscitation and empiric antibiotics.

▶ Most common sources of fever without localizing signs/symptoms vary by stage of disease:
  • CD4 counts > 500: in general, causes similar to immunocompetent individuals.
  • CD4 counts 200–500: early bacterial respiratory infections.
  • CD4 counts < 200: early *Pneumocystis carinii* pneumonia, central line infection, MAC, TB, CMV, drug fever, sinusitis; less common causes include endocarditis, lymphoma, *Histoplasma*, *Cryptococcus*.

▶ Consultation with an infectious disease specialist and sometimes others with expertise in HIV infection is often necessary when managing various manifestations of HIV.

▶ Individual patient presentation can vary widely, based on the stage of the disease, and, therefore, clinical impression is crucial in determining ED management and disposition.

PNEUMOCYSTIS CARINII PNEUMONIA

▶ Currently, most common opportunistic infection among AIDS patients.

▶ However, incidence has decreased since HAART and use of prophylactic medications.

▶ Generally, *Pneumocystis carinii* pneumonia does not occur until the CD4 count < 200.

Clinical Presentation

▶ Generally has gradual onset, characterized by fever (79–100%), cough (95%), and progressive dyspnea (95%); other symptoms include fatigue, chills, chest pain, and weight loss. Approximately 7% of patients are asymptomatic.

▶ Most common exam findings are fever (84% of patients with temperature > 38.1° C), tachypnea (62%), and, often, crackles/rhonchi, but normal breath sounds occur in 50% of cases.

▶ CXR are initially normal in up to 25% of patients with *Pneumocystis carinii* pneumonia, but most common radiographic abnormalities are diffuse, bilateral interstitial or alveolar infiltrates.

- Two most common abnormal lab values are a CD4 count < 200 and an elevated LDH.
- ABG usually shows hypoxemia and an increase in the A-a gradient.
- *Pneumocystis carinii* pneumonia should be suspected if a patient demonstrates a decrease in pulse oximetry with exercise/exertion.
- Specific diagnosis of *Pneumocystis carinii* pneumonia requires documentation of the organism in respiratory specimens—not typically done in the ED.

Management

- HIV patients with CD4 counts < 200 may already be on prophylaxis for *Pneumocystis carinii* pneumonia, generally consisting of SMX-TMP in various dosing regimens; other possible prophylactic regimens include dapsone and aerosolized pentamidine.
- Patients with *Pneumocystis carinii* pneumonia are normally treated for 21 days with anti-*Pneumocystis* therapy:
  - For both oral and IV therapy, SMX-TMP is considered regimen of choice.
    - Oral: 2 double-strength tablets (= 320 mg TMP/1600 mg SMX) q8h
    - IV: SMX-TMP, 4–5 mg/kg q6h (dosed based on TMP component)
  - Pentamidine at 4 mg/kg IV per day for those with a sulfa allergy.
- Use of concurrent corticosteroid treatment:
  - Indicated in patients with more severe illness:
    - ABG on room air showing a $PO_2 < 70$ mmHg or A-a gradient > 35 mmHg
    - Patients who are not prescribed steroid therapy initially but later develop progressive respiratory distress
  - Recommended regimen: prednisone, 40 mg PO bid × 5 days; prednisone, 40 mg PO qd × 5 days; prednisone, 20 mg PO qd × 11 days
- Those with respiratory failure should be supported with mechanical ventilation.
  - Note that there is an increased risk of PTX in those with *Pneumocystis carinii* pneumonia.
- Those hospitalized for *Pneumocystis carinii* pneumonia should be isolated from other immunocompromised patients.

KAPOSI'S SARCOMA

▶ Most common tumor arising in HIV-infected persons and is an AIDS-defining illness.

▶ In the U.S., KS is > 20,000 times more common in those with AIDS than in the general population, and > 300 times more common than in other immunosuppressed patients.

▶ Found more often in homosexual men than in other risk groups.

Clinical Presentation

▶ Has a variable clinical course, ranging from minimal disease presenting as an incidental finding to explosive growth resulting in significant morbidity and mortality.

- Skin involvement is most common means of diagnosing, consisting of painless, raised brown-black or purple papules and nodules that do not blanch.
- Common cutaneous sites are the face, chest, genitals, and oral cavity.
- Oral cavity involvement in approximately one-third of all patients and initial site of the disease in about 15%; lesions may become easily traumatized during normal chewing, causing pain, bleeding, ulceration, and secondary infection.
- GI tract is involved in approximately 40% of patients with KS at initial diagnosis.
  - May be asymptomatic or cause weight loss, abdominal pain, nausea/vomiting, upper or lower GI bleeding, malabsorption, intestinal obstruction, diarrhea
- Pulmonary involvement is seen in up to one-third of patients with KS.
  - Can present with SOB, fever, cough, hemoptysis, chest pain, or as an asymptomatic finding on CXR

▶ Skin biopsy can confirm the diagnosis of cutaneous manifestations.

▶ Endoscopy or bronchoscopy can be used to determine GI/respiratory involvement.

Management

▶ There is no known cure for KS.

▶ Goal of treatment is palliation.

▶ Consists of a wide range of therapy from initiation of HAART and local/topical treatments to various chemotherapeutic agents.
  • Not typically instituted in the ED
▶ ED concerns regarding KS include GI bleeding and airway compromise in the form of hemoptysis—these should be managed in the usual manner.

DISSEMINATED *MYCOBACTERIUM AVIUM* OR *MYCOBACTERIUM INTRACELLULARE* COMPLEX

▶ Consists of disseminated infection to bone marrow, liver, spleen, lungs, GI tract

Clinical Presentation

▶ Occurs predominantly in those with CD4 counts < 100.
▶ Symptoms consist of persistent fever, night sweats, weight loss, diarrhea, malaise, and anorexia.

Management

▶ Diagnosis made by isolation of the organism in culture, usually of the blood or lymph node—not typically available in the ED.
▶ Lab abnormalities frequently include anemia and elevated alkaline phosphatase and LDH.
▶ Treatment is with clarithromycin, 500 mg PO bid, combined with ethambutol, 15 mg/kg PO qd, and possibly the addition of oral rifabutin.

TUBERCULOSIS

▶ Incidence of TB among AIDS population at 200–500 times general population

Clinical Presentation

▶ Frequently occurs in patients even with CD4 counts in the 200–500 range.
▶ Classic respiratory symptoms include cough, hemoptysis, night sweats, fevers, weight loss, and anorexia.
▶ Should maintain high index of suspicion for TB among AIDS patients with respiratory symptoms in the ED.

▶ CXR may show classic upper lobe involvement and cavitary lesions, although less frequent among advanced HIV disease patients.

▶ Definitive diagnosis requires isolation of organism in stain/culture of sputum or bronchoscopy biopsy.

Management

▶ Consider isolation.

▶ Treatment requires a four-drug therapy to cover multidrug-resistant TB.

CYTOMEGALOVIRUS

▶ Most common cause of serious opportunistic viral disease in HIV-infected individuals.

▶ Disseminated disease commonly involves GI tract, pulmonary, and CNS systems.

▶ Most important manifestation of local CMV infection is retinitis.

Clinical Presentation

▶ Usually requires CD4 counts < 50.

▶ CMV retinitis is leading cause of blindness in AIDS patients.

▶ Presentation is variable—may be asymptomatic initially, but progress to changes in visual acuity, field cuts, photophobia, scotoma, eye redness, pain.

▶ Findings on funduscopic exam include fluffy perivascular lesions and areas of hemorrhage within them.

Management

▶ Disseminated CMV is treated in general with IV foscarnet or ganciclovir; oral ganciclovir is used for prophylaxis.

▶ CMV retinitis can be treated with several options, including IV ganciclovir or foscarnet, IV cidofovir, oral valganciclovir, or an intra-ocular ganciclovir implant.

▶ Consultation with an ophthalmologist is recommended.

NEUROLOGIC COMPLICATIONS

▶ Most commonly consisting of AIDS dementia, toxoplasmosis, and cryptococcosis, but also can include bacterial meningitis,

histoplasmosis, CMV infection, PML, HSV infection, neuro-syphilis, TB, CNS lymphoma.
► Toxoplasmosis is the most common cause of focal encephalitis in patients with AIDS.

Clinical Presentation
► Common presentations indicating CNS involvement include seizures, altered mental status, headache, meningismus, focal neurologic deficits.

Management
► ED evaluation should include, when appropriate, a head CT followed by LP.
► Especially in patients with CD4 counts < 200, consider sending additional CSF studies to the typical set, such as India ink stain, viral culture, fungal culture, toxoplasmosis and crypto-coccosis antigen, and coccidioidomycosis titer, and, if possible, excess CSF should be held for additional testing at a later date.

GI COMPLICATIONS
► Oral candidiasis and thrush affect more than 80% of AIDS patients.
► Esophageal involvement can occur with *Candida*, HSV, CMV.
► Causes of diarrhea in the HIV population include bacteria, parasites, viruses, fungi, and antiretroviral drug side effects, and, in up to 20–30% of cases, no pathogen is found.

Clinical Presentation
► The tongue and buccal mucosa are commonly involved in thrush and can be distinguished from hairy leukoplakia using a potassium hydroxide smear.
► Esophagitis is suspected with a complaint of odynophagia and dysphagia plus evidence of oral thrush, especially in patients with CD4 counts < 100.

Management
► Oral candidiasis and thrush should be treated with clotrimazole or nystatin suspensions and can be managed as an outpatient.

► Treatment of esophagitis in the ED must be with systemic therapy and is usually presumptive and typically for *Candida*, which accounts for 50–70% of infections—generally start with oral fluconazole, 100–200 mg PO qd for 14–21 days.

► Evaluation of diarrhea can include stool for leukocytes, ova, and parasites, acid-fast staining, stool culture—results typically not available in the ED.

► ED management of diarrhea includes repletion of fluids/electrolytes and, if bacterial infection suspected, empiric treatment with ciprofloxacin can be used.

► Non-toxic patients with diarrhea who tolerate orals can be discharged home with appropriate follow-up.

CHAPTER 171

ELECTROLYTE DISTURBANCES

Matthew J. Greenberg

▶ In general, chronic disturbances are better tolerated despite having a more drastic laboratory appearance.
▶ Acute electrolyte changes are poorly tolerated and require rapid intervention.

SODIUM

▶ Sodium is the primary cation found in the extracellular space.
▶ Derangements of sodium actually tend to be issues of water balance. Too much free water leads to hyponatremia. A lack of free water appears as hypernatremia.

Hyponatremia

▶ Defined as a sodium concentration < 135 mmol/L
▶ Caused by
  • Excessive water intake or
  • Renal inability to excrete free water (Table 171-1)
▶ Associated with hypotonic, normotonic, or hypertonic states
▶ Dilutional hyponatremia
  • Most common form of hyponatremia.
  • Free water input exceeds output with relative dilution of all serum solutes, including sodium.
▶ Translational hyponatremia
  • Shift of free water from the intracellular compartment to extracellular due to a solute load in the extracellular compartment.
  • Commonly seen in DKA; high glucose concentration draws water from within the cells.
    ○ Correction factor: add 1.6 to measured [Na$^+$] for every 100 mg/dl of glucose above 100 mg/dl to estimate serum [Na$^+$].

TABLE 171-1.
CAUSES OF HYPONATREMIA

Hypotonic hyponatremia	Hypervolemic
Hypovolemic	CHF
Diuretics	Cirrhosis
Vomiting, diarrhea	Nephrotic syndrome
Blood loss	Renal failure
Excessive sweating	Pregnancy
Third spacing	**Isotonic hyponatremia**
Bowel obstruction	Pseudohyponatremia
Burns	Hyperlipidemia
Euvolemic	**Hypertonic hyponatremia**
Thiazide diuretics	Hyperglycemia
Adrenal insufficiency	Mannitol
SIADH	
Cancer	
CNS disorders	
Drugs	

Clinical Presentation
▶ Nausea, vomiting, headache, cognitive impairment, lethargy, restlessness, confusion, seizures, and coma
▶ More uncommonly: rhabdomyolysis, muscle cramps, and non-cardiogenic pulmonary edema

Treatment
▶ Correct the underlying etiology.
▶ Fluid restriction.
▶ Replace sodium in symptomatic patients.
  • Correction of not more than 8–12 mmol/L per day or 1–2 mmol/L per hour for the first few hours is recommended.
  • Only treat to a corrected [Na^+] of 125 or until seizing stops.
  • Can usually be replaced with NS.
  • Consider hypertonic saline (3%) if seizing.

Central Pontine Myelinolysis
▶ Rare and dreaded complication of the treatment of hyponatremia.
▶ If the [Na^+] is corrected too quickly, brain shrinkage may result, leading to demyelination of the pontine neurons.
▶ Symptoms may be permanent and include quadriplegia, pseudobulbar palsy, seizures, coma, and death.

Hypernatremia
▶ See Table 171-2.

TABLE 171-2.
CAUSES OF HYPERNATREMIA

Net water loss	Hypertonic sodium gain
Unreplaced insensible loss	Sodium bicarbonate administration
Hypodipsia	Hypertonic feeding preparations
Neurogenic diabetes insipidus	Sodium chloride ingestion/infusion
Post-traumatic	Primary hyperaldosteronism
Tumors	Cushing's syndrome

▶ Defined as a sodium concentration > 145 mmol/L.
▶ Indicative of a free water deficit from either net hypertonic sodium gain or free water loss.
- Sodium gain is most often associated with clinical interventions (i.e., sodium bicarbonate administration).
- Maintenance of hypernatremia requires loss of thirst response or lack of access to water.
- Most commonly affecting infants, the elderly, or the mentally impaired.
▶ Clinical manifestations in infants: muscle weakness, restlessness, high-pitched cry, insomnia, lethargy, and coma.
▶ Elderly have fewer symptoms: thirst, muscle weakness, confusion, or coma.

Treatment
▶ Correct underlying etiology.
▶ 0.45% NaCl guided by calculation of water deficit:

$$\text{Water deficit in liters} = 0.6 \times \text{weight (kg)} \times (\text{Na} - 140)/140$$

▶ If patient hypotensive, start resuscitation with 0.9% NaCl.
▶ Acute hypernatremia can be corrected at a rate of 1 mmol/L per hour.
▶ Too rapid a correction of chronic hyponatremia may result in cerebral edema.

POTASSIUM
▶ Total body potassium stores are tightly regulated.
- 98% of potassium located intracellularly to maintain the sodium potassium gradient.

TABLE 171-3.
CAUSES OF HYPOKALEMIA

Inadequate intake (< 40 mEq per day)	Diarrhea or laxative abuse
High-dose glucocorticoids	Renal loss
Renal tubular acidosis types 1 and 2	Loop and thiazide diuretics
Familial hypokalemic periodic paralysis	Vomiting
Mineralocorticoid excess	

▶ Potassium is particularly important in the creation and maintenance of the electrical cardiac cycle.

Hypokalemia

▶ See Table 171-3.
▶ Defined as serum potassium of < 3.5 mmol/L.

Clinical Presentation

▶ Generalized weakness, paralytic ileus, cardiac arrhythmias, ascending paralysis, and rhabdomyolysis
▶ ECG changes: flat or inverted T waves, ST depression, or U waves

Treatment

▶ Oral replacement of 20–80 mEq.
▶ IV potassium replacement of 10 mEq/hour (up to 20 mEq/hour) can be performed under continuous ECG monitoring.
▶ Potassium chloride is the usual salt utilized for replacement.
▶ Potassium phosphate may also be utilized if hypophosphatemia is present.
▶ Hypomagnesemia should be treated concomitantly, as it will impair potassium replacement.
▶ Excluding intracellular shifting, a drop in serum potassium of 0.3 mEq/L represents a depletion of approximately 100 mEq of total body stores.

Hyperkalemia

▶ See Table 171-4.
▶ Defined as serum potassium > 5.0 mmol/L.

Clinical Presentation

▶ Fatigue, weakness, paresthesias, paralysis, and palpitations.

TABLE 171-4.
CAUSES OF HYPERKALEMIA

Factitious	Massive tissue trauma/burns
Hemolysis	Rhabdomyolysis
Thrombocytosis (platelets > 10^6/ml)	Blood transfusion
Leukocytosis (WBC > 10^5/ml)	Drugs
Renal insufficiency/failure	Potassium-sparing diuretics
Tumor lysis syndrome	ACE inhibitors
Insulin resistance or deficiency	Angiotensin receptor blockers
Acidosis	

▶ Cardiac arrhythmias include AV conduction blocks, VF, and asystole.

▶ ECG changes begin with peaked T waves, decreased P waves, prolonged PR interval, and BBBs.

▶ Typical ECG progression with slowing and widening of the QRS into an idioventricular rhythm leading to a sine wave pattern, VF, and eventual asystole.

Treatment

▶ Maintain continuous ECG monitoring.

▶ Immediate treatment should begin with any ECG changes or a serum K^+ > 6.0 mmol/L.

▶ Be prepared for arrhythmias and the need for defibrillation.

▶ Monitor potassium levels and be prepared to administer additional medications.

▶ Attempt to recognize and correct the underlying cause (Table 171-5).

CALCIUM

▶ Calcium ions are tightly regulated, as they play an important role in intracellular second messenger systems, particularly those associated with muscle contraction.

▶ 98% of total body calcium is sequestered in bone.

▶ Biologically active ionized serum calcium represents 50% of total serum calcium.

- 40% of the remainder is protein bound.
- Total calcium is, therefore, inherently linked to protein levels, specifically albumen.

TABLE 171-5.
TREATMENT OF HYPERKALEMIA

Three-tiered approach to treatment:
1. IV calcium, 10–20 ml of 10% calcium gluconate or chloride to rapidly reverse the cardiac conduction abnormalities.
   Calcium is contraindicated in the setting of digoxin toxicity.
   $CaCl_2$ provides three times as much elemental calcium per volume as the gluconate salt.
   $CaCl_2$ is much more toxic to tissue if extravasated.
   $CaCl_2$ will precipitate if administered with sodium bicarbonate.
2. Temporary shifting of potassium intracellularly.
   Regular insulin, 10 units IV with 50 ml D50.
      Onset 15–20 minutes.
      Expect plasma potassium to fall by 0.5–1.5 mmol/L.
   Sodium bicarbonate in patients with acidosis.
   Nebulized albuterol, 10–20 mg.
      Onset in 30 minutes.
      Expect plasma potassium to fall by 0.6–1.0 mmol/L.
3. Remove potassium from body.
   Sodium polystyrene sulfonate resin (Kayexalate), 15–30 g PO/NG/per rectum.
      May also be given as a retention enema with onset in 1 hour.
      Orally will take 4–6 hours to work (has to get to colon, which is site of action).
   Hemodialysis.

Hypocalcemia

▶ See Table 171-6.

▶ Onset of symptoms generally occurs as ionized calcium levels drop below 2.8 mg/dl (0.7 mmol/L), which generally correlates to a total calcium of 7.0 mg/dl (1.8 mmol/L).

Clinical Presentation

▶ Muscle weakness, wasting, myalgias, fatigue, distal extremity and perioral paresthesias, dysphagia, abdominal pain, constipation, confusion, irritability, anxiety, or frank psychosis.

TABLE 171-6.
CAUSES OF HYPOCALCEMIA

Hypoparathyroidism	Vitamin D deficiency	Decreased bone resorption
DiGeorge syndrome	E.g., malnutrition, mal-absorption	Sepsis
Rhabdomyolysis		Burns
Tumor lysis syndrome	Drugs (e.g., phenytoin)	Pancreatitis

► Common exam findings:
  • Hyperreflexia, tetany, carpopedal spasms, Chvostek's and Trousseau's signs.
  • Seizures, laryngospasm, bronchospasm, and papilledema may also be seen.
  • Cardiac manifestations include CHF, bradycardia, and ventricular arrhythmias.
► Typical ECG finding is ST-segment and QT-interval prolongation.
► Chvostek's sign: tapping over the facial nerve causes spasms of the facial muscles.
  • Present in 10–30% of normal population
  • Contraction of eyelid with maneuver almost diagnostic
► Trousseau's sign: inflation of a BP cuff for 3–5 minutes or compression over the median nerve causes carpospasms.

Treatment
► Administration of calcium
  • Parenteral calcium as either the chloride or gluconate salt.
  • Chloride salt provides more elemental calcium but has more side effects (see hyperkalemia treatment above).
  • Consider concomitant vitamin D replacement, especially if utilizing oral supplementation.

Hypercalcemia

► See Table 171-7.
► Defined as a serum ionized calcium > 2.7 mg/dl or total calcium of 10.5 mg/dl.

Clinical Presentation
► Fatigue, weakness, anorexia, depression, nausea, vomiting, abdominal pain, and constipation.

TABLE 171-7.
CAUSES OF HYPERCALCEMIA

Milk alkali syndrome	Paget's disease
Lithium toxicity	Hyperparathyroidism
Thiazide diuretics	Malignancy
Hypothyroidism	Sarcoidosis
Immobilization	Vitamin D intoxication

TABLE 171-8.
TREATMENT OF HYPERCALCEMIA

Hydration with crystalloid.
Increase urinary excretion with diuretics.
 Lasix: start at 20–40 mg IV every 2 hours after appropriate fluid
  resuscitation.
Inhibit osteoclast activity with bisphosphonates.
 Zoledronic acid, 4 mg IV over 15 minutes.
 Pamidronate, 60–90 mg IV over 24 hours.
 Etidronate, 7.5 mg/kg IV over 4 hours.
Calcitonin, 4 IU/kg SC or IM.
Treat any underlying cause.
Consider corticosteroids if granulomatous disease or lymphoma is
 suspected etiology.
Consider hemodialysis for severe hypercalcemia (18–20 mg/dl).

▸ Cognitive changes including hallucinations, psychosis, stupor,
 and coma can be seen.
▸ Peptic ulcers and pancreatitis can be induced by severe eleva-
 tions of calcium.
▸ Renal disease, such as nephrogenic diabetes insipidus, type 1
 renal tubular acidosis, and nephrolithiasis, can be seen.
▸ ECG changes:
 • QT interval shortening, ST depression, and widened T waves.
 • Rarely bradyarrhythmias, BBB, and second-degree and com-
  plete heart block can occur.

Treatment
▸ See Table 171-8.

CHAPTER 172

WOUND CARE AND TETANUS

Joseph H. Hartmann

▶ Wound healing involves three overlapping phases: inflammation, tissue formation, and tissue remodeling, which can extend up to a year.

▶ Tensile strength after repair is 5–10% of original at 1 week, gaining about 10% each successive week until 8–10 weeks when it reaches 80% of original.

▶ Lacerations never attain same tensile strength as intact skin (usually 75–80% of original).

▶ Recognize, document, and discuss with patient comorbidities that may relate to repair and outcome: diabetes, obesity, advanced age, malnutrition, immunosuppression, steroid use, and anticoagulant use.

ANESTHESIA

▶ Lidocaine, 1% or 2% most commonly used, with onset in 2–4 minutes and duration of 45–60 minutes.
  • Using solution with epinephrine doubles the duration of action while aiding hemostasis during closure.
  • Avoid use of epinephrine-containing solutions on digits, ears, nose, or penis due to possible ischemic complications.

▶ Bupivacaine or mepivacaine provides significantly longer duration of action, not uncommonly lasting ≥ 12 hours.

▶ Pain of local infiltration is reduced by using small-bore needle (27- to 30-gauge), warming solutions, buffering solutions, slowing rate of injection, SC rather than intradermal injection, and pre-treatment with topical anesthetics [triamcinolone acetonide cream (TAC), LAT, EMLA].

CLEANSING

▶ Do not shave hair surrounding laceration because this does not reduce infection rate.

▶ Do not shave eyebrows; they may not grow back or may do so abnormally.
▶ Much debate surrounding choice of cleansing agent, but irrigation with either NS solution or tap water is okay.
▶ Optimal irrigation pressures obtained with 30–60 ml syringe with 19-gauge needle angiocatheter or use of splash shield system.
▶ If wound is highly contaminated, consider use of Shur-Clens with high-porosity sponge.
▶ Most FBs (even glass) can be visualized with radiography; sonography can be of use if needed.

WOUND CLOSURE

▶ Explore wound to document extent of injury and presence or lack of FBs.
▶ Debride devitalized tissue, if present.
▶ Ideally, wounds are closed in < 4–6 hours, usually acceptable in < 12 hours. Occasionally, wounds are closed in > 12 hours, depending on cosmetic deformity and degree of contamination.

CLOSURE OPTIONS

▶ Surgical tape
  • Pro: rapid application, patient comfort, lowest infection rate
  • Con: frequently falls off, leading to wound dehiscence
▶ Staples
  • Pro: rapid application, low tissue reactivity
  • Con: less meticulous closure than sutures, can interfere with some imaging modalities (CT, MRI)
▶ Suture
  • Pro: meticulous closure, greatest tensile strength, lowest dehiscence rate
  • Con: slowest application, greatest tissue reactivity
▶ Tissue adhesives
  • Pro: rapid application, patient comfort, no anesthesia required, cosmesis equal to sutures, can be used for 25–33% of lacerations

- Con: lower tensile strength than sutures, cannot get wet, for topical use only; use on hands, feet, and around eyes relatively contraindicated

POST-CLOSURE CARE

▶ Topical antibiotic application post-staple or suture repair can inhibit bacterial growth, can increase rate of re-epithelialization, and may prevent scab formation.

▶ Do not use topical antibiotic after topical adhesive closure as this will loosen the adhesive, risking wound dehiscence.

▶ Gentle cleansing after 24–48 hours is indicated for stapled and sutured wounds.

- Patients may shower with tissue adhesives but should not otherwise cleanse wound, bathe, or swim.

▶ Suture removal:

- Face: 5 days
- Low-tension areas: 7–10 days
- High-tension areas: 10–14 days

▶ Oral antibiotics not generally indicated except in bites (human, dog, cat).

- See Chap. 173.

▶ Review tetanus immunization status.

- See below for tetanus.

▶ Minimize scar by avoiding sunlight/tanning booths, use sun block for 1 year, and use topical vitamin E and/or aloe.

▶ Even with best management, wound infection will occur in < 5% of patients.

- Provide warning signs of infection.

TETANUS

Pathophysiology

▶ *Clostridium tetani* is an anaerobic gram-positive bacillus.

▶ Tetanospasmin, a potent neurotoxin, is responsible for clinical manifestations of excessive, uncontrolled muscle contraction.

- Binding of toxin at synapse is irreversible and cannot be neutralized with anti-toxin. Recovery of nerve function requires growth of new nerve terminals, accounting for long recovery period.

▶ Population at risk (North America and Western Europe):
- Geriatric population, immunocompromised, and immigrants

Clinical Presentation

▶ Tetanus-prone wounds:
- Wounds contaminated with soil, feces, or saliva; puncture or crushing wounds; GSWs; burns; and frostbite
- Tetanus-potential wounds
  ○ Corneal abrasions, corneal burns (chemical, welder's flash), decubitus ulcerations, diabetic ulcerations, abscesses [chronic abscesses, IV drug abuse (skin-popping) abscesses]

▶ Incubation period 3–14 days.

▶ Trismus (lockjaw): masseter muscle involvement is presenting symptom (75%).

▶ Mandibular, facial, and neck muscular rigidity occurs within 24–48 hours (risus sardonicus).

▶ Generalized muscular rigidity (tetany) follows (opisthotonos).

▶ Additional signs and symptoms:
- Irritability, dysphagia, laryngeal spasms, hydrophobia, excessive orotracheal secretions

▶ Reflex spasms can be triggered by minimal external stimuli, including noise, light, and touch.

▶ Complications:
- Asphyxia, apnea, dislocations, fractures, rhabdomyolysis

▶ Diagnosis based on clinical symptoms.
- No specific lab studies
- Wound cultures unreliable

Management

Prophylaxis

▶ Primary immunization requires three doses of tetanus toxoid to confer adequate protection, then booster at 10-year intervals to maintain immune status.

▶ Prophylaxis for unknown immunization history or less than three prior doses:
- Clean, minor wounds
  ○ Td/DTP: yes; TIG: no
- All other wounds
  ○ Td/DTP: yes; TIG: yes

► Prophylaxis for patient with history of three or more doses:
  • Clean, minor wounds
    ○ Td/DTP: no*; TIG: no
  • All other wounds
    ○ Td/DTP: no†; TIG: no
► Dosages:
  • DTP for children < 7 years of age: 0.5 ml IM
  • Td for person ≥ 7 years of age: 0.5 ml IM
  • TIG: 250 units IM
  • 500 units in high-risk wound < 24 hours old

Treatment of Tetanus
► Eradication of organisms
  • Metronidazole, 500 mg IV q6h
  • Alternatives: erythromycin, tetracycline, chloramphenicol, and clindamycin
► Neutralization of circulating toxin
  • TIG, 3000–6000 units IM (some evidence that as little as 500 units IM as a single dose may be adequate) and
  • Tetanus toxoid (DTP or Td), 0.5 ml IM at presentation, 6 weeks, and 6 months after presentation
► Supportive care
  • Minimize CNS effects of toxin.
  • Control muscle spasm with midazolam, lorazepam, or diazepam.
  • Intubation and ventilatory care.

---

*Yes, if last dose was > 10 years ago.
†Yes, if last dose was > 5 years ago.

CHAPTER 173

WOUND CARE: SPECIAL CONSIDERATIONS

Joseph H. Hartmann

SCALP

▶ Between periosteum and galea aponeurosis lies a potential space in which hematoma and/or infection can form and spread via this space, involving the entire scalp.
- Repair galeal defects to minimize hematoma formation and prevent a widened depressed appearance of final scar.
- Apply pressure dressing for first 24 hours if extends to galea to prevent hematoma formation.

▶ Forehead laceration:
- Skin tension lines always perpendicular to underlying muscles.
- Approximate skin tension lines and hairline precisely.

EYE

▶ Never shave or clip eyebrows: they provide valuable landmarks and may not grow back.

▶ Eyelids offer little protection from penetrating globe injuries.

▶ Defer to ophthalmologist if involvement of inner surface of lid, tarsal plate, lid margins, lacrimal duct, or wound causes ptosis.

NOSE

▶ Avoid use of injectable anesthetic containing epinephrine, but use of topical anesthetic with epinephrine is acceptable.

▶ Always examine for septal hematomas.
- Small unilateral hematoma is aspirated with 18-gauge needle.
- Large unilateral hematoma is incised horizontally at base.
- Pack nose to prevent accumulation (48–72 hours).
- Prophylactic antibiotic for 3–5 days to prevent cartilage infection.
- Large bilateral hematomas go to OR.

LIP

▶ Greatest concern with lip laceration is precise approximation of vermilion border with first suture prior to infiltration with anesthetic; even a single millimeter error will lead to cosmetically displeasing result.

▶ Through-and-through laceration of lip requires layered closure of inner mucosa, orbicularis oris muscle, and skin.

CHEEK

▶ Laceration of cheek requires special attention to possible facial nerve, parotid gland, and/or Stensen's duct involvement.

EAR

▶ All hematomas require evacuation to prevent subchondral extension leading to "cauliflower ear" cosmetic defect.

▶ Avoid use of anesthetic containing epinephrine; consider regional anesthesia by auricular block.

▶ Do not debride comminuted cartilaginous injury as it may be necessary for reconstructive surgery later.

▶ Through-and-through lacerations of auricle involving underlying cartilage can be repaired with one or two 6-0 nylon sutures to approximate cartilage margins (bury the knots).

▶ Circumferential head dressings incorporating the injured ear are important to prevent auricular hematoma and further deformity.

EXTREMITIES

▶ Because of mobility of extremities, consider the position at time of injury as well as mechanism of injury when evaluating for underlying anatomic structure involvement.

▶ Peripheral nerve motor function:
  • Radial: extension of wrist and digits
  • Ulnar: abduction of fingers and adduction of fingers and thumb
  • Median: abduction, flexion, opposition of thumb
  • Superficial peroneal: eversion of foot
  • Deep peroneal: inversion of foot, dorsiflexion of ankle
  • Tibial: plantar flexion of ankle

▶ As a general rule, flexor tendon injuries require a more aggressive repair than extensor tendon injuries, but location does influence this somewhat.

▶ Unless one is specifically privileged for tendon repair, this is better left to the appropriate surgical specialist.

  • Delayed repairs are not uncommon, particularly for extensor tendon injuries.

FOREIGN BODIES

▶ Present in small percentage of wounds but contribute to significant number of malpractice claims.

▶ Consider mechanism of injury, type of object causing injury, and type of laceration, such as puncture wounds. If patient reports a sensation of "something in my cut," they are often correct.

▶ Explore wound by direct visualization. Extend margins of puncture wound if necessary; do not blindly probe.

▶ Most metal, glass, and plastic is inert, causing a limited inflammatory response.

  • Vegetative FBs (wood, thorns, spines) cause most severe inflammatory reactions.

▶ Plain radiography with an under-penetrated soft tissue technique detects 80–90% of FBs. Most glass ≥ 2 mm is visible, and even glass 0.5–2.0 mm is visualized in > 50% of cases.

▶ Ultrasound has a wide variation in sensitivity, specificity, and overall accuracy dependent on object size and operator skill.

▶ Migration can occur, sometimes to surprising distances.

▶ Prophylactic antibiotic benefit is unproven for most but justified for contaminated wounds, particularly if tendon, joint, or bone involvement has occurred.

PUNCTURE WOUNDS

▶ Generally, incidence of infection is twice that of non-punctate wounds but can be significantly higher if immunocompromised.

▶ *Staphylococcus* and streptococcal species are most common etiology for infection.

▶ *Pseudomonas aeruginosa* most frequent in post–puncture wound osteomyelitis.

► Low-pressure irrigation (0.5 psi) recommended for cleansing.
► Debridement or block dissection (coring) has not been shown to reduce infection rate.
► Prophylactic antibiotics not indicated for clean, non-plantar puncture wounds.
► Plantar puncture wounds located in the forefoot, particularly in high-risk patients, should be treated with a fluoroquinolone.
► *Pseudomonas* osteochondritis ("sweaty tennis shoe syndrome"):
  • Plantar puncture wound through rubber-soled shoe (hence its name), most often located at or distal to metatarsal neck (forefoot).
    ◦ Lab: CBC, ESR, CRP
    ◦ X-ray: often normal early; may show periosteal reaction or bone/cartilage erosion
    ◦ MRI or bone-scan diagnostic
► Antibiotic treatment:
  • Ciprofloxacin, 750 mg PO bid × 6 weeks, or cefepime, 1 g IV bid × 4 weeks

NEEDLE-STICK INJURY

► Risk of infection:
  • Hepatitis A: negligible
  • Hepatitis B: 10%
  • Hepatitis C: 2%
  • HIV: 0.3%
► Prophylaxis:
  • Pre-exposure: hepatitis A and B vaccines
  • Post-exposure
    ◦ Hepatitis A: immune serum globulin
    ◦ Hepatitis B: HBIG
    ◦ Hepatitis C: none to date
    ◦ HIV: combination antiviral therapy
► Consult current hospital protocol as recommendations are complex and changing.

RABIES

► Dog, cats, ferrets:
  • If healthy and available for 10-day observation, no prophylaxis indicated unless animal shows clinical signs of rabies.

- If animal unavailable for observation, consult local public health officials.
▶ Skunks, raccoons, bats, foxes, and most carnivores:
  - Regard as rabid unless animal proven negative by lab testing.
▶ Squirrels, hamsters, guinea pigs, gerbils, chipmunks, mice, rats, rabbits, and hares:
  - Almost never require post-exposure prophylaxis.
  - Consult local public health officials.
▶ Post-exposure rabies prophylaxis:
  - Human diploid cell vaccine (HDCV), 1 ml IM, days 1, 3, 7, 14, 28.
  - Use anterior thigh of child, deltoid muscle of adult.
▶ Passive immunization provides immediate protection.
  - Human rabies immunoglobulin (HRIG), 20 IU/kg infiltrated around wound site and give the rest IM in gluteal muscle

BITE WOUNDS
Pathophysiology

▶ Usually polymicrobial with aerobic and anaerobic flora from mouth of human or animal.
▶ Often difficult to reliably culture the offending organisms from wound.
▶ Human bites often present as clenched fist injury or fight bite.
  - Not unusual to have multiple organisms contaminating wound.
  - Human bite much more likely to become infected than animal bites.
▶ Dog bites account for 80–90% of all animal bites but are less likely than cat bites to become infected.
  - Usually involving dominant extremity in adults and extremity and/or face in children.
▶ Cat bites, being more likely to be puncture-type wounds, carry higher infection rate, though offending organisms differ little from those found in dogs.
  - Almost always polymicrobial infections
    ○ *Pasteurella* species (particularly *Pasteurella multocida*), streptococci and staphylococcal species, and *Bacteroides* species

Clinical Presentation

▶ Findings consistent with cellulitis unless abscess formation has occurred.

Management

▶ Wound management with particular attention to copious irrigation to cleanse.

▶ Recommend radiographic study to exclude presence of FBs (teeth) or fractures.

▶ Tetanus and/or rabies prophylaxis may be indicated.

▶ Generally, puncture wounds should be left to heal by secondary intention.

▶ Splint and elevate hand.

▶ Antibiotic therapy:
  • Ampicillin-sulbactam, 1.5–3.0 g IV as initial loading dose; consider short stay admission for patients at risk with dosing q6h over 24 hours, followed by amoxicillin-clavulanate, 875 mg PO bid × 10 days.
  • If penicillin allergic: clindamycin and ciprofloxacin (clindamycin and SMX-TMP for children < 16 years old).

▶ Squirrels, hamsters, guinea pigs, gerbils, chipmunks, mice, rabbits, and hares:
  • No antibiotic or rabies prophylaxis indicated

▶ Rat bite:
  • Ampicillin or tetracycline; rabies prophylaxis not indicated

▶ Skunk, raccoon, bat, or fox:
  • Ampicillin or tetracycline; rabies prophylaxis indicated

CHAPTER 174

REGIONAL ANESTHESIA

Brad J. Uren

▶ Four types of blocks frequently used in the ED: local infiltration, digital blocks, dental blocks, and hematoma blocks.

LOCAL INFILTRATION

▶ The most commonly used local anesthesia.
▶ Used frequently for laceration repairs, I&D, and wound exploration.
▶ Local infiltration to the tissue surrounding the wound, abscess, or area to be explored.
▶ Injection generally more comfortable through the lacerated tissue.
▶ Inject just enough anesthetic to cause the tissue surrounding the injection site to raise a small wheal and blanch.
▶ If sufficient anesthetic to cause analgesia would distort the tissue enough to complicate repair, consider a field or digital block.

DIGITAL BLOCKS

▶ Can achieve anesthesia to the entire digit with proper use
▶ Can allow for nail removal, laceration repair, joint reduction, abscess/paronychia drainage, drainage of a felon

Procedure

▶ Neurovascular bundle runs along the medial and lateral aspect of the digits.
▶ Base of the digit identified by finding the proximal head of the phalanx by palpation.
▶ Typically, injection is from the dorsal aspect perpendicular to the palm both lateral and medial to the bone, as close as possible without striking the bone.

▶ Once adjacent to the bone, inject anesthetic (lidocaine 2% without epinephrine) into both the medial and lateral base of the digit, about 1 cc per side.

DENTAL BLOCKS

▶ Numerous teeth can be anesthetized using regional dental anesthesia.

▶ Blocks are much more effective in the mandible than in the maxilla.

Alveolar Nerve Block Anatomy

▶ Can anesthetize the entire side of the mandible being injected, including the lip and portions of the chin.

▶ Allows several hours of analgesia permitting patient to seek dental care.

▶ Easiest with the patient seated upright, and the operator standing to the contralateral side.

▶ Retract the cheek with the thumb and forefinger laterally.

▶ Identify the groove in the mucosa making up a triangle in the mucosa behind the last molar of the mandible.

▶ Insert the needle into the groove, approximately 1 cm above the top of the molar, just under the surface of the tissue.

▶ Adjust the angle of injection such that the syringe is directed laterally, and the barrel of the syringe points toward the contralateral canine.

▶ Advance the needle carefully until bone is encountered.

▶ Aspirate to ensure that the needle is not intravascular.

▶ Inject approximately 2–4 cc of anesthetic; may use either short- or long-acting anesthetics, though a mix of both is ideal.

HEMATOMA BLOCKS

▶ Although these have been used alone for fracture reduction, they generally are used as an adjunct to the analgesia for reduction.

▶ Sterile skin preparation.

▶ Insert needle into the hematoma surrounding the fracture site, and inject anesthetic. The amount will vary based upon the size of the bone/area fracture (e.g., humerus requires more anesthetic than a radial fracture). Typically, 10–20 ml will be used.

▶ Diffusion allows for reasonable analgesia within 15–20 minutes.

TOXICITY

▶ Toxic dose of local lidocaine without epinephrine is 4–5 mg/kg and 7 mg/kg in lidocaine with epinephrine.
  • For a 70-kg patient, toxic dose is 350 mg, which is 35 cc of 1% lidocaine (10 mg/cc) or about 17 cc of 2% lidocaine (20 mg/cc)
▶ Bupivacaine toxic dose is 2.5 mg/kg.
▶ Initial toxic symptoms of lidocaine toxicity include
  • Headache, tinnitus, facial twitches, lightheadedness, a metallic taste, and numbness of the lips and tongue
▶ In higher doses, there may also be seizures, unconsciousness, apnea, and cardiovascular collapse.

◑ **PEARLS AND PITFALLS**
  • Always aspirate before injecting anesthetic to ensure that the needle is not intravascular.
  • Limit the amount of injection during digital blocks to prevent ischemia from a tourniquet effect.
  • Epinephrine should not be used in digits, nose, ear, penis, or other appendage in which vasoconstriction may result in ischemia.

CHAPTER 175

PROCEDURAL SEDATION AND ANALGESIA

Michael Lutes and Ari Leib

OVERVIEW AND PREPARATION

▶ No matter what drugs are chosen, certain practices should be routinely undertaken.
- Informed consent should be obtained when feasible.
- Airway assessment using Mallampati score, mouth opening, neck flexion and extension, and thyromental distance.
- Pre-oxygenation for 3–5 minutes (this allows for 1–3 minutes of apnea without O_2 desaturation in patients without pulmonary disease).
- Cardiac and respiratory monitoring with pulse oximetry.
- At least one functional IV line in place (preferably 18-gauge or larger).
- Oral suction at the bedside.
- Bag valve mask readily available.
- ET intubation equipment in the room.
- Crash cart with defibrillator and resuscitation medications in the room.
- Ample supply of the chosen medications.
- Reversal medications for the chosen medications in the room.
- Hospital policies on documentation, monitoring, medication administration, and personnel training should be followed.

SPECIFIC AGENTS

▶ Methohexital (Brevital)
- Mechanism of action: ultra–short-acting barbiturate that acts on GABA receptors as a direct stimulator; has no analgesic effect.
- Common uses: brief procedures requiring deep sedation, such as dislocated joint reduction.

- **Dosing:** 1 mg/kg IV bolus (0.5 mg/kg titrated up to effectiveness should be considered for elderly patients and those with underlying cardiac or pulmonary disease).
- **Duration of action:** typically 8–10 minutes.
- **Contraindications:** caution should be used in patients with hepatic impairment as this drug is metabolized solely by the hepatocytes.
- Adverse reactions: hypotension, respiratory depression, myocardial depression, and laryngospasm.
- Attractive features: immediate onset, short duration, and provides strong amnesia of event.

▶ Etomidate
- Mechanism of action: ultra–short-acting sedative agent (non-barbiturate that directly binds and stimulates GABA receptors); has no analgesic properties
- Common uses: RSI, elective cardioversion, and LP (is rapidly gaining favor for joint dislocation reduction and other ED procedures)
- **Dosing:** 0.1–0.15 mg/kg IV bolus
- Onset of action: approximately 1 minute
- **Duration of action:** very short; 3–5 minutes
- **Contraindications:** underlying severe pulmonary disease
- Adverse reactions: respiratory depression/apnea, vomiting, myoclonus (little clinical significance), and transient adrenal suppression
- Attractive features: short onset, very little if any hemodynamic compromise, and consistent duration of action

▶ Ketamine
- Mechanism of action: dissociative anesthetic that provides both analgesia and amnesia
- Common uses: pediatric procedural sedation for intubation, LP, and joint manipulation
- **Dosing:** 1–2 mg/kg IV, 4 mg/kg IM in adults
- Onset of action: 1–2 minutes IV, 3–8 minutes IM
- **Duration of action:** 5–15 minutes IV, 12–25 minutes IM
- **Contraindications:** head injury, eye injury, cardiovascular disease, and known CNS malformations
- Adverse reactions: increased ICP, increased IOP, hallucinations, and vivid and sometimes unpleasant dreams (only in adults)

- Attractive features: combined analgesic and amnestic agent, rare respiratory depression, IV or IM availability, quick onset, and moderate duration of action for predicted slightly longer procedures

▶ Midazolam (Versed)
- Mechanism of action: a benzodiazepine that increases the duration of GABA binding to receptor sites; provides no analgesia.
- Common uses: procedures in elderly patients with COPD and hemodynamic compromise.
- **Dosing:** in healthy patients < 60 years of age, 0.5–2 mg IV over at least 2 minutes (2.5 mg maximum over 2 minutes); dose may be repeated every 2–3 minutes to achieve desired effect with total dose usually 2.5–5 mg. In patients > 60 or with underlying cardiopulmonary disease, 0.5–1 mg IV over 2 minutes (1.5 mg maximum over 2 minutes); up to 1 mg doses may be repeated every 2–3 minutes to achieve desired effect with total dose usually < 3.5 mg.
- Onset of action: 1–5 minutes.
- **Duration of action:** 30 minutes–2 hours.
- **Contraindications:** sensitivity to benzodiazepines.
- Adverse reactions: respiratory depression, hypotension, vomiting, and over-sedation.
- Attractive features: titratable for elderly patients and those with underlying disease; has sedative, anxiolytic, muscle relaxation, and anti-convulsant properties.
- Reversal agent: flumazenil, 0.2 mg IV q1min as needed to reverse sedation (maximum 3 mg/hour).

▶ Fentanyl
- Mechanism of action: full opioid agonist that acts on each of the different types of opioid receptors to provide analgesia; no true amnestic effect.
- Common uses: the most commonly used adjunct to sedative amnestics in procedural sedation for nearly all procedures.
- **Dosing:** 0.5–1 mcg/kg IV over 2 minutes; may dose every 3–5 minutes as needed for pain. Total is not to exceed 2–4 mcg/kg.
- Onset of action: 2–4 minutes.
- **Duration of action:** approximately 30 minutes.

- **Contraindications:** severe liver or renal insufficiency, hypersensitivity to fentanyl, severe respiratory depression, and increased ICP (relative contraindication).
- Adverse reactions: hypotension, bradycardia, respiratory depression/apnea, and chest wall rigidity.
- Reversal agent: Narcan, 0.1–0.2 mg IV q2–3min PRN.
- Attractive features: highly lipophilic nature yields short onset of action, powerful analgesia (100 times more potent than morphine and 1000 times more potent than meperidine), short duration of action, minimal histamine release compared to other narcotics, and less respiratory depression and minimal hemodynamic effects compared to other opioids.

▶ Propofol (Diprivan)

- Mechanism of action: general anesthetic sedative agent that potentiates GABA by increasing its binding to receptors; has no analgesic effects.
- Common uses: should be used in brief, painful procedures where repeated dosing is not expected to be necessary (often used for abscess I&D).
- **Dosing:** 0.5–1 mg/kg bolus.
- **Duration of action:** 3–10 minutes (dose dependent).
- **Contraindications:** patients with prior anesthesia reactions and patients with known dysrhythmias.
- Adverse reactions: include hypotension, respiratory depression, dysrhythmias, rash, and injection site pain.
- Attractive features: rapid onset, potent sedation, and rapid recovery.

CHAPTER 176

CHRONIC PAIN AND ADDICTION

Stefanie Simmons and Samuel A. McLean

▶ 20% of the population has chronic pain that is regional in location.
▶ 10% of the population has chronic pain that is widespread.
▶ Most chronic pain syndromes have a significant neuropathic component.
▶ The amount of pain an individual is experiencing is not proportional to structural abnormalities (e.g., how bad it looks on visual inspection or MRI).
▶ Many patients with chronic pain receive sub-optimal outpatient treatment.
  • Opioids and NSAIDs are over-utilized; TCAs, anti-epileptic drugs, and non-pharmacotherapeutic modalities such as exercise and physical therapy are under-utilized.
  • Consider recommending that patients discuss possibility of alternate drug trial with their primary care physician if their pain regimen is not mechanism based.

TERMINOLOGY AND EPIDEMIOLOGY OF SUBSTANCE ABUSE

▶ Drug abuse in the U.S. is common: 10.5% of Americans have a current drug or alcohol use disorder (2002 National Epidemiologic Survey on Alcohol and Related Conditions).
▶ Rate of narcotic addiction among chronic pain population no higher than general population rate.
▶ **Dependence:** physiologic state in which abrupt cessation of drug results in withdrawal symptoms.
  • Found with many drugs, including beta-blockers, clonidine, opioids, and alcohol.
▶ **Tolerance:** neuro-adaptation to the effects of chronically administered substances necessitating higher doses for the same effects.
▶ **Addiction:** persistent pattern of dysfunctional use; use despite negative consequences of a substance, including continued use in the absence of functional gains from pain medication.

▶ **Opiophobia:** inappropriate concerns about the safety of opiate medications when compared to NSAIDs or other modalities for treating pain that results in their under-use by physicians.

ADDICTION RISK FROM OPIOID USE

▶ Risk of addiction from opioid use < 1% from short-term exposure to opioids in non-addicts; increases to approximately 45% with long-term opioid use in patient with history of addiction.

▶ Risk of addiction in most ED narcotic use for self-limited conditions (e.g., fracture) in patient without addiction history is essentially zero.

▶ Control of an acute exacerbation of chronic pain in the ED most often requires the use of opioids.

LONG-TERM OPIOID TREATMENT OF PATIENTS WITH HISTORY OF ADDICTION

▶ Best practice includes maximally structured outpatient program of frequent visits, long-acting opioids with low street value, limited supply, and urine testing. Refer patients to primary care physician or pain clinic for this treatment.

▶ **Distinguishing between patients who are addicted/looking for a high and those who are really in pain often is difficult.**

- Many chronic pain syndromes, including their acute exacerbations, exhibit no radiographic or physical evidence.

- The patient's description of his or her pain and its course may be the only information available to make treatment decisions.

- Under-treatment of chronic pain can lead to drug-seeking behaviors such as seeking multiple prescribers, requests for early refills, and dramatization of pain symptoms not motivated by inappropriate drug use but from inadequate treatment.
  - ○ This phenomenon was first described in patients with cancer pain and has since been recognized in other syndromes of chronic pain, including sickle cell anemia.

- Often cannot be differentiated on a single visit to the ED.

- Small supply of narcotics with close follow-up is often the best strategy.

CHAPTER 177

CONVENTIONAL EXPLOSIVES AND BLAST INJURIES

Dan B. Avstreih

▶ The vast majority of terrorist events involve conventional explosives.

▶ Similar mechanisms involved in industrial accidents, structural fires, and methamphetamine lab explosions.

PATHOPHYSIOLOGY

▶ Two types of explosives: high-order and low-order.

▶ High-order explosives include TNT, C4, and ammonium nitrate fuel oil; low-order explosives include pipe bombs, gunpowder, and aircraft fuel (Table 177-1).

CLINICAL PRESENTATION

▶ Clinical presentation varies based on the nature of the incident and patient location.

▶ Specific factors such as type of explosive/device, confined vs. open space, and victim distance from the blast are all predictive of injury type.

▶ Injuries are typically a combination of blunt and penetrating trauma, often with quaternary blast injury such as burns.

▶ Symptoms of concurrent nuclear, biological, or chemical (NBC) exposure (e.g., anticholinergic toxidrome) may also be present in victims of terrorist attacks.

▶ The clinician must be aware of the unique injuries present in high-order explosive patients:
- Blast lung
  - Spectrum of primary blast injury from pulmonary petechiae to hemopneumothorax.

TABLE 177-1.
TYPES OF BLAST INJURIES

Blast injury	Mechanism	Typical injury patterns
Primary	Impact of over-pressurization wave on tissue interfaces. Only present in high-order explosives.	Gas-filled structures such as the lungs, bowel, and middle ear are the most susceptible, though there are reports of non-traumatic globe rupture and concussion as well.
Secondary	Impact of projectiles and bomb fragments.	Extensive blunt and penetrating trauma. Shrapnel wounds behave as low-velocity GSWs.
Tertiary	Victim is thrown by super-heated blast wind against stable objects.	Primarily blunt trauma, though penetrating injury can be seen if victim is thrown onto protruding objects.
Quaternary	Any injury not caused by the first three mechanisms.	Burns, smoke inhalation, CO/cyanide poisoning, angina, COPD exacerbations, psychological.

- ○ Symptoms include chest pain, dyspnea, and cough.
- ○ Classic triad is apnea, bradycardia, and hypotension.
- Acute gas embolism
  - ○ Air embolism secondary to pulmonary AV fistulas caused by barotraumas.
  - ○ Presents with acute ischemic symptoms, especially in brain and spinal cord.
- Abdominal injury
  - ○ Over-pressurization impact on gas-filled sections of bowel can cause acute perforation and hemorrhage.
  - ○ Mesenteric shear injuries and solid organ rupture are also seen.
  - ○ Abdominal primary blast injury is much more common if incident occurs underwater.
- Ear trauma
  - ○ TM rupture is most common primary blast injury.
- White phosphorous burns
  - ○ Common in military munitions.
  - ○ Causes severe burns when exposed to air.
  - ○ Can lead to hypocalcemia and hyperphosphatemia.

- ○ Phosphorous pentoxide by-product is a severe pulmonary irritant.
- Concussion
  - ○ Mild traumatic brain injury can result from blast trauma, even in the absence of direct head trauma.

EMERGENCY DEPARTMENT MANAGEMENT

Diagnosis

▶ The diagnosis of blast injury is made primarily from history.

▶ Diagnostic testing should be guided by the nature of the specific incident and presenting signs and symptoms.

▶ Intact TMs do not rule out pulmonary or abdominal blast trauma.

▶ Frequent re-assessment and re-triage of blast victims, particularly those with shrapnel wounds.

- The path of shrapnel is often unpredictable, and these potentially salvageable patients can have critical but initially unapparent injury.

▶ Maintain a high index of suspicion for NBC contamination.

▶ Secondary or unexploded devices can be inadvertently transported to the ED in patient belongings or clothing.

Treatment

▶ Explosions are often mass casualty incidents; early activation of the hospital disaster plan is indicated.

▶ As in all cases of trauma, the ABCs are paramount.

▶ Early involvement of trauma surgery.

▶ Most blast injuries are treated in the standard fashion (e.g., blunt trauma like MVAs or falls, and penetrating trauma like GSWs).

▶ The blood loss from multiple deep soft-tissue shrapnel injuries can lead to hypothermia and coagulopathy, significantly increasing operative mortality; some experts recommend aggressive wound packing during the secondary survey.

▶ Prophylactic tube thoracostomy before general anesthesia or air transport of patients with blast lung.

▶ Acute gas embolism is treated with 100% O_2, left lateral recumbent position, and hyperbaric O_2 (HBO).

► White phosphorous–contaminated wounds should be copiously irrigated and rinsed with a 1% copper sulfate solution, and then have the particles manually removed.

Disposition

► Varies by specific mechanism and catalogue of injuries.
► Victims of open-space explosions sustaining only minor soft-tissue injuries with normal vitals and normal lung and abdominal exams can generally be discharged after 4–6 hours of observation.
► Because primary blast injury can be difficult to diagnose, observation of patients with pulmonary or GI complaints may be indicated.

◐ **PEARLS AND PITFALLS**
- Early implementation of disaster plan is essential for successful management of mass casualty incidents.
- Primary blast trauma can be difficult to diagnose and represents a major cause of mortality.
- Do not discount the possibility of blunt and tertiary blast trauma, such as C-spine injury, even if patients arrive by private vehicle.
- Be alert for NBC contamination and for secondary or non-detonated devices on patients.

CHAPTER 178

NUCLEAR, BIOLOGICAL, AND CHEMICAL TERRORISM

Dan B. Avstreih

▶ The increasing threat of terrorism presents a growing challenge to ED physicians.

▶ Although less common, incidents involving nuclear, biological, or chemical (NBC) terrorism are potentially the most complex and demanding.

NUCLEAR AND RADIOACTIVE WEAPONS

▶ The most likely nuclear terrorism scenarios are dispersion of nuclear-contaminated materials by a conventional explosion (dirty bomb), destruction of a nuclear power plant, or the detonation of a Cold War–era "suitcase" nuclear weapon.

Clinical Presentation

▶ Radioactive dispersal device victims will suffer primarily from blast trauma and are at low risk for acute radiation syndrome (ARS).

▶ Nuclear weapons and power plant incidents can precipitate ARS (see Chap. 132).

▶ Nuclear weapons also cause thermal burns and blast trauma.

Management

▶ Early activation of hospital disaster plan.

▶ ABCs and aggressive decontamination are paramount.

▶ Staff must frequently assess and decontaminate themselves (e.g., change gloves and gowns).

▶ Blast trauma and burns are treated in the standard fashion, though wounds need aggressive decontamination.

▶ In patients with ARS, operative intervention for trauma and burns should occur within the first 48 hours or be delayed 2–3 months.

▶ Treatment of ARS is primarily supportive (see Chap. 132).
▶ Potassium iodine (KI) is the treatment for radio-iodine exposure.
▶ KI must be given within 4 hours of exposure to be effective.

BIOLOGICAL WEAPONS

▶ Uniquely challenging due to the delay between exposure and symptom development and due to the non-specific and common nature of many early complaints.
▶ Emergency physicians need to be alert for the clinical patterns of uncommon diseases as well as for non-specific clusters.

Anthrax (*Bacillus anthracis*)

▶ An aerobic, gram-positive, spore-forming bacillus.
▶ In non-weaponized exposure, infection is primary zoonotic, with 95% cutaneous and 5% via the respiratory or GI mucosa.

Clinical Presentation
▶ Incubation period is typically 1–6 days.
▶ Cutaneous anthrax presents with the characteristic malignant pustule.
▶ Pulmonary anthrax presents with
  • 2–3 days of non-specific constitutional symptoms: malaise, fatigue, and myalgias, followed by a sudden onset of progressive respiratory distress.
▶ CXR typically shows characteristic mediastinal widening and pleural effusions.

Management
▶ Ciprofloxacin is the preferred agent for all forms of anthrax infection.
  • Ciprofloxacin, 500 mg PO qd × 60 days
▶ Doxycycline can also be used.

Plague (*Yersinia pestis*)

▶ Highly virulent zoonotic infection: 1–2 organisms can cause disease.
▶ Infection is usually from flea carriers, resulting in bubonic and/or septicemic plague.
▶ Bio-weapon dispersion would most likely employ infectious aerosol, causing epidemic pneumonic plague.

Clinical Presentation

▶ Bubonic plague
  • 1- to 8-day incubation period
  • Acute constitutional symptoms, followed 6–8 hours later by a painful suppurative lymphadenitis, producing the characteristic bubo
▶ Septicemic plague
  • Can develop from untreated bubonic plague
  • Symptoms typical of gram-negative sepsis
▶ Pneumonic plague
  • Inhalation or hematologic spread.
  • Acute productive cough, often with hemoptysis.
  • Bilateral alveolar infiltrates are the most common CXR finding.

Management

▶ Early and aggressive treatment is required for survival.
▶ Diagnosis is made via bubo aspiration or by blood, sputum, or CSF cultures.
▶ Cultures are often negative until 48 hours, so DFA antigen testing is often useful.
▶ Isolate the patient and advise the lab staff that will handle the cultures.
▶ Gentamicin or streptomycin is the drug of choice.
▶ Add chloramphenicol if there is meningitis or shock.

Tularemia (*Francisella tularensis*)

▶ Aerobic, gram-negative facultative intracellular coccobacillus.
▶ Zoonotic agent usually transmitted through infected rabbits.
▶ Highly virulent: 10 organisms can cause infection.

Clinical Presentation

▶ Ulceroglandular tularemia presents with characteristic skin lesions and lymph nodes > 1 cm.
▶ Skin lesions are generally single, painless, and chancre-like. These ulcers can be pharyngeal in aerosol exposures.
▶ Typhoidal tularemia does not have the skin and lymphatic findings.
▶ Both forms present with diffuse flu-like symptoms.
▶ Pneumonia occurs in 80% of typhoidal cases, even though CXR is often unremarkable.

Management
▸ Diagnosis is made by serology.
▸ Streptomycin is the drug of choice; gentamicin is also effective.
▸ Tetracycline and chloramphenicol can also be employed.

CHEMICAL WEAPONS
▸ Chemical weapon agents are the most likely non-conventional terrorist weapon.
▸ Knowledge and ingredients for production are readily available.
▸ Sarin used by the Aum Shinrikyo cult in Japan in 1994 and 1995.

Nerve Agents (Sarin, VX, Organophosphate Pesticides)
▸ Phosphorylate and inactivate AChE.
▸ Acetylcholine accumulates in synapses, inhibiting cholinergic neurotransmission.
▸ Also affect nicotinic receptors and CNS, GABA, and NMDA receptors.

Clinical Presentation
▸ SLUDGE syndrome: *s*alivation, *l*acrimation, *u*rination, *d*efecation, *G*I pain, *e*mesis.
▸ Miosis is a common but not universal finding due to nicotinic stimulation.
▸ Altered mental status and seizures are also seen.

Management
▸ Decontamination and early triage.
▸ Respiratory compromise is the most common cause of death.
▸ Aggressive airway management, especially suctioning.
▸ Treatments:
  • Atropine, 2–4 mg q5–15min until pulmonary secretions decrease; may need continuous drip
  • Pralidoxime (2-PAM), 1–2 g over 15 minutes, then 500 mg/hour IV gtt until improved
▸ Benzodiazepines for seizure prophylaxis if > 4 mg atropine is used.

Vesicants/Blister Agents (Mustards, Lewisite)
▸ Mustard agents generate a highly toxic sulfonium ion, which irreversibly alkylates DNA, RNA, and protein.

▶ The mechanism of organic arsenicals (lewisite, ethyldichloro-arsine, methyldichloroarsine, phenyldichloroarsine) is unknown but is likely similar.

Clinical Presentation
▶ Garlic, horseradish, or mustard odor.
▶ Progressive irritation, blistering, and burns of skin, eyes, and respiratory tract.
▶ Severe GI irritation leads to abdominal pain, vomiting, and diarrhea.
▶ Bone marrow suppression, most commonly leukopenia.

Management
▶ Immediate decontamination, especially of asymptomatic patients, is essential.
▶ Early intubation for patients with respiratory complaints.
▶ Mucolytics are also useful.
▶ Mustard burns do not require as much fluid replacement as thermal burns; use urinary output as a guide.
▶ British antilewisite (BAL) or dimercaprol can be used for lewisite exposure.
▶ There is no antidote for mustard agents.

Pulmonary/Choking Agents (Phosgene, Diphosgene)
▶ White cloud with characteristic "fresh hay" odor.
▶ Respiratory tract primarily affected
▶ Reacts with intracellular water to form hydrochloric acid.

Clinical Presentation
▶ Dose-dependent effects.
▶ Low concentrations cause cough, mild dyspnea, and chest discomfort.
▶ High concentrations can trigger laryngospasm and sudden death or cause ARDS.
▶ CXR may show "bat-wing" infiltrates.
▶ Non-cardiogenic pulmonary edema can be silent, especially in children.
▶ Symptoms may be delayed, sometimes as much as 72 hours.

Management
▶ CXR at 0 and 4–6 hours.

- ▶ LDH levels correlate with serious phosgene exposures.
- ▶ Bronchodilators for wheezing.
- ▶ ARDS treated in standard fashion with ventilatory support and PEEP.
- ▶ Victims who are asymptomatic at 6 hours with normal CXRs may be discharged with close follow-up.
- ▶ All patients with symptoms require admission.

CHAPTER 179

EMTALA

Brad J. Uren

- ▶ Referred to alternatively as COBRA due to the parent act, or the "anti-dumping law," after the common name of the practice it was intended to stop.
- ▶ The Emergency Medical Treatment and Labor Act (EMTALA), enacted in 1986, is a federal law, which is part of the COBRA of 1985 (42 USC §1395dd).
- ▶ EMTALA requires that EDs evaluate and treat all patients regardless of their insurance or ability to pay.
- ▶ Covers all ED patients and makes special provisions for patients in labor.
- ▶ Outlines guidelines for treatment and transfer of ED patients.
- ▶ This is achieved by placing significant financial penalties for physicians and hospitals that do not follow the principles established by EMTALA.

PROVISIONS OF EMTALA

- ▶ Three basic requirements of EMTALA:
  - Mandates a medical screening exam to determine whether an emergency medical condition exists.
  - If an emergency medical condition exists, the ED must provide treatment (within the capability of the hospital) until the patient is stabilized, or if they do not have the capability, transfer the patient to another hospital.
  - Tertiary hospitals with specialized capabilities have an obligation to accept transfers if they have the capabilities to treat them.

Emergency Condition

- ▶ Defined largely by the patient
- ▶ Condition that includes severe pain or that can be reasonably thought to result in death, injury, or loss of function to body or organ system

713

▶ Specifically includes pregnancy and labor, or the belief that one is in labor

Screening Exam
▶ Not specifically requiring a physician exam, though a physician exam virtually ensures compliance with this portion of the statute.
▶ Triage assessment is to establish when the patient is seen by the physician, not if the patient needs to be seen by the physician.

Additional Requirements
▶ Care cannot be delayed due to insurance/payment or by questions about methods of payment or insurance coverage.
▶ EDs must notify their patients and visitors in writing by means of posted signs of their rights to a medical exam and to receive treatment.
▶ EDs can request insurance information, but this can only be done **after** the patient has been informed of his or her rights and has had medical evaluation started.

WHEN EMTALA ENDS
▶ If no emergency condition exists after screening exam.
▶ If patient has been treated and condition stabilized for discharge.
▶ With admission; there are separate rules for inpatients regarding transfer.
▶ With transfer, if the patient requests transfer or if the hospital is unable to provide treatment for the patient's condition.
▶ If a patient refuses to stay, though care should be taken to document that the patient knows his or her EMTALA rights and has waived them.

TRANSFER RULES
▶ Patients should be transferred if the patient requests it or if the hospital cannot provide adequate care.
▶ Referring physician must speak with the accepting hospital to arrange transfer and obtain permission to transfer.
▶ Sending physician selects the mode of transport/en route care and maintains responsibility until the patient arrives at the other facility.

- ► Sending facilities must stabilize the patient to the extent that their capabilities allow, and they must attest to this fact at the time of transfer.
- ► Records including labs, radiology, and other studies and documentation must be sent with the patient.

PENALTIES

- ► Both CMS and OIG have substantial financial penalties for EMTALA violations.
  - Termination of the hospital's Medicare provider agreement.
  - Hospital fines of $25,000–$50,000 per violation (lower penalties for smaller hospitals with < 100 beds).
  - Physicians can be fined up to $50,000 per incident.
  - Individual physicians can be disqualified from participation in Medicare.
  - Hospital can be found accountable in civil court.
  - Suit can be brought by the receiving hospital against the sending hospital if damages result from a non-compliant transfer.

○ **PEARLS AND PITFALLS**
  - Do not forget the waiting room; patients in the waiting room are ED patients and cannot be transferred without screening and appropriate transfer arrangements.
  - Whenever possible, patients leaving the ED AMA or leaving the waiting room prior to evaluation should be given the opportunity to sign a statement acknowledging their EMTALA rights.
  - Documentation of transfers, accepting physicians, discussion with consults, treatment provided, and the patient's consent to transfer is critical. Many EMTALA judgments suffer from lack of documentation.

CHAPTER 180

BILLING AND REIMBURSEMENT

Lynn Nutting

- ▶ Standard terminology is used when referring to matters that describe billing and reimbursement.
- ▶ **Professional billing:** services performed and billed by physicians, nurse practitioners, and physician assistants.
- ▶ **Facility billing:** room charge; procedures performed by physicians, nurse practitioners, physician assistants, nurses, and other hospital staff; equipment used during the care of the patient; and medications supplied. Reimbursement is remitted to the institution or health care facility, not the physician.
- ▶ **Current Procedural Terminology (CPT):** a publication by the American Medical Association describing various types of office visits and procedures. Each office visit or procedure is assigned a five-digit numeric code and is used to report services to insurance carriers. The American Medical Association updates the manual annually and accepts requests from providers to create new procedures as they evolve. Example:
  - 12001: simple repair of wounds to scalp, neck, genitalia, trunk, and/or extremities
- ▶ **Evaluation and management (E&M):** CPT codes that are used to report office visits or consults. There are three sets of E&M codes used in the ED: ED visit codes (CPT 99281–99285), critical care (CPT 99291–99292), and observation (CPT 99217–99220 and 99234–99236).
  - E&M charges related to the specialty of emergency medicine are billed using an ED visit, observation, and/or critical care CPT code.
  - Critical care is the only E&M charge that is based on time spent with the patient and defined activities related to patient care, excluding procedures and resident teaching time.
- ▶ **HCPCS:** similar to CPT codes, HCPCS codes are used to report facility services. They consist of medication, medical and surgical supplies, durable medical equipment, and procedure codes.

▶ **ICD-9:** a publication by the CMS that assigns numeric codes to diagnoses. The code is used to report both physician and facility services to insurance carriers. CMS updates the manual annually. The primary diagnosis reported on an emergency medicine claim is the reason chiefly responsible for care provided to a patient. Example:
  • 883.0: open wound of finger(s), nail, subungual
▶ Observation and ED visit levels are determined by the assessment of six components associated with provider documentation:
  • **Chief complaint**
    ○ Why the patient is seeking treatment; signs or symptoms related to encounter
  • **History of present illness**
    ○ Description of location, context, quality, timing, duration and severity, modifying factors, associated signs and/or symptoms related to the chief complaint
  • **Review of systems**
    ○ Positive or negative responses to a review of body systems that could be a factor in diagnosing the patient's chief complaint.
    ○ Body systems include allergic/immunologic, constitutional, cardiovascular, endocrine, ENT, GI, GU, lymphatic, integumentary, musculoskeletal, neurologic, psychiatric, and respiratory.
  • **Past, family, and social history**
  • **Physical exam**
    ○ A count of body systems or areas examined: systems include cardiovascular, constitutional, ENT, endocrine, eyes, GI, GU, respiratory, musculoskeletal, neurologic, lymphatic, integumentary, and psychiatric; body areas include abdomen, back, chest, extremity, genitalia, head, and neck.
  • **Medical decision making**
    ○ Elements include diagnosis and treatment options, data reviewed, and the amount of risk to the patient
▶ Facility billing consists of a room charge plus medication, procedures, and/or equipment.
▶ Room charges are reported to insurance carriers using the CPT codes for professional ED levels 1–5 (CPT 99281–99285), critical care (CPT 99291), and observation services; however, the leveling criteria are not the same.

- CMS allows hospitals to individually define leveling criteria as long as the criteria are consistently applied to all cases. Currently under development is a standardized facility leveling system.

▶ **Point system**
  - Used to calculate room levels by assigning points to each intervention.
  - For instance, triage assessment (5 points), X-ray transport (10 points), patient admitted to ICU (100 points). The level is selected based on total points.

▶ **ACEP facility leveling criteria**
  - Levels are defined through a description of interventions, indications, and discharge instructions, e.g., respiratory illness; two or fewer NMTs equal a level 4 ED visit.

▶ Procedures, medication, and equipment can be billed in addition to a room charge.

▶ Procedures performed by anyone, including the physician, can be reported.

▶ The goal is to report services that result in a direct facility expense.
  - Examples of procedures include infusion, injection, LP, suture repair, intubation, etc.

▶ Physician practices and hospital patient accounts departments are often evaluated on the indicators listed below.
  - **Payer mix**
    ○ Percent of charges by payer.
    ○ An unusually high mix of Medicaid would indicate an overall decrease in reimbursement.
  - **Payer contracts**
    ○ Contracts that outline payer reimbursement provisions such as percent of charge, fee schedule (Medicare, Medicaid, Blue Cross Blue Shield, and other commercial insurance carriers), or capitated rate (a per member per month reimbursement rate utilized by health maintenance organizations)
  - **Days in accounts receivable**
    ○ The number of days it takes to collect on an unpaid account
  - **Aged accounts receivable**
    ○ References the total uncollected dollars in various aging categories such as > and < 90 days, > 180 days, and > 360 days

- **Net collection rate**
  - Percent collected, including adjustments
- **Gross collection rate**
  - Percent collected on actual dollars received
- **Bad debt rate**
  - Percent of uncollectible revenue that is written off or adjusted
- **Total accounts receivable**
  - Total dollar amount of billed, unpaid claims
- ▶ Billing and reimbursement guidelines are ever-changing; however, the fundamentals remain the same.
- ▶ Bill for no more or less than services provided.
- ▶ Maintain thorough documentation of the patient encounter, foster ownership of the billing and reimbursement process, and maintain compliance to CMS regulations.

BIBLIOGRAPHY

Adams HP Jr., et al. *Guidelines for the early management of patients with ischemic stroke: a scientific statement from the Stroke Council of the American Stroke Association*. Dallas: American Heart Association, 2003;34(4):1056–1083.

American Heart Association. *ACC/AHA 2002 guideline update for the management of patients with unstable angina and non-ST-segment elevation myocardial infarction*. Dallas: American Heart Association, 2002;40:366–374.

Anderson DR, et al. Management of patients with suspected deep vein thrombosis in the emergency department: combining use of a clinical diagnosis model with D-dimer testing. *J Emerg Med* 2000;19(3):225–230.

Attia J. The rational clinical examination. Does this adult patient have acute meningitis? *JAMA* 1999;282(2):175–181.

Bracken MB, et al. A randomized, controlled trial of methylprednisolone or naloxone in the treatment of acute spinal-cord injury. Results of the Second National Acute Spinal Cord Injury Study. *N Engl J Med* 1990;322(20):1405–1411.

Clinical policy: evidence-based approach to pharmacologic agents used in pediatric sedation and analgesia in the emergency department. *Ann Emerg Med* 2004;44:342–377.

Clinical policy for children younger than three years presenting to the emergency department with fever. *Ann Emerg Med* 2003;42:530–545.

DeGans J, et al. Dexamethasone in adults with bacterial meningitis. *N Engl J Med* 2002;347:1549–1556.

eMedicine web site. Available at http://www.emedicine.com.

Expert Panel Report 2: guidelines for the diagnosis and management of asthma. Bethesda, MD: U.S. Department of Health and Human Services, Public Health Service, National Institutes of Health, National Heart, Lung and Blood Institute, 1997;Jul. 146 pp.

Goldfrank LR, et al. *Goldfrank's toxicologic emergencies*, 7th ed. New York: McGraw-Hill, 2002.

Hasbun R. Computed tomography of the head before lumbar puncture in adults with suspected meningitis. *N Engl J Med* 2001;345(24):1727–1733.

Hoffman JR, et al. Validation of a set of clinical criteria to rule out injury to the cervical spine in patients with blunt trauma. *N Engl J Med* 2000;343:94–99.

Marx JA, Hockberger RS, Walls RM, eds. *Rosen's emergency medicine: concepts and clinical practice*, 5th ed. Vol. 3. Philadelphia: C.V. Mosby, 2002.

Pollack CV Jr., et al. 2004 American College of Cardiology/American Heart Association guidelines for the management of patients with ST-elevation myocardial infarction: implications for emergency department practice. *Ann Emerg Med* 2005;45(4):363–376.

Roberts JR, Hedges JR. *Clinical procedures in emergency medicine*, 4th ed. Philadelphia: Elsevier, 2004.

Stiell IG, et al. The Canadian C-spine rule for radiography in alert stable trauma patients. *JAMA* 2001;286:1841–1848.

Swaroop VS, Chari ST, Clain JE. Severe acute pancreatitis. *JAMA* 2004;291(23):2865–2868.

Tintinalli JE, et al. *Emergency medicine, a comprehensive study guide*, 6th ed. New York: McGraw-Hill, 2004.

Tissue plasminogen activator for acute ischemic stroke. The National Institute of Neurological Disorders and Stroke rt-PA Stroke Study Group. *N Engl J Med* 1995;333(24):1581–1587.

Trobe JD. *The physician's guide to eye care*, 2nd ed. San Francisco: The Foundation of the American Academy of Ophthalmology, 2001.

INDEX